Common Medical Problems
in the Tropics

Common Medical Problems

in the Tropics

Christopher R. Schull

MB BS (Qld), DPH (Eng), FRACP

Formerly Specialist Medical Officer (Physician), Madang and Honorary Senior Lecturer and Clinical Tutor (Internal Medicine) College of Allied Health Sciences, Madang, Papua New Guinea

MACMILLAN

First published 1987
Reprinted 1990, 1991, 1992 (twice), 1993 (twice), 1995

Published by MACMILLAN EDUCATION LTD
London and Basingstoke
*Associated companies and representatives in Accra, Banjul,
Cairo, Dar es Salaam, Delhi, Freetown, Gaborone, Harare,
Hong Kong, Johannesburg, Kampala, Lagos, Lahore, Lusaka,
Mexico City, Nairobi, São Paulo, Tokyo*

ISBN 0-333-41973-1

Printed in Hong Kong

A catalogue record for this book is available from the
British Library.

TALC and the Tropical Child Health Unit of the
Institute of Child Health, London, received
assistance in the production of this book as a low
cost edition from the Australian Development
Assistance Bureau and the Swedish International
Development Authority

Contents

Preface

If you are a health worker in a rural health centre in a tropical or developing country, this book was written specifically for you. If you are a health worker in a small provincial hospital, an urban health centre, or the outpatients' department of a large hospital, this book was written especially for you also. If you are a health worker of any other sort interested in the promotion of good health, prevention of disease and treatment of medical problems of adults in tropical and developing countries, this book was written for you too.

Most of you will be paramedical workers such as Health Extension Officers, Medical Assistants, Nurses and similar workers. Some of you will be Medical Officers working outside a large well-equipped hospital. Most of you will be doing most of the work which most medical 'general practitioners' in the industrialised western countries do. This book was written in the way it is as you usually (1) work without direct or easy contact with a Medical Officer in a well-equipped hospital; (2) cannot easily and quickly get pathology tests done in a reliable laboratory; but you (3) can refer or transfer patients to a Medical Officer in a hospital – if this is needed. An important feature of this book is helping you to make decisions based on clinical findings without waiting for laboratory help. It is very important for you to be able to do this, as experience in a number of countries has taught that even when laboratory services are supposed to be available, they are in fact not available or give very unreliable results which are misleading or even dangerous. Another important feature of this book is helping you to decide if and when a patient of yours should be referred or transferred to a Medical Officer in a hospital.

If you are a Medical Officer and especially if you are a consultant physician (in internal medicine), this book was written in the hope you also could use it – summarise it, expand it, or alter it, to make it specific and more useful for the health workers in the area in which you live and practice medicine. It is hoped you can do this without your having to first do all the groundwork to get basic information together and then make it relevant to the above health workers and the people in tropical and developing countries.

When you read this book, especially if you are a Medical Officer, please remember that some things stated as facts and some explanations given are so started and so given for the Health Extension Officers, Medical Assistants and Nurses who have only a very short training in the basic medical sciences and pathology. Discussion of controversial subjects and patho-physiological explanations can be found in standard texts and journals.

This book grew out of work and teaching done with Health Extension Officers and Nurses in Papua New Guinea in the 10 years up to 1982, and also time previously spent in Nigeria and other places. The author worked for a year in a rural health centre without hospital facilities in post-war Nigeria and for another year in a rural health centre in Papua New Guinea. After these years, from a new position as consultant physician for an area as well as hospital, the author regularly visited health centres and their staffs of paramedical workers and discussed with the staff all their patients and also any of their other problems. Also, all the adults with medical problems transferred by the health workers from health centres were received into the author's hospital ward. Also, about half the author's time each day was spent teaching paramedical workers in the half of the hospital ward which was run (with the aid of the trainee paramedical workers and their tutors) as a health centre and not a hospital ward. (All new urban patients were admitted to and managed in the health centre ward, and were transferred to the medical officer section of the ward only if transfer to medical officer and hospital care became necessary.) (Patients transferred from rural health centres were admitted directly to the medical officer section of the ward.) Half of most nights and the majority of most weekends were spent by not only the author but also his wife, devising the management regimes, the indications for transfer or referral of patients and all the other things which went into the preparation of books such as this. These regimens and books were then tried out by the health workers locally and later in all of Papua New Guinea; and then in the light of the usefulness or otherwise of parts of them, modifications were made and new editions of books produced. Many parts of these books, which some Medical Officers said should be removed, were left in because Health Extension Officers and Nurses repeatedly asked for that information and were certain it should not be removed.

This present book is modification of the final reference book produced for Papua New Guinea *Adult Internal Medicine in Papua New Guinea – A Reference Book for Health Workers in Health Centres and Hospital Outpatients Departments*, 1984, C. R. Schull, published by the Government Printer, Port Moresby, Papua New Guinea. The author was asked to try to make the Papua New Guinea book useful to paramedical workers in other parts of the world. The author realised that he was not knowledgeable enough or experienced enough to do this adequately. It was clear, however, after searching in vain for a similar book for the rest of the world through all available libraries, that no one else had felt qualified or experienced enough to write it; or if they had, they had not been motivated enough to do it. Although there were books for paramedical workers on Child Health, Surgery and Obstetrics and Gynaecology, there were none along these lines in Adult Internal Medicine for senior paramedical workers. Hence this book.

This book is a reference book. It is not meant to be all learned. It is meant to be read during the years of student life when training to be a health worker; and then to be then referred to during working life to help when problems arise. The book is therefore large and has many words to try to explain things as clearly as could be done.

It is hoped that supervising or teaching Medical Officers in each country, who do not have time to prepare all the books needed by paramedical workers, may be able to take the parts from this book which apply to their country, simplify and summarise those parts (and alter or amplify or add to other parts if needed), and produce perhaps two other more useful books.

One book probably needed would be a 'summary' i.e. a book with just those things which the student and health worker must *know,* i.e. be able to recite orally or write, interpret on patients and use in practice to solve the problems of patients and the common health problems of the area. Such a book for Papua New Guinea is '*Common Medical Problems of Adults in Papua New Guinea – A Summary*', 1979, C.R. Schull, Kristen Pres Inc., Madang, Papua New Guinea.

The other book which is probably needed is a small book that can be carried in the health worker's pocket all the time and which has the details of the management of the common health problems in that area including drug doses (and it is much safer to look these up than to try to remember them and perhaps make a fatal mistake). Of course the health worker must be taught actually to look up the book when he is seeing the patient. Such a book is *Diagonsis and Treatment of Common Health Problems of Adults in Papua New Guinea*, 1980, C.R. Schull, Kristen Pres Inc., Madang, Papua New Guinea.

Experience with Health Extension Officers and Nurses has taught that only one part of the book is likely to be consulted at any one time. Experience has also taught that repetition is a good teacher. The above will also partly explain some of the repetition in the book.

After the introductory chapter most chapters are set out using the following plan (modified as needed). At first there is a short description of the anatomy and physiology of the system. Then there is a list of the symptoms and signs which can be caused by abnormal structure or function of that system. This section includes details of how to examine the patient to find these signs. Next there is a section which includes the common conditions and diseases of the system. Finally, there is a section which summarises the causes of and management of the common symptoms and signs caused by disorders and diseases of the system.

Although this is a reference book, the health worker student should become familiar with it before graduating. During student life you should read the following.

1. All of the first *eleven* chapters including

diagnosis of disease, management of a patient and control and prevention of disease.

2. All sections of Anatomy, Physiology, Pathology, Symptoms and Signs in chapters which have these discussed.

3. The sections on all the common important diseases in the country in which he is working.

These will include the following in almost all countries –

(1) Severe bacterial infections including septicaemia (Chapter 12).

(2) Malaria (Chapter 13).

(3) Tuberculosis (Chapter 14).

(4) Leprosy (Chapter 15).

(5) The common infectious diseases which occur almost everywhere (Chapter 16).

(6) Any of the other infectious diseases which occur in your area (Chapter 17 and 18).

(7) Syphilis, gonorrhoea, and amoebic ulcer (Chapter 19).

(8) Otitis of various types, the common cold, influenza, acute bronchitis, pneumonia, asthma and chronic bronchitis; and causes of cough, sputum, haemoptysis, shortness of breath and pain in chest (Chapter 20).

(9) Anaemia, Tropical Splenomegaly Syndrome and, if it occurs in your area, Sickle Cell Anaemia (Chapter 21).

(10) Filariasis (Chapter 22).

(11) Gastro-enteritis, intestinal parasites and peptic ulcer; and causes of vomiting, haematemesis, diarrhoea and dysentery (Chapter 23).

(12) Jaundice, hepatitis, liver abscess, hepatoma and cirrhosis (Chapter 24).

(13) Meningitis of all types, cerebral malaria and other types of 'encephalitis', convulsions, epilepsy, paralysis, unconsciousness and headache (Chapter 25).

(14) Urinary tract infections, causes of urinary frequency and pain, nephrotic syndrome, chronic kidney failure and causes of proteinuria (Chapter 26).

(15) Osteomyelitis and pyomyositis (Chapter 28), acute bacterial arthritis, 'tropical arthritis', tuberculous arthritis and osteoarthrosis (Chapter 29).

(16) Foreign bodies in the eye, conjunctivits, corneal ulcer and iritis (Chapter 31).

(17) Tinea, impetigo and scabies and the principles of treatment of all skin conditions (Chapter 32).

(18) Snakebite (Chapter 33).

(19) Swallowed poisons (Chapter 34).

(20) Acute and chronic organic psychoses, schizophrenia, manic-depressive psychoses, acute psychotic reactions, anxiety states and 'acting out' states (Chapter 35).

(21) Some important symptoms and signs including fever, general oedema, general wasting, dehydration, abdominal pain, abdominal tenderness – guarding – rigidity, abdominal masses and abdominal distension.

(22) Resuscitation including artificial ventilation (Chapter 37) and treatment of shock (Chapter 27).

Any other diseases which are common in the area in which the health worker is, must be added to this list.

Malnutrition is not only a cause of disease, but also interacts with infection in a number of ways. Malnutrition decreases immunity or resistance to infection. Malnutrition makes any infection present more serious, and makes it less likely for the body to overcome that infection, even when correct treatment of the infection is given. Infection in a person who already has malnutrition makes that malnutrition even worse. As these conditions are even more important for children than adults, and as they are dealt with at length in the books on child health and children's diseases, malnutrition has not been discussed in a separate chapter in this book and the interaction of malnutrition and infection has not been emphasised. This is not meant to indicate that malnutrition and its relation to infection and its prevention and its treatment are not important for adults – they are. For detailed discussions of these, however, see books on child health and children's diseases; but remember that these things apply to adults also.

If the health worker does decide to purchase some other books in adult internal medicine, the first three to consider are:

Davidson, S. and Macleod, J., (latest; edition), *The Principles and Practice of Medicine*, London, Churchill Livingstone. (ELBS ed).

MacLeod, J., (latest edition), *Clinical Examination*, London, Churchill Livingstone, (ELBS ed).

Lawrence, D., (latest edition), *Clinical Pharmacology*, Edinburgh and London, Churchill Livingstone. (ELBS ed).

All of these books are available in cheap ELBS editions. The latest edition should, of course, be obtained.

The author is only too well aware of the many imperfections in this book. If the book is to be improved, advice on how to do this is needed from those who use it. If Health Extension Officers, Medical Assistants, Nurses, Tutors and Medical Officers who use this book in any way for any purpose would be kind enough to write to the author and tell him of errors or omissions noted or things which are hard to understand, etc. and also make specific suggestions for improvements, this would greatly help. PLEASE WRITE.

It is hoped that what is in this book will show how health workers using only simple and cheap items (available in most health centres and hospital outpatients departments), are able to manage almost all of the medical health problems of adults safely and effectively.

C.R. Schull
Senior Specialist,
Respiratory Medicine/Intensive Care,
Repatriation General Hospital,
Newgate Street,
Greenslopes, 4120,
Australia.

1987

Acknowledgements

This book was prepared with the help of many of my friends and colleagues. So many helped in so many ways over so many years it is now no longer possible to record all the people who helped – even in major ways.

Foremost among those who made this book possible were my wife and children. They not only went without many things so that this and the other books for Papua New Guinea could appear; they also gave encouragement and help and my wife did all the typing for the numerous Papua New Guinean drafts and editions.

Many of my colleagues in Papua New Guinea gave encouragement and help. In particular Doctors John and Narelle Stace helped in very many ways and in every way they could. Dr Brother Andrew SSF contributed significantly to the chapter on mental illnesses. Professor George Wyatt made valuable suggestions and Dr Greg Lawrence read the whole of the Papua New Guinean edition and made numerous suggestions for improvement. Papua New Guinean health workers, and in particular Dr Puka Temu and HEO Tutor Mr Mika Kenas gave invaluable guidance. Of course, many of the ideas in the book came from observation of what happened to patients and other situations which arose during health centre work and then discussion of these with the staff involved.

For the International edition, Dr F.J. Wright of Edinburgh kindly and helpfully checked the various chapters with diseases with which the author had not had significant practical experience. Dr C.J. Eills of Birmingham then read through the text and made many valuable suggestions. Both of these doctors have had vast experience in tropical and developing countries and are internationally recognised authorities in tropical diseases. The author is very grateful to them for their invaluable advice.

Two editors, at first Mrs Jennifer Gamel and later (for the bulk of the work) Mrs Sheila Jones, did a large amount of important work in preparing and improving the text for publication.

As the author did not plan to publish any works for distribution outside Papua New Guinea until he was requested to do so just before he had to leave Papua New Guinea to return to Australia, and as there was no copyright law in Papua New Guinea, no particular record of the origin of diagrams and descriptions of laboratory procedures etc. collected for use of health workers was kept. Most of these which the author did not produce in Madang were obtained from slides or photographs in the Medical Learning Resources Unit of the University of Papua New Guinea in Port Moresby, and most of these were not documented as to origin. If, therefore, there are any parts of the book, and especially any diagrams, which have been inadvertantly reproduced without appropriate acknowledgment made, the author apologises for this and would make such acknowledgment if permission for the use of these were granted for any future edition, and the publishers would make the necessary arrangements.

Money to assist in travel for library research and typing of the International text was kindly supplied by the Damian Foundation, Belgium, Boehringer Ingelheim Australia and the World Health Organization, Geneva. Large grants were then given by both the Swedish International Development Authority and the Australian Government's Australian Development Assistance Bureau to Teaching Aids at Low Cost, London, to provide money for the printing and sale of the book by Macmillans at a price well below the normal price for a book of this size. The author has and will accept no payment of any kind in a further attempt to keep the price as low as possible. It is only through the generous assistance of the above charitable, company and government bodies, however, that it has been possible to produce and distribute this book.

Despite all the above help, however, the production of this and the other books has been an 'after hours' effort by a clinician who considers himself in no way an academic or an author. Responsible for errors and omissions, therefore, rest with the author, and not those who helped in so many ways.

To all the people, as well as the above, who helped the author, he gives his thanks. The author knows these people well enough to be certain that if this book helps improve the health of people in tropical and developing countries then those who contributed to the production of this book will be thanked enough.

C.R.S.

The author and publishers are grateful to the World Health Organization and Pan American Health Organization for permission to reproduce maps showing the distribution of diseases.

Figure 18.7 is produced by courtesy of Professor D.H. Molyneux, University of Salford and Taylor and Francis, London.

Figure 19.18 is from Pictorial Handbook of Common Skin Diseases by Prof. A.N. Okoro, University of Nigeria, Nsukka, (Macmillan, 1981).

The author and publishers wish to acknowledge, with thanks, the following photographic sources:
Dr A. Buck p 360 (from A Colour Atlas of Tropical Medicine and Parasitology by W. Peters and H.M. Gilles, Wolfe Medical Publications Ltd)
Dr Rod Hay, School of Hygiene and Tropical Medicine, London p 355
Dr D.M. Minter p 118 top (from A Colour Atlas of Tropical Medicine and Parasitology by W. Peters and H.M. Gilles, Wolfe Medical Publications Ltd)
St. Bartholomew's Hospital, Department of Medical Photography pp 137 left; 137 right (photograph Morris Sydney); 356 bottom (photograph Roy Gray)
Tropix Photograph Library pp 116; 118 bottom
C. James Webb pp 119 left; 180; 188; 367
WHO pp 119 right; 365 (photograph J. Abcede); 366 (photograph D. Deriaz); 366 (photograph E. Mandelmann); 369
All other photographs are courtesy of the author.
Cover photographs courtesy of the author, Tropix Photograph Library and C. James Webb

1

The Purpose of the Health Worker

The Health Worker, has three aims:
1. to promote good health,
2. to prevent disease,
3. to treat disease,
in both individuals and the whole community.

When you treat disease, again you have three aims:
1. to cure the patient, (this is not always possible);
2. to relieve the patient's symptoms (this is almost always possible);
3. to reassure and encourage the patient and his relatives (this is always possible).

It is very easy to spend all your time treating disease and so have no time to prevent disease and promote health. This is not the best way to spend your time. Of course you must treat patients with disease. This helps the patient and his relatives. It also shows the community that you know how to help them and that you do want to help them. It is only when the community discovers this that they will take any notice of your work to prevent disease and promote health. Unless you really do prevent disease and promote good health, your work in treating the sick will not help the community very much. It is no good curing a

patient if you do not prevent the patient getting the same disease again when he goes home. His family and friends may also get the disease. So:
1. You must use some of your time to treat patients with disease.
2. You must use some of your time to prevent disease.
3. You must use some of your time to promote good health.

You will often find it difficult to leave your work in the health centre and go out into the community to prevent disease and promote health. But you must do this. You can also do a lot to control and prevent disease in the health centre. When a person comes to you in the health centre and you diagnose his disease, you can give the patient and his family and friends education about how to control and prevent disease, and about other things which would improve their health. Remember two things:
(1) When people are well they usually take no notice of health education as they feel they will not get a disease. But when they are sick, the patient and his family and friends will often take notice of health education, as they then know they can get the disease.
(2) Most cases of undiagnosed infectious diseases such as leprosy and tuberculosis are in the family and friends of patients with these diseases. Therefore before you go out of the health centre to look for these sorts of disease in the whole community, first make sure you educate and examine all the family and friends who have come (with the patient) to you in the health centre.

This does not mean you should stay in the health centre all the time. It means you should never miss the chance to control and prevent disease and promote health when a sick person comes to the health centre.

You, the Health Worker, must also remember that what you *do* to treat and prevent disease and promote health will have much more effect than what you *say* about these things. Your effectiveness as a Health Worker will depend on what sort of person you really are and the way you live and work.

2

Some Clinical Definitions

Do not try to learn these definitions until you have:
(1) read more about them in later chapters,
(2) talked about them with your teachers and
(3) used the things they are about in your practical work.

Anatomy
Anatomy is the science of the *structure* of the body; or *how the body is made*.

Physiology
Physiology is the science of the normal *function* of the body; or *how the living body works*.

Definition of a disease
In this book the definition of a disease is a short statement about the nature of the disease; or what kind of disease it is.

Frequency
The frequency is how often the disease occurs. There are more accurate terms. These include the following:
Prevalence: This is the *total* number of persons with the disease at a *stated* time in a *stated* population.
Incidence: This is the number of *new* persons developing the disease during a *stated* time in a *stated* population.

A classification and the causes of disease (aetiology)
There are ten common kinds or classifications of disease (congenital, traumatic, inflammatory (4 types), neoplastic, degenerative, chemical-induced, malnutrition, psychological, body system failure (especially vascular) and others including unknown). The causes of many of these classifications of diseases are known (see Chapter 4). In fact, some of the classifications are based on the cause of disease. However, there are also causes which are not yet known about. For example, it is said that a patient's disease may be degenerative (or due to the body wearing out); but it is not known why the body, which can repair itself, eventually wears out. The most common causes of disease in tropical and developing countries are infections with organisms, trauma and malnutrition. (See Chapter 4.)

Pathology
The cause of the disease can make changes in the normal anatomy and physiology of the body. These changes are called pathology. See Chapter 3.

Epidemiology
Epidemiology gives the known answers to the questions:
(1) *who* gets a particular disease and *how many* people get it?
(2) *when* and *where* do these persons get the disease? and
(3) *how* and *why* do they get the disease? (See Chapter 5.)

Symptoms
Symptoms are *what the patient feels*.
The patient *tells* you his symptoms when he talks to you about what he *feels*.
You can usually discover symptoms when you take a *medical history* from the patient. When you take a medical history you must ask about:
1. General information.
2. The patient's symptoms and how long he has had each one. (Record these in the patient's own words.)
3. The history of the present illness (or the story of how the patient went from being well to sick).

4. The specific questions (or specific interrogation) that you must ask to discover if there are also symptoms of a disease of any other system of the body (as well as those the patient has already talked about).
5. The past history – you ask the patient about the drugs he has taken, treatment he has been given by traditional healers, previous attacks of this illness, other illnesses, operations, accidents and previous and present pregnancies, etc.
6. The family and contact history – you check if an illness in the family or in one of his contacts could be affecting the patient.

There are three other things you must do when you take a medical history.
(1) If the patient may have a mental condition, take the history again from a relative or another witness.
(2) Check the patient's outpatient card for any history in it.
(3) Tell the patient a summary of the history and ask him to correct anything wrong.

Signs
Signs are what you find (see, feel, percuss, hear, etc.) when you examine the patient.

You do the *clinical* or *medical* or *physical* examination to discover all the patient's signs. You must do it systematically (or in a special order) in 9 sections, so that you never forget anything.
1. Basic observations. These help you decide if the patient is 'sick' or not. They also help you to look for common diseases (even if the patient does not complain of their symptoms). If you find these diseases while they are still not serious and you can treat them and prevent them from getting worse. These observations include: level of consciousness and signs of meningeal irritation; temperature; pulse rate; respiration rate and type of respiration; blood pressure; weight with observations about dehydration, oedema, malnutrition or chronic wasting illness; and colour, especially anaemia.
2. Head and neck including ear, nose, throat, lymph glands and thyroid.
3. Chest, including spine.
4. Abdomen.
5. Skin.
6. Muscles, bones, joints.
7. Ear, nose and throat (if not done before).

8. Any special examinations, if needed.
9. Examination of mental state (psychiatric examination), if needed.

See Chapter 6 page 18.

Course and complications
The course is what usually happens to a person who has the disease. Complications are other things which do not usually happen in the course of the disease. Complications are other clinical conditions which can happen on top of the original clinical condition.

Tests or investigations
You do tests for 3 reasons:
1. to help you decide between different possible diagnoses,
2. to confirm a diagnosis, and
3. to provide a baseline by which you can judge if the patient is getting better or worse.

There are 3 groups of tests:
1. Those you can do at the health centre. e.g. haemoglobin, urine tests, lumbar puncture, etc.
2. You take a sample at the health centre, but send it to the hospital laboratory to be examined there, e.g. 'serum tests', malaria smear, sputum smears, etc. (In some large health centres there is a medical laboratory assistant who can do some of these tests at the health centre.)
3. If you cannot do the test or take a sample at the health centre, you must send the patient to the hospital for the test. e.g. X-rays, etc.

See Chapter 6 page 21.

Differential diagnosis
The differential diagnosis (DD) is the list of all the diseases *which could* be causing the patient's main symptoms and signs. See Chapter 6 page 21.

Diagnostic features
In this book diagnostic features are the most typical things about the disease (in a short list). These features are nearly always present if that disease is present.

Provisional diagnosis
The provisional diagnosis (PD) is the disease (or diseases) you think the patient really has. You

decide this after eliminating all the other diseases in the differential diagnoses because they do not fit the patient's symptoms and signs as well as the provisional diagnosis does. When you have made a provisional diagnosis, you manage the patient for this disease. See Chapter 6 page 21.

Management

Management is not only the treatment of the patient. A patient who has a disease creates problems for many people. To manage these problems you must do at least these four things:

1. treat the patient;
2. notify or advise certain other people;
3. control the spread of the disease, if necessary;
4. prevent other members of the community from getting the disease and the patient from getting it again.

These things are considered separately below. See also Chapters 7, 8 and 9.

Treatment of the patient

Treatment includes the following nine things:

1. *Decision on outpatient treatment or admission for inpatient treatment.*
2. *Nursing care* of many types including at times, bed rest, special positions, special care of respiratory tract, eyes, bladder, pressure areas etc., isolation, observations, food, fluids, etc.
3. *Specific treatment* to attempt to *cure* the disease e.g. drugs, fluids, food, surgery, dressings, plasters, physiotherapy and psychiatric counselling.
4. *Symptomatic treatment*, to attempt to relieve the patient's symptoms and make him *feel* better e.g. drugs, etc. as in 3 above; nursing care as in 2 above.
5. *Giving an explanation, reassurance and comfort to the patient and relatives.*
6. *Giving health education* about control and prevention of the disease to the patient and to the relatives.
7. *Consultation about the patient with the Preventive Medicine/Administrative Health Officer or hospital Medical Officer* (sometimes). This can be for advice or about transfer of the patient to medical officer care or referral of the patient to the next visiting medical officer.
8. *Discharging the patient* and giving final health education.

9. *Following the patient up*, if needed.

See Chapter 7.

Indications for consultation, transfer or referral

Some symptoms and signs mean that you should do one of the following three things:

1. Describe the patient's condition to the Health Officer or hospital Medical Officer by telephone or radio, and ask for advice (that is 'consult').
2. Transfer
   (a) Transfer the patient to the hospital as an emergency case for urgent treatment by a medical officer as soon as you can find a plane or car or boat to take him there, i.e. 'urgent transfer'.
   (b) Transfer the patient to the hospital as a non-emergency case using the next available usual transport, i.e. 'non-urgent transfer'.
3. Ask the next medical officer who visits the health centre to see the patient, i.e. 'referral'.

See Chapter 7 page 27.

Prognosis

The prognosis is what the likely result of a condition will be (e.g. cause the patient's death, get better quickly, last for a long time, etc.)

See Chapter 6 page 21.

Notification

1. You must notify certain diseases to the Health Officer or Health Department by telegram if they occur. Some have to be notified immediately if any new case occurs. Some have to be notified immediately if an epidemic occurs. This second group and another group usually have to be notified monthly if any cases occur.
2. You must notify certain cases to the coroner or (patrol) officer in charge of the station and the police. These include all cases of 'sudden and unnatural death' and cases when you do not know the cause of death, including persons who are 'dead on arrival'. Notify all fights, accidents, alleged poisoning, etc. if the patient is ill.
3. You should notify relatives and friends (and sometimes other people) and advise them of the

patient's condition, treatment and probable future.

See Chapter 8.

Control
Control is what you must do to stop the disease spreading. You need to know the epidemiology of the disease so that you can choose the best means of control. These means may include one or more of the methods:
1. inactivating the specific (or causative) agent in the reservoir (usually killing a parasite in the body of the original host);
2. blocking the means of spread of the specific (or causative) agent from the reservoir to susceptible persons;
3. increasing the resistance of the susceptible persons; and
4. giving prophylactic treatment to susceptible persons who are probably infected.

See Chapter 9.

Prevention
Prevention is what you need to do to stop the disease occurring. You need to know the epidemiology of the disease so that you can choose the best means of prevention. The means used for prevention are the same as for control. (See above and Chapter 9.)

Acute
Any condition which comes suddenly and lasts a short time may be called 'acute'. This often means less than one month.

Chronic
Any condition which lasts a long time may be called 'chronic'. It usually starts slowly, but an acute condition may become a chronic condition. This usually means more than one month.

Subacute
A subacute condition is one which is somewhere between acute and chronic.

Lesion
Lesion is a general or non-specific term for a pathological change in a body tissue. It is often used to mean damage to the structure of part of an organ, especially damage caused by an injury or infection.

Syndrome
Syndrome is the name given to a *group of symptoms and/or signs*. When these symptoms and signs *all occur together* this means that a certain pathological process is present. There may be a number of causes of this syndrome.

Curative or clinical medicine
Curative medicine or clinical medicine are terms sometimes used for the processes of seeing a patient, taking a history, doing an examination, doing tests, making a diagnosis and treating the patient.

Note on prefixes and suffixes

Certain words or syllables may be added to the beginning of a word (prefix) or the ending of a word (suffix) to form a new word with a different meaning. Some of the prefixes and suffixes often used in medicine are listed below.

Common prefixes
hypo- less than normal or under.
 e.g. hypothermia: temperature less than normal.
 hypodermic: under the dermis or skin.
hyper- more than normal or above.
 e.g. hyperthyroidism: thyroid makes more hormone than normal.
an- without.
 e.g. anuric: without urine or no urine made.
exo- outside.
 e.g. exopthalmos: eye pushed out.
endo- within or inside (not to the outside).
 e.g. endocrine: gland which secretes into the blood.
macro- large.
 e.g. macroscopic: large enough to be seen by the naked eye.
micro- small.
 e.g. microscopic: so small can be seen only with the aid of a microscope.

Common suffixes
-aemia or -emia   refers to the blood.
 e.g. anaemia: without normal amount of blood.

-uria   refers to the urine.

    e.g. haematuria: blood in the urine.

-pathy   disease.

    e.g. encephalopathy: disease of the brain.

-itis   inflammation of.

    e.g. conjunctivitis: inflammation of conjunctivae.

-oma   tumour of organ.

    e.g. meningioma: tumour of meninges.

SI units

The International System of Units (SI) is based on the units: metre, kilogram, second, ampere, kelvin, candela and mole. It is already used by many countries as their only legal system.

Names and Symbols for basic SI units

Physical quantity	Name of SI unit	Symbol for SI unit
length	metre	m
mass	kilogram	kg
time	second	s
thermodynamic temperature	kelvin	K
amount of substance	mole	mol

Prefixes for SI units

Prefixes can be used to show decimal fractions or multiples of the basic (or derived) SI units.

Fraction	Prefix	Symbol
$\frac{1}{10}$ or 10^{-1}	deci	d
$\frac{1}{100}$ or 10^{-2}	centi	c
$\frac{1}{1000}$ or 10^{-3}	milli	m
$\frac{1}{1000000}$ or 10^{-6}	micro	μ

Multiple	Prefix	Symbol
$\times 10$ or 10^1	deca	da
$\times 100$ or 10^2	hecto	h
$\times 1000$ or 10^3	kilo	k
$\times 1000000$ or 10^6	mega	M

Length

The SI unit of length is the metre (m).

1 micron (μ) (obsolete) = 10^{-6} m = 1 μm.

1 inch (in) = 2.54 cm = 0.254 m.

1 foot (ft) = 0.3048 m.

1 yard (yd) = 0.9144 m.

Volume

The SI unit of volume is the cubic metre (m^3); but since this is inconveniently large for most measurements in medicine, the litre (l) has beeen kept as an alternative to the cubic decimetre (dm^3).

    1 m^3 = 1000 l.

    1 fluid ounce (oz) = 28.41 ml.

    1 pint = 20 fluid oz. = 568 ml.

    1 gallon = 4.55 l.

Mass

The SI unit of mass is the kilogram (kg).

    1 kg = 1000 grams (g).

    1 grain = 64.8 mg.

    1 ounce (oz) = 28.35 g.

    1 pound (lb) = 16 oz = 453.6 g.

    1 ton = 2240 lb = 1016 kg.

    1 tonne = 1000 kg = 0.984 ton.

Amount of substance

Where the molecular weight of a substance is known, its amount should usually be expressed in terms of the mole (mol). One mole of a substance is that amount of the substance which contains the same number of particles (whether atoms, molecules, ions or radicals) as 12 g of carbon 12. In short, 1 mole is the particle weight (such as atomic weight or molecular weight) expressed in grams.

    The 'equivalent' is now not used. It was used to express the amount of an ionised substance; it is the number of moles multiplied by the valency. Thus 10 mol Na^+ = 10 equiv.; but 10 mol Ca^{++} = 20 equiv.

Concentration and osmotic pressure

Concentrations of substances in biological fluids should be expressed in molar terms if the molecular weight is known and in terms of mass if not. Thus plasma glucose is expressed as mmol/l while plasma albumen is expressed as g/l. In each case the reference unit of volume is the litre. A special exception is haemoglobin whose concentration in blood is expressed as g/dl.

    Osmotic pressure is expressed as osmolarity (moles per litre of solution) or osmolality (moles per kilogram of water).

Pressure

The SI unit of pressure is the pascal (Pa); this is the pressure exerted by 1 newton acting on an area of a square metre ($1 \text{ Pa} = 1 \text{ N m}^{-2}$).

    1 cm H_2O = 98.1 Pa.

    1 mm Hg = 1 torr = 133.3 Pa = 0.1333 kPa.

    1 kPa = 7.50 mm Hg = 10.1 cm H_2O.

    1 normal atmosphere = 760 mm Hg

    = 101.3 kPa.

Temperature

The SI temperature scale is the kelvin scale (K) but this is inconvenient to use in medicine and the Celsius (formerly 'centigrade') scale (°C) has been retained.

    Degree Celsius = K − 273.15.

Conversion from the Fahrenheit scale to the Celsius scale can be carried out with either of these formulae:

$$\frac{9}{5} C = F - 32$$

$$\frac{9}{5} (C + 40) = F + 40$$

Where F is the temperature in degrees Fahrenheit and C is the temperature in degrees Celsius.

Time

1 hour (h) = 60 minutes (min) = 3600 seconds (s).

The use of hertz (Hz) for frequency to replace cycles per second is recommended provided it is not used for the timing of discontinuous events, i.e. not, for example, for the frequency of passing urine or the dispensing of doses of medicine. It should not be used for frequency of rotation.

Abbreviations

The following abbreviations are in common use in some places and are sometimes used in this book.

b.d.	Two times each day.
BP	Blood pressure.
C°	Temperature in degrees Celsius or Centigrade.
IMI	Intramuscular injection.
IM	Intramuscularly.
IVI	Intravenous injection.
IV	Intravenously.
nocte	At night; each night.
oral	By mouth.
PR	Pulse rate.
p.r.n.	If needed; if necessary.
q.d.s.	As for q.i.d. (see below) but should be used only for things which are taken (swallowed).
q.i.d.	Four times each day (e.g. before morning meal, in the middle of the day, before evening meal and at night before going to sleep).
RR	Respiration rate.
SCI	Subcutaneous injection (into the fat under the skin).
stat	Immediately, straight away.
T°	Temperature.
t.d.s.	As for t.i.d. (see below) but should be used only for things which are taken (swallowed).
t.i.d.	Three times a day (e.g. before morning meal, before evening meal and at night before going to sleep; *or* before morning meal, in the middle of the day and before evening meal).
>	Greater than; more than.
<	Smaller than; less than.

3

Pathology

The normal human body is made in a certain way. This is called its structure or its *anatomy*. The normal human body works in a certain way. This is called its normal function or *physiology*. Many things can damage the normal anatomy of the body or upset the normal physiology of the body and cause changes in the anatomy and/or the physiology. These are called *pathological changes*.

> Pathology (or pathological change) is the change in the normal anatomy and physiology made by the cause of disease.

The pathological changes (and sometimes the causes of them) show themselves as the symptoms, the signs and the abnormal tests of disease.

When a part of the body is attacked by things which may damage it (see Chapter 4 page 10) this can cause many different types of pathological change. Three very important pathological changes are:
1. death of part or all of the body,
2. inflammatory reaction (or inflammation), and
3. neoplasm (or 'cancer' formation).

Inflammation

Inflammation is the change which happens in a tissue when it is injured, if the injury does not completely destroy the tissue.

Some causes of inflammation are:
1. trauma,
2. infection,
3. chemicals,
4. allergy (see Chapter 4 page 10).

There are two main types of inflammation:
1. acute,
2. chronic.

The type and amount of inflammation depends on the cause. Acute serious injury or infection with some organisms causes acute inflammation. Chronic mild injury or infection with other organisms (especially those which cause leprosy and tuberculosis) causes chronic inflammation.

Acute inflammation
In acute inflammation more blood flows to the area. This is because the blood vessels become wider. Fluid (containing white blood cells, antibodies and other proteins from inside the blood vessels) goes through the capillary walls into the tissues of the area. The fluid can dilute the thing that is damaging the body. White blood cells can surround the thing and try to digest it. Proteins can make a wall around the area so that bacteria cannot spread. Antibodies can attach themselves to the thing that is injuring the body and destroy it or make it easier for white cells to digest it. Immune white cells can attach themselves to the thing that is injuring the body and destroy it. Pus consisting of dead cells and destroyed tissue, etc. can appear in the area.

Some of the symptoms and signs of acute inflammation are:
1. swelling,
2. redness or shinyness,
3. heat,
4. pain and tenderness,
5. loss of function,
6. sometimes, fluid or pus in the area.

Chronic inflammation
Chronic inflammation can happen because of the type of the cause (chronic mild injury or some types of bacteria) or because an acute inflammation has been in the area for a long time and the body has not quite been able to destroy the cause.

In chronic inflammation the blood vessels become only a little wider and fluid, protein and cells escape only slowly into the area. However, the cells normally present in the area are slowly killed and replaced by fibrous tissue. As the fibrous tissue gets older, it shrinks and causes scarring. The tissue in the area of the chronic inflammation is slowly destroyed. Pus may be made if many white cells are killed.

Symptoms and signs of chronic inflammation in an area include:
1. swelling but not usually very much;
2. redness is not usual;
3. heat but only slight;
4. pain and tenderness but not usually very much;
5. loss of function is usual;
6. there can be fluid or pus.

Chronic inflammation will stop if the cause is removed. Healing will then happen. However, if the organ has been badly damaged or if the area of the body has been very scarred, it may never function properly again.

General (whole body) effects of inflammation

In both acute and chronic inflammation, *certain toxins and other chemicals are put into the blood*. Some of these chemicals are made by the body to help the defensive inflammatory reaction. Some of these chemicals cause more white blood cells to be made, fever, fast pulse rate, etc. Some of these chemicals may be from the thing that is causing the inflammation, especially if it is an organism. Some of these chemicals may be toxins which cause high fever, damage to blood vessels with bleeding, wasting of the body (muscles get thin and weak), damage to the bone marrow and blood cells with anaemia etc.

In acute inflammation, more acute changes are caused – high fever, shivering (rigors), fast pulse, bleeding, etc.

In chronic inflammation less acute changes are caused – low fever, wasting, anaemia etc.

Neoplasm (also called newgrowth or tumour or cancer)

Normal body cells grow only where and when they are needed, e.g. during growth of a child, or to repair a wound, or to make new parts for the body to replace worn out parts. These normal cells stop growing after they have done their work.

A neoplasm is the growth of *abnormal body cells* which *keep on growing either where or when they are not needed*. The body cannot stop them growing.

The cause of some neoplasms is not known. Known causes of neoplasm include:
1. Chemicals, e.g. tobacco smoke causes lung cancer. Betel nut and lime causes mouth cancer.
2. Some drugs, but not those used by most health workers.
3. Probably some viruses.
4. Too much sunlight in people with light coloured skins (or albinos) causes skin cancer.
5. Radiation from atomic bombs etc. causes blood cancers.

There are two types of neoplasm:
1. Benign (or simple) neoplasms. The cells of benign neoplasms stay in the place where they started to grow and do not spread to other organs.
2. Malignant neoplasms. The cells of malignant neoplasms not only grow at the place where they started to grow. These cells also spread directly or in the blood or in the lymph to other parts of the body where they also start to grow. Malignant neoplasms can therefore be of two types:
   (a) Primary – the neoplasm at the place where it started,
   (b) Secondary – the neoplasm at the place it has spread to from the primary neoplasm.

Neoplasms damage the body in many ways:
1. Destruction of the tissue in which it is growing, e.g. neoplasm in the liver causes liver failure with jaundice.
2. Obstruction of the organ in which it is growing, e.g. neoplasm in the intestine causes intestinal obstruction with abdominal pain, constipation and vomiting.
3. Pressure on other important structures, e.g. Burkitt's tumour in the face pushes an eye out so that the lids cannot close.
4. Ulceration of the surface with bleeding or infection, e.g. stomach cancer causes vomiting of blood and anaemia.
5. Wasting and malaise (not feeling well).

4

A Classification of Disease – the causes of diseases

Diseases can be grouped or classified in many different ways. One good way to classify diseases in a health centre is by a *combination* of cause and pathology and clinical findings. Like this:

Congenital

These are diseases or abnormalities that were present when the patient was born. There are three sub-groups:

1. inherited or hereditary, i.e. passed on from the mother or the father – these diseases are in the family (e.g. thalassaemia);
2. damage done to the baby while it was in the mother's womb (e.g. blindness or congenital heart disease from an attack of rubella (German Measles) in the mother);
3. unknown (e.g. talipes or club foot).

Traumatic

These are injuries. *Causes* include:

1. mechanical injuries (e.g. cuts, bruises, fractures),
2. heat (e.g. burns).

Inflammatory

Inflammation is a reaction of part of the body to things which can injure it but do not completely destroy it. The most important part of the inflammatory reaction is that the blood vessels become wider and bring much more blood to the area. The blood vessels then allow fluid, proteins and cells to go into the area to fight the thing that is attacking the body (see Inflammation, Chapter 3).

Causes include:

1. Infection with organisms including: viruses, bacteria, protozoa, rickettsiae, fungi, worms and insects (called 'infestations').
2. Trauma: mechanical, heat.
3. Chemicals, especially: toxins, bites, stings and venoms (e.g. insect stings, stone fish sting).
4. Allergic reactions.
   Allergy is an inflammatory reaction of part of the body caused by some foreign substance on or in the body. This substance does not cause inflammation in the body of normal people. But if a person develops allergy to this substance, he develops abnormal antibodies (see Chapter 10) to this substance. When this substance comes in contact with the body again there is a reaction between the substance and the abnormal antibodies which causes an inflammatory reaction.
   (a) Allergy can be caused by substances touching the skin, e.g. skin rash due to streptomycin powder in some nurses.
   (b) Allergy can be caused by substances being inhaled (i.e. breathed in) e.g. asthma and hay-fever from house dust in some people.
   (c) Allergy can be caused by substances being injected, e.g. skin rash, asthma or shock in some people after penicillin injection or certain insect bites.
   (d) Allergy can be caused by substances being swallowed, e.g. skin rash in some people after swallowing aspirin tablets or cows' milk.

Neoplastic (also called tumours, cancers, newgrowths, or growths)

Neoplasms are made of abnormal body cells. These cells grow both when and where they are not needed. They cause damage to the normal parts of the body where they are growing.

They may be:

1. simple or benign,
2. malignant, either
   (a) primary where the neoplasm started, or
   (b) secondary where the noeplasm has spread to.

(See Neoplasm, Chapter 3).

Causes include:

1. viruses, e.g. EB virus together with malaria infection causes Burkitt's tumours;
2. chemicals, e.g. tobacco smoking causes lung cancer, lime and betel nut chewing causes mouth cancer;
3. some drugs, e.g. immunosuppressive drugs can cause lymphomas;
4. excess radiation, e.g. sun on skin of albino causes skin cancer;
5. hereditary factors;
6. other and as yet unknown causes.

Degenerative

These diseases are a wearing out of part of the body.

Causes include:

1. Old age, e.g. cataracts cause blindness in old people.
2. Habits or events during life can cause parts of the body to wear out more quickly that others, e.g. osteoarthritis when men play football and damage their knee joints many times.
3. Amyloid disease. This is an unusual condition in which an abnormal protein is put into the tissues and stops organs working properly. It happens in old age and sometimes in chronic inflammatory diseases (e.g. leprosy) and sometimes for no known cause.

Chemicals – drugs, poisons, toxins, venoms

These may have been given purposely or accidently. They may have been given for good or bad reasons. They may have been given by the health worker, the employer, an enemy or the patient himself.

1. Drugs should be given only by those who know the risks of their unwanted bad effects as well as their wanted good effects. These persons include health workers and patients who are instructed in the use of certain drugs, e.g. antimalarials. Drugs given by health workers and patients to treat one disease are a very common cause of another disease.

   The patient may also give himself other drugs – alcohol, tobacco and lime with betel nut. These are very common causes of disease – accidents, chronic bronchitis and cancer of the mouth (respectively).
2. Poisons may be added to a person's food or drink by an enemy; but this in fact is very rare.

Poisons may be taken by the patient himself to attempt suicide or attempt to treat a condition (e.g. unwanted pregnancy); but most commonly by accident (e.g. kerosene left in a soft-drink bottle).

3. Toxins may be formed by bacterial in food. When eaten, the toxins cause 'food poisoning'.
4. Venoms may be injected by insect or snake bites. They may cause various changes including pain, paralysis of muscles and abnormal bleeding.

Malnutrition

Not enough food, or not enough of some foods, or too much of some foods can cause disease, e.g.:

- marasmus from not enough food,
- kwashiorkor from not enough protein,
- anaemia from not enough iron or folic acid,
- obesity from too much food.

Psychological

Situations causing worry, stress and anxiety often cause disease, e.g. tension headaches, and 'hysterical' paralysis.

Failure of an organ or system of the body
(especially blood vessels)

Some conditions or diseases of parts of the body are caused by the failure of other parts of the body.

The most common of these conditions are those caused by the failure of the blood vessels. If an artery becomes narrow or blocked, then little or no food and oxygen can go to the part of the body supplied by the artery. That part is then damaged and cannot function properly and may die. If veins become blocked then blood pumped into part of the body cannot go out of that part. That part then swells up, is damaged and cannot function properly. Such conditions have *vascular* causes.

Failure of one body system may cause other conditions:

1. *Blood failure* may cause shock (not enough blood volume); shortness of breath, fainting, dizziness (anaemia); bleeding (platelets or clotting protein abnormal), etc.
2. *Heart failure* may cause oedema, enlarged liver, etc.
3. *Respiratory* (*lung*) *failure* may cause wasting, cyanosis, abnormal behaviour, heart failure, etc.

4. *Liver failure* may cause wasting, oedema, bleeding, abnormal behaviour, jaundice, etc.
5. *Endocrine gland failure* (e.g. pancreatic failure) may cause wasting, passing a lot of urine, unconsciousness, etc.

All body systems must be considered; but especially important are vascular, blood, heart, respiratory, kidney, liver and endocrine.

Others

Other groups do exist but are not as common as the 9 groups discussed above. Some have known causes. Some have causes not yet discovered.

Summary

When a disease or disability is discovered in a patient and the diagnosis is not obvious, answer the following questions:

Is this condition:
1. Congenital?
2. Traumatic?
3. Inflammatory, caused by:
   (a) trauma?
   (b) infection?
   (c) toxins or bites or venoms?
   (d) allergy?
4. Neoplastic?
5. Degenerative?
6. Caused by chemicals – drugs, poisons, toxins, venoms?
7. Caused by malnutrition?
8. Caused by psychological causes?
9. Caused by the failure of an organ of the body – especially blood vessels?
10. Caused by other causes known or unknown?

5

Epidemiology

It is not enough to know only the causes of illnesses.

The presence of the cause of a disease (usually called the 'specific agent') does not mean that disease will always be caused. All people have the organisms which cause pneumonia (the specific agent of pneumonia) in their respiratory tracts sometimes. But few get pneumonia. Some, however, do. Why? Smoking tobacco causes lung cancer. But many people smoke all of their lives and do not get lung cancer. Some, however, do. Why? There are certain things about the specific agent, or about the person who has the specific agent acting on him, or in the environment, that determine if disease will or will not happen.

The study of the distribution of disease in the community (i.e. when it occurs, where it occurs and who gets it) and all the things that determine if disease will or will not happen, is called epidemiology.

> Epidemiology is the study of *who* gets a particular disease, *where* and *when* these persons get the disease, and *how* and *why* they get the disease. (See Figures 5.1 and 5.2).

Epidemiology gives the known answers to these questions about a disease.

1. *Who* (including how many) }
2. *When* } are the people affected?
3. *Where* }
4. *How* does the whole process including the means of transfer of the specific agent (or 'cause') happen?
5. *Why* – or what are the factors (reasons) in:
   (a) the specific agent (i.e. the 'cause'); or
   (b) the means of transfer of the specific agent; or
   (c) man; or
   (d) the environment
   which determine if the disease happens or not.

Accurate terms to describe how often a disease occurs (or the *frequency* of a disease) include:
* *prevalence* of a disease is the *total* number of persons with the disease at a certain time in a certain population.
* *incidence* of a disease is the number of *new* persons getting the disease during a certain time in a certain population.

See Chapter 9 for other definitions and explanations.

Epidemiology has many uses. Many of these uses are not useful in your day-to-day work. Some, however, are.

If you know the epidemiology of a disease, it will help you in the differential diagnoses (see Chapter 6) of a patient who is sick. Some diseases do not affect some groups of people but may be common in other groups of people. By knowing which group of persons your patient is in and what diseases are common in his group, it is much easier to decide which disease your patient has.

If you know the epidemiology of a disease it will help you to understand that there is often more than one 'cause' of a person getting sick. There may be more than one thing which you need to do, therefore, to make the patient well again.

If you know the epidemiology of types of diseases, this may help you to find the reason for an outbreak of a disease in your community.

If you know the epidemiology of a disease it will help you control and prevent a disease. You may have to try to kill or remove the specific agent which can cause the disease. You may have to change the environment to stop its means of spread. You may have to increase the resistance of or, in more detail:

Figure 5.1 Diagrams showing how disease may be caused.

Figure 5.2 A diagram showing the things that are studied in epidemiology.

14

the person who is susceptible to the specific agent. It is only if you know the epidemiology of the disease, that you can decide which of these things is the best to do.

If you really want to improve the health of the people in your community, you need to use the methods of epidemiology to make a 'community diagnosis' of your own community. You need to find out who makes up your community and how many men, women and children there are. You need to know what illnesses really do affect these people. You need to know which members of the community have these illnesses. You need to know when and where and how and why these people get these illnesses. It is only when you have used epidemiological methods to make your own community diagnosis that you will be able:

1. to make the best use of epidemiological methods in diagnosing and treating individual patients, and
2. to give the best advice for disease prevention and health promotion to all the people of the community.

6

Diagnosis of Disease

Remember: you must diagnose before you can treat.

You must first diagnose what condition or disease a patient has before you can choose the proper treatment to help the patient. The only treatment which will help the patient is the proper treatment for the condition or disease which the patient really has. Treatment (even good treatment) for a condition which the patient does not have will not help the patient.

Taking a medical history

If you know what questions to ask you can take a full history in about 2–5 minutes in most ordinary cases.

If you make the patient give you a good history, you will often hear the patient tell you a story which you recognise. The story may be one you have heard before or it may be a story that you have read about in your medical books. In either case, you will recognise the patient's story as the story of a disease about which you know. Even if you do not recognise the story of a disease, you will hear about important symptoms which you can use in making the differential diagnosis.

Also the history will often tell you how you need to examine the patient.

The medicial history is in 9 parts (the medical examination is in 9 parts too):

To make the correct diagnosis you must do all of the following 6 things:
1. Take a medical history.
2. Do a medical or physical examination.
3. Make a differential diagnosis (or make a list of the diseases which *could* be causing the patient's main symptoms and signs).
4. Do or order any tests that are needed:
    (a) to find out which of the diseases in the differential diagnosis the patient really has; *or*
    (b) to confirm a diagnosis; *or*
    (c) to give a 'baseline' to see if the patient gets better or worse.
5. Make a provisional diagnosis and decide:
    (a) which disease (or diseases) is most likely to be causing the patient's symptoms and signs;
    (b) how severe this disease is;
    (c) how quickly this disease is getting better or worse.
6. Decide on the prognosis of the patient.

1. general information and admission notes;
2. complaints and their duration;
3. history of the present illness;
4. specific questioning (or specific interrogation);
5. past history;
6. family and contact history;
7. if the patient may have a mental condition, take the history again from a relative or another witness;
8. check the patient's outpatient card for any history in it;
9. tell the patient a summary of the history – ask him to correct anything wrong.

1. General information and admission notes
Write down:
    Date.
    Patient's name and address, etc.[1]
    With whom patient lives and the address.[1]
    Reason for admission.
    Who referred patient.

---

1 The patient's exact present address and also a friend's or relative's name and address are most important. If you do not write this down it will not be possible to find the patient later if it is necessary. You may need to find the patient if he has an infectious disease (e.g. tuberculosis) and does not come for treatment.

2. Complaints and their duration (or how long they have lasted).[2]

Write down:
> Only the main problems.[3]
> Only short descriptions.
> Only the patient's own way of describing them.

3. History of present illness (HPI)

Ask questions like these and write down the answers:
> How long ago was it that something first went wrong with you?
> What was this first thing that went wrong?
> What was the next thing that happened?
> When did this happen?
> What happened next?... When?...

You should also:
> (a) Ask for a full description of pain or any other symptom.
> (b) Ask about *all* the symptoms of *all* the body systems in which the patient has symptoms.
> (c) Ask about the presence or absence of all the symptoms of any possible disease.
> (d) Ask what treatment has already been given.

4. Specific interrogation (SI) or specific questioning

Ask the patient about (unless already talked about in the HIP):[4]
> Fever.
> Cough. Sputum. Haemoptysis.
> Pain in the chest.
> Chronic cough.
> Shortness of breath.

---

2 When you have ordered treatment, look back at this list to make sure you have done something for the patient's complaints.

3 Make sure the patient tells you all of his complaints. He may leave the most important one till last.

4 You must always get answers to all of these questions. If you already know the answers from the HPI, do not ask the questions again. You cannot think that the patient does not have these symptoms only because the patient has not told you about them. He may not think they are important. He may not want to talk about them. These questions are about the main symptoms caused by the main pathological processes in each of the major body systems. You must find out about each one of them. In some places where there are special diseases, other questions may have to be added to this list.

> Eating well. Vomiting. Diarrhoea.
> Pain in the abdomen.
> Urinary pain, urinary frequency, abnormal colour of urine. Blood in the urine.
> Date of last menstrual period.
> Getting fatter or thinner or staying the same weight.
> What the patient thinks is wrong.
> What the patient thinks is the cause.

If the patient is *pregnant* also ask about:
> Oedema? Treatment?
> High blood pressure? Treatment?
> Vaginal bleeding? Treatment?
> Anaemia? Treatment?
> Labour pains started? When?
> Vaginal show or bleeding? When?
> Membranes ruptured? When?

5. Past history (PH)

Ask about:
> Drugs:
> (a) given today,
> (b) given for the treatment of this illness before today,
> (c) given regularly,
> (d) alcohol and tobacco – how much, how often.
> Treatment given by traditional healers? What?
> Previous attacks of this illness? When? What treatment?
> Previous other serious illnesses or operations or accidents? What? When?

If the patient is *pregnant*, also ask about:
> How many births? Dates?
> How many miscarriages? Dates?
> How many still births or neonatal deaths? When? Why?
> Any difficult deliveries (Caesarian section, symphysiotomy, vacuum extraction, very long labour (> 24 hours)? Which births?
> Any post-partum haemorrhage or retained placenta? Which births?

6. Family history and contact history (FH, CH)

This is especially important for those who live in the same house. Ask if there is:
> anyone with this illness,
> anyone with other serious illness,

anyone with tuberculosis (or cough for more than 4 weeks),
anyone with leprosy.

7. *If the patient may have a mental problem or condition, take all history again from a relative or other witness*

8. *Look at the patient's outpatient card* for any HPI, SI, PH, FH etc. in it. (Return the card to the patient.)

9. *Tell the patient a summary of the history obtained. Then ask him to correct anything wrong*

If pain (or another symptom) is present it will often help the health worker to ask about:
1. The site (or where it is).
2. The radiation (or if it spreads to any other place and where).
3. The character or type (e.g. constant [stays the same all the time] or colic [comes and goes again and again in minutes]).
4. The severity (or how bad it is).
5. The frequency (or how often it comes).
6. The duration (or how long it lasts).
7. Any special times it comes.

Performing a medical or physical examination

The medical examination is in three parts. The *first part or basic observations* should *always* be done on *all* patients for at least two reasons.
1. It will show you if the patient is 'sick' or not. This is not done by intuition (a feeling or an idea). This is done by observation during examination.
2. It is a simple test for the common and fatal diseases. You may need to add some other observations to this list in places where there are special diseases. The following diseases are suggested by the 'basic observations':
   • Meningitis is suggested by the change in the level of consciousness and the stiff neck.
   • Malaria is suggested by a high temperature.
   • Pneumonia is suggested by a fast and abnormal type of respiration.
   • Gastro-enteritis is suggested by the weight loss and signs of dehydration.
   • Malnutrition or wasting is suggested by the signs of malnutrition and wasting.
   • Anaemia is suggested by the colour.

Therefore, even if a patient has only a simple laceration, you should still do the 'basic observations' so that you can do any necessary preventive medicine. Diseases may be found while they are still mild. Treatment will stop these diseases becoming severe or causing death.

The *second part* is the examination of the part of the body which the symptoms suggest is diseased.

The *third part* of the examination is the examination of the whole body. You must examine the whole of the body if:
1. The patient is 'sick'.
2. The disease you think the patient may have could affect more than one part of the body.
3. You are not certain of the diagnosis.

In each part of a clinical examination you usually do these five things:
1. Inspection – look and see.
2. Palpation – feel and touch with hands.
3. Percussion – tap and listen (and feel).
4. Auscultation – listen (usually with stethoscope).
5. Measurement – not often done in a health centre.

It is not always possible to do all these things. But you should do them all, in this order, if possible.

The medical examination is in 9 parts.
1. Basic observations.
2. Head and neck including the ears, nose and throat, thyroid and lymph glands.
3. Chest and spine.
4. Abdomen.
5. Skin and hair.
6. Muscles, bones, joints.
7. Head and neck etc. (if not done before).
8. Any special examinations suggested by previous history and examination.
9. Mental state.

1. Basic observations

Signs of meningeal irritation (drowsiness, or irritability or fitting, stiff neck, stiff back, Kernig's sign positive).

Does the patient have signs of meningitis or cerebral malaria?

temperature (T°)
pulse rate (PR)
blood pressure (BP) (if needed)
respiration rate (RR) and
   type of respiration
weight
} 5 vital signs

Does the patient have signs of malaria or pneumonia or shock or weight change?

dehydration
  – eyes sunken, mouth dry,
    inelastic skin, pulse fast,
    weight loss
oedema (limbs, back, face)
malnutrition
wasting
colour
  – anaemia, jaundice,
    cyanosis
} 5 general conditions

Does the patient have any of these 5 signs?

Is the patient 'sick'?

2. Head and neck including ears, nose and throat, thyroid and lymph glands in the neck and axilla

(See also Chapter 20 page 149, Chapter 30 page 330, Chapter 22 page 198.)
These may be left until 7.

3. Chest

(See also Chapter 20 page 150).
Look for:
(a) rate of respiration,
(b) type of respiration,
(c) deformity of spine or chest.

Feel for decreased movement of:
(a) all of the chest,
(b) part or parts of the chest.

Percuss for:
(a) dullness or
(b) increased resonance
} in { all of the chest, or, part or parts of the chest.

Listen for:
(a) amount of breath sounds
(b) breath sounds normal or bronchial
(c) crackles or crepitations
(d) wheezes or rhonchi
} in { all of the chest, or part or parts of the chest.

Ask the patient to cough – listen to the cough.
Look at sputum (is there any pus?).
Does the patient have pneumonia or tuberculosis or obstruction of bronchi?

4. Abdomen

(See Chapter 36 page 402, Chapter 21 page 181, Chapter 22 page 198, Chapter 23 page 212.)
Look at:
(a) size (distension),
(b) shape (herniae, masses,)
(c) surface (scars),
(d) movement when breathing

Feel for:
(a) tenderness, rebound tenderness, guarding, rigidity;
(b) liver, spleen, uterus and bladder;
(c) lumps, including hernia and lymph glands.

Percuss, if needed, for:
(a) organs or masses,
(b) fluid (e.g. ascites).

Listen, if needed, for bowel sounds.

Pelvic examination through the rectum (PR), if needed, for:
(a) tenderness
(b) enlarged organs
(c) masses
(d) faeces, blood or pus in rectum.

Pelvic examination through the vagina (PV), if needed, for:
(a) tenderness
(b) enlarged organs

(c) masses

(d) blood or pus in vagina.

Does the patient have signs of 'peritonitis' or an enlarged organ, or an inflamed organ or an abnormal mass?

If the patient is *pregnant*, also:
Palpate for:
(a) size of uterus (height of fundus);
(b) lie of fetus; what is presenting part.
Auscultate for fetal heart rate.

If the patient is in *labour*, also:
Palpate for:
(a) size of uterus (height of fundus);
(b) lie of fetus, what is presenting part, engagement of head;
(c) frequency, duration and strength of contractions.
Auscultate for fetal heart rate.
Do pelvic examination PV for:
(a) state of cervix and start cervicograph;
(b) membranes ruptured or intact;
(c) level of head (above or below spines);
(d) caput.

5. Skin and hair
(See also Chapter 32.)
Look for:
scabies,
infections,
other rashes,
scars.

Does the patient have scabies or impetigo or leprosy?

6. Muscles, bones and joints
(See also Chapter 28.)
Look and feel for:
(a) deformity
(b) tenderness
(c) swelling

Does the patient have fracture, osteomyelitis, arthritis or absess?

7. Head and neck, ENT, thyroid, lymph glands (if not done)

8. Any special examination indicated by previous history and examination
Five important examinations which you may need to do:
(a) If gynaecological disease is possible, do pelvic examination PV (see Chapter 26 page 282).
(b) If leprosy is suspected, do examinations for nerve enlargement and tenderness and for loss of sensation and for paralysis (see Chapter 18 page 77).
(c) If there is pain in the eye or loss of sight, examine for iritis and corneal ulcer and corneal foreign body (see Chapter 31 page 335).
(d) If there is a wound, check that nerves, tendons and blood vessels are all working.
(e) If there is oedema or if heart failure is suspected, examine for raised jugular venous pressure (see Chapter 27 page 301).

9. Mental state
(See also Chapter 35 page 387.)
(a) Ability to communicate (hear, see, move, talk, etc).
(b) Level of consciousness.
(c) Memory – recent past – distant past.
(d) Orientation: person, time, place.
(e) Intelligence.
(f) Thoughts by:

(g) Mood by:

(h) Insight.

If you carry out a good examination you will often see in the patient a 'picture' or 'pattern' which you recognise. The 'picture' or 'pattern' may be one you have seen before in another patient or it may be one you recognise from reading about it from your medical books. In either case, you will have recognised the 'picture' or 'pattern' as a disease which you know about. Even if you do not recognise a 'picture' or 'pattern' of a disease, you will have found important signs to use in making the differential diagnosis.

Making a differential diagnosis (DD)

The patient's symptoms and signs are caused by, (a) an abnormality of the structure and/or function of a part of his or her body and (b) the cause of this abnormality.

A number of different conditions can cause the same symptom or sign. These different conditions, however, usually have other symptoms or signs or tests as well, which are not all the same. The different conditions which cause the same symptom or sign can be separated by using these other symptoms and signs and tests.

The differential diagnosis is a list of the conditions any one of which could be causing the patient's main symptoms and signs.

Write down the patient's main symptoms and signs in a row across the top of a page of paper. Then under each of these symptoms and signs, write down the list of conditions which could cause these symptoms and signs. The differential diagnosis is all the conditions in all the lists.

Next, look for a disease (or diseases) which is in each list (as a cause of each symptom and sign). This is the condition which is most likely to be the cause of the patient's condition. If there is more than one condition in all of the lists, then tests will probably be needed to find out which of the conditions is the real cause of the patient's problems.

Doing or ordering tests (or investigations)

You may need a test:
1. to decide between the possible diagnoses in the DD;
2. to confirm a diagnosis;
3. to give a base line to be able to judge if a patient is getting better or worse.

See Appendix 1 (page 22) for how to take and send blood for tests in the hospital laboratory.

Making a provisional diagnosis (PD)

The provisional diagnosis (PD) is the condition you think the patient really has.

You decide the PD after considering all the conditions in the differential diagnosis that could cause the patient's main symptoms and signs. Reject the other conditions in the list if:
1. these conditions do not cause all of the patient's symptoms and signs; and
2. these conditions have other symptoms or signs or tests which do not fit the patient.

Choose the condition as the PD which:
1. is a cause of all the patient's symptoms and signs; and
2. has other symptoms and signs and tests all of which do fit the patient.

In this book, the PD of most of the common symptoms and signs is set out.

The prognosis

The prognosis is what you think will happen to the patient because of the condition you have diagnosed, e.g.
- die or live,
- improve quickly or slowly,
- not improve at all.

The prognoses of the common diseases are set out in this book.

The signature of health worker and date should always be written after any of the above are written into the patient's notes.

Summary

Diagnosis of disease includes:
1. Taking a medical history (9 parts).
2. Doing a clinical examination (9 parts).
3. Making a differential diagnosis.
4. Doing or ordering any tests needed.
5. Making a provisional diagnosis.
6. Deciding the prognosis.

You must practice doing medical histories and examinations again and again until all of the things in this chapter can be done is 5–10 minutes.

Appendix 1:

Method of taking blood for tests. Making blood smears and sending pathology specimens to the hospital laboratory.

Collection of blood

Skin puncture (capillary blood)
1. In adults use the patient's finger or the lobe of the ear, choosing a site free from disease.
2. In infants use the heel.
3. Squeeze or flick the ear, finger or heel a few times. Clean it with spirit or antiseptic and allow to dry.
4. Make a good prick with a quick motion, using a sterile, dry, sharp lancet.
5. Try not to squeeze the finger or ear after you have pricked it because this spoils the specimen for some methods.
6. Make a blood film straight from the drop of blood or fill a blood pipette with it.
7. Label the specimen clearly.

Venepuncture (venous blood)
1. The syringe and needle *must* be clean, dry and *sterile*. Check that the syringe will suck. Fit a sharp sterile needle.
2. Place the tourniquet around the arm above the elbow; ask the patient to open and close his hand several times.
3. Clean the skin over the veins at the fold of elbow with iodine or spirit.
4. Pull the skin tight over the vein with the thumb of the left hand. With a quick push, puncture the skin and vein with the needle which has the bevel upwards.
5. Do not move needle or syringe after the needle is in the vein.
6. Withdraw blood by pulling on the plunger of the syringe.
7. When ready to remove syringe, put a small piece of sterile, dry cotton-wool over the needle. Remove tourniquet and withdraw needle from vein. Ask the patient to hold the cotton-wool on the needle puncture for 2–3 minutes.
8. Remove needle from syringe and gently empty blood into a sterile test tube to clot; or into a bottle containing an anticoagulant, mixing gently to prevent clotting.

9. Keep stopper in bottle to prevent evaporation.
10. Wash syringe and needle at once with cold water to remove blood before it clots.
11. The bottle containing the EDTA blood must be mixed for 3 minutes immediately before using the blood for a test.
12. Label the specimen clearly.

Anticoagulant used in haematology

1. It is necessary to have the correct proportion of blood to anticoagulant to prevent shrinkage of the cells which would give incorrect results.
2. *8% EDTA Solution*
   (a) Pipette 0.1 ml of EDTA solution into small screwtop bottles. Allow the water to evaporate completely at room temperature. Fix the screwcaps and label them.
   (b) This amount of EDTA prevents 4 ml of blood from clotting. It is important to try to add just 4 ml of blood to the bottle.

Preparation of thin blood films

To make a good thin blood film the slides must be perfectly clean; so first wash the slides in detergent and then clean water and store them in methylated spirit or 70% alcohol. Before use, wipe the slide dry with a clean cloth or paper (toilet paper will do). *Always hold the cleaned slide by the edges.*

Preparation of spreader
Break off the corners of a glass slide, making sure that the edge of the slide is smooth. *It must not be chipped or rough* because this will spoil the blood film.

NO chipped or rough edge

spreader

YES smooth edge

Figure 6.1

Making the film

1. Place a small drop of fresh blood, about 1 cm ½ inch from the end of the clean slide.

2. Hold the spreader so that it slopes backwards.
3. Place the spreader just in front of the drop of blood, then move it back till it touches the blood. The blood will then spread along the edge of the spreader.
4. Push the spreader forward smoothly and quickly.
5. Immediately, hold the slide by the edges and wave it in the air quickly until the blood film dries.
6. Write the patient's name on the end of the slide with a marking pencil, or write in pencil the patient's name on the blood film.
7. Always wash the spreader with water after use, then dry it with soft paper.

Figure 6.2

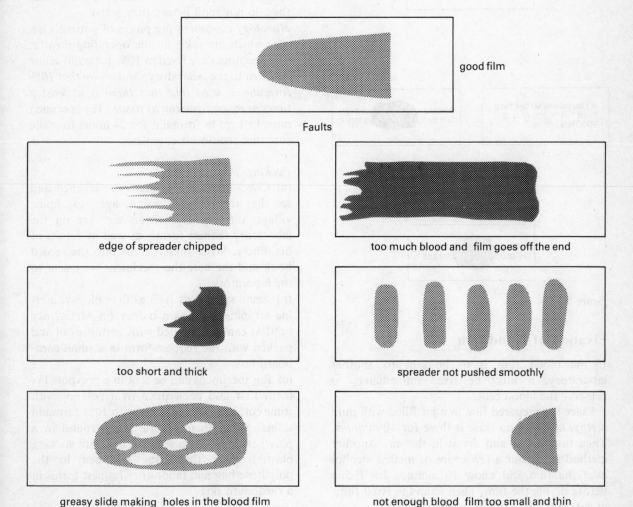

good film

Faults

edge of spreader chipped

too much blood and film goes off the end

too short and thick

spreader not pushed smoothly

greasy slide making holes in the blood film

not enough blood film too small and thin

Figure 6.3

Preparation of thick blood film

1. Place a drop or 3 small drops of fresh blood in the centre of a clean slide.
2. Spread the blood with the corner of a slide, making sure that it is spread evenly, until you can just see the print of a newspaper or book through it.
3. Leave the slide flat and allow to dry, protecting from flies and insects.

IF YOU CAN READ THE TYPE. THEN THE BLOOD FILM IS TOO THIN

IF YOU CA[...]THE TYPE. THE BLO[...]O THICK

IF YOU CA[...]THE TYPE. THE BLOO[...]CORRECT

Figure 6.4

Fixation of blood film

If the blood film is to be sent to another laboratory, it must be fixed immediately to preserve the blood cells.

Place the prepared film in a jar filled with *pure methyl alcohol* and leave it there for 10 *minutes*. Then take it out and dry it in the air. Another method is to pour a few drops of methyl alcohol over the film and allow 10 minutes for fixing before drying the film. Then wrap the fixed films in soft paper (e.g. toilet paper) and pack.

Make 2 films in case one is broken or damaged.

Details of how to take other tests are found in the appropriate chapters

Urethral smears for gonococci Chapter 19 page 131.
Smears for Donovan bodies Chapter 19 page 136.
Skin smears for AFB (leprosy) Chapter 15 page 87.
Skin biopsies Chapter 15 page 90.
Sputum smears for AFB (tuberculosis) Chapter 14 page 69.
Etc.

Sending specimens to laboratory

1. Some specimens must be sent from a health centre to a laboratory. It is very important that specimens are packed and sent properly so that they do not spoil before they arrive.
2. *Histology specimens* are pieces of patient's tissues which are taken in the operating theatre. The specimens are fixed in 10% formalin saline and sent to the laboratory. *Make sure that 10% formalin is used and that there is at least 5 times as much formalin as tissue*. The specimen must be kept in formalin for 24 hours to make sure that fixation is complete.

   Packing
   (a) Check that all specimens are labelled and see that the patient's name, age, sex, home village and census division etc. are on the laboratory request forms, as well as details of his illness. Write these details into the record book and the date the specimens were sent to the laboratory.
   (b) Small specimens such as liver biopsy, uterine scrapings and skin biopsy (in McCartney bottles) can be wrapped with cotton-wool and packed with the request form in a small cardboard box.
   (c) Big specimens can be sent in a polypot. Fix them first and pack them in a polypot with some cotton wool made wet with 10% formalin saline. Wrap them several times round in a polythene bag. Then seal this bag with sticking plaster. Pack the tissue wrapped in the polythene bag and laboratory request forms in a cardboard box.
3. *Bacteriology specimens*. Send specimen in a universal container packed in a cardboard box

(see above). Swabs for culture should be sent in 'Stuart's transport medium' available from the Hospital Laboratory.

4. *Haematology, biochemistry and serology specimens*

(a) Blood specimens such as serum, EDTA blood and thin blood films may need to be sent. Fix the films by pouring a few drops of methyl alcohol over the films, allow 10 minutes for fixing, then dry them. Write on the laboratory request form that they are fixed with methyl alcohol. Wrap the slides separately with toilet paper and pack with the request forms in a small cardboard box.

(b) Wrap the serum and EDTA specimens carefully in cotton wool and put them inside a plastic bag. Seal the plastic bag with sticking plaster and pack with laboratory request forms in a cardboard box. Write '*BLOOD SAMPLES*' and '*Notify the department on arrival*' on top of the parcel.

(c) It is very important that all blood specimens should be sent by air freight or other quick delivery and *not* by ordinary post.

(d) *Specimens for biochemistry and serology.* Always send *serum*, never *whole blood*. The only time you send whole blood is for blood sugar which is collected into the special fluoride oxalate bottle. (These special bottles can be obtained from the hospital.)

7

Treatment, Drugs and Pain Relief

1. Decide on outpatient treatment or admit for inpatient treatment.
2. Order the proper nursing care.
3. Give specific treatment to cure the disease.
4. Give symptomatic treatment to relieve the symptoms.
5. Give explanation and comfort to the patient and to the relatives.
6. Give health education to the patient and to the relatives about control and prevention of the disease.
7. Consult with the medical officer *or* transfer the patient to medical officer care *or* refer the patient to the next visiting medical officer if necessary.
8. Discharge the patient and give final health education.
9. Follow-up the patient if necessary.
   Treatment of a patient may include any or all of these things.

Treatment of the patient

Only when you have made a provisional diagnosis of the patient's problem can you decide how to treat the patient and manage the problem caused by the disease. Treatment of the patient only is not enough. You must do four things when you diagnose a disease:

1. Treat the patient (see this chapter).
2. Notify the necessary authorities and relatives (see Chapter 8).
3. Control the spread of the disease if necessary (see Chapter 9).
4. Prevent the disease occurring again in the patient and in the community if possible (see Chapter 9).

There are nine things you must do to treat a patient properly:

1. Treat as outpatient or admit for inpatient care

2. Order proper nursing care (if necessary).
(a) Rest – in bed; in special position, etc.
(b) Special care of respiratory tract, mouth, eyes, ears, bowels, bladder, limbs, pressure areas, etc.
(c) Special fluids – orally or intravenously.
(d) Special diet.
(e) Special observations.
(f) Isolation.
(g) Collection of specimens for tests.

3. Give specific treatment (to cure).
(a) Drugs. Which drugs; by what route; how much; how often; for how long?
(b) Surgery. What surgery; who will do it; when?
(c) Dressings, plasters, etc.
(d) Physiotherapy.
(e) Fluids – oral or intravenously. Food or diet.
(f) Psychiatric counselling.

4. Give symptomatic treatment (to relieve symptoms).
(a) To make the patient *feel* better (i.e. to relieve his symptoms, especially pain).
(b) 'Rule' treatment, e.g. 'Give anti-malarials to every patient with a fever'. (There are different 'rule' treatments for different places and different countries.)

Symptomatic treatment may include any of the things in 2 and 3 above, especially:
(a) drugs,
(b) surgery,
(c) dressings,
(d) diet,
(e) psychiatric counselling,
(f) nursing in special positions,
(g) special nursing care of parts of the body.

5. Give explanation and comfort

Give explanation and comfort to the patient and to his relatives.

6. Give health education

Give health education about control and prevention of the disease to the patient and relatives.

7. Consult – Transfer – Refer (if necessary).

Consult with the medical officer (by phone or radio if necessary) if you are not sure of the diagnosis or what the management should be.

Transfer of patient to medical officer care in a hospital if necessary. Transfers are of two types: urgent (emergency); or non-urgent (routine).

Arranging transfer includes the following:
(a) Get permission from medical officer if, when, where, how to transfer.
(b) Get written permission of patient or relative for any necessary treatment.
(c) Tell the hospital when the patient should arrive.
(d) Arrange for drugs, dressings, fluids, oxygen, splints, stretcher, pillow, blanket, etc.
(e) Arrange for a suitable person to accompany the patient.
(f) Arrange transport.
(g) Provide a letter.

Refer problem cases who are non-urgent to next visiting medical officer.

8. Discharge the patient

Arrange for patient to return for review on completion of treatment if necessary.

Write up patient's outpatient health record and give it to him.

Give final health education.

9. Follow-up the patient (if necessary).

> Management of the problem caused by the diagnosing of a case of a disease includes:
> 1. Treat the patient (9 things may be necessary) (see above).
> 2. Notify the necessary authorities and relatives.
> 3. Control the spread of the disease if necessary.
> 4. Prevent the disease occurring again in this patient and in the community if possible.

Drug treatment

A *drug* is any substance which can change the body or pathological states of the body.

Drugs act by changing the function or structure of parts of the body, or by changing the structure or function of organisms or substances which have entered the body.

Always use the *'approved'* or *'official'* name for a drug. Do not use the trade names given by companies to their brands of the drug, as the health department changes the brands of the drug supplied from time to time.

Drugs may be given by a number of different ways (or routes):

1. By mouth (orally).

Drugs are usually given by mouth. Drugs are not given by mouth if they would not be absorbed, because of any of the following reasons:
(a) Their structure is such that they are not able to be absorbed from the gastro-intestinal tract.
(b) Vomiting and/or diarrhoea.
(c) Shock (with little blood going to the gastro-intestinal tract).
(d) Swallowing not possible (e.g. unconscious).
(e) The patient is not willing, or is not reliable enough, to swallow the drug.

2. By injection.

Injections may be of different types:
(a) intravenous injection (IVI),
(b) intramuscular injection (IMI),
(c) subcutaneous injection (SCI),
(d) intradermal injection (IDI),
(e) injection into special structures (e.g. intra-pleural injection).

Drugs are given by injection for any of the following reasons:
(a) They may not be absorbed from the gastro-intestinal tract because of vomiting, diarrhoea, shock or the drug being of a structure not able to be absorbed.
(b) Oral administration is not possible – patient is not reliable enough, or is not conscious, etc.
(c) Treatment needs to be effective quickly.
(d) A high concentration in special structures in the body is needed.

3. Rectally, by suppository.
4. Through the blood vessels in the lung by inhalation.

Drugs do not all go to all parts of the body. A drug has to be chosen which will go to the parts of the body where it is needed, but not go to parts of the body where it could cause damage.

Most drugs are destroyed ('*inactivated*' or '*metabolised*') *and got out of the body* ('*excreted*') by either the liver or the kidney. In liver or kidney diseases, therefore, drug doses may have to be lower than normal.

All drugs have unwanted side effects. These may include the following:

1. Effects which are normal actions of the drug other than the one action wanted for this patient.
2. Allergy (see Chapter 10 page 37) and other effects which do not normally occur, but do occur in a few special persons.
3. Damage to an unborn child in the uterus.

Give a drug only if its possible bad effects are less than the risk of the untreated disease.

Drug treatment of pain – analgesia

The best treatment for pain is to remove the cause of the pain. While this is being done or if this is not possible, use one of the following groups of pain relieving drugs called analgesics.
1. General anaesthetics, e.g. ketamine.
2. Narcotic or opiate drugs, e.g. morphine, pethidine, codeine phosphate.
3. Non-narcotic analgesic and anti-rheumatic drugs, e.g. aspirin, paracetamol.
4. Other systemic drugs with various actions, e.g. chlorpromazine.
5. Local anaesthetics, e.g. lignocaine, procaine, amethocaine, local cooling agents.

Choice of analgesic

For mild pain, give aspirin or paracetamol tablets.

If aspirin or paracetamol is not enough, use compound analgesic tablets also called codeine compound tablets ('Codeine Co') which are a combination of aspirin and a small dose of codeine phosphate. Paracetamol and codeine tablets are also available.

For bowel colic, use codeine phosphate.

For severe pain use pethidine tablets or injection. If pethidine is not enough, use morphine injection. Do *not* use these drugs for chronic pain unless the patient is expected to die soon.

Use chlorpromazine in small doses together with the usual dose of pethidine or morphine to make these drugs more effective and last longer; but only in special cases.

For very severe pain, give a general anaesthetic, usually a ketamine injection.

For some pains in only one part of the body (e.g. a sting from a 'stone fish') you can use an injection of a local anaesthetic around the painful area.

Morphine, pethidine and codeine

These are dangerous drugs. They are also called narcotic or opiate drugs. There are special rules for storing and using them. Effects and precautions include:
1. Pain is relieved. *Never use them in abdominal pain until the cause is definitely diagnosed and proper treatment started. Otherwise, when pain and tenderness is gone, diagnosis may not be possible.*
2. Breathing and coughing is less. *Never use in chronic obstructive lung disease or asthma or if the patient might have any difficulty in breathing. Otherwise the patient might completely stop breathing.*
3. Diarrhoea is stopped and constipation can be caused. They are very effective treatment for severe diarrhoea.
4. Vomiting is caused sometimes.
5. Itch occurs sometimes.
6. Sleepiness and change in consciousness is caused. *Never use if the patient has a head injury as level of consciousness is then difficult to interpret.*
7. Happiness is often caused. Addiction occurs quickly. *Never use for chronic pain or for more than a few days unless the patient is soon to die.* However, they are good treatment for pain in the dying patient.

Overdose is treated with artificial ventilation and nalorphine or naloxone.

Aspirin

Effects include the following:

1. Pain is relieved (mild pain only).
2. Temperature is lowered. However, treatment of the cause of the raised temperature is much more important.
3. Anti-inflammatory effects occur if large doses are given regularly. This is done for arthritis and leprosy reactions.
4. Indigestion, peptic ulcer and gastro-intestinal bleeding can occur. Do not give aspirin if the patient possibly has a peptic ulcer or any bleeding.
5. Allergic reactions can occur.

The dose of aspirin is 300–1200 mg (1–4 tabs) each 4–6 hours.

Give aspirin when required for pain.

Give aspirin regularly for its anti-inflammatory effect.

If the dose of aspirin is too high, the patient may get:

1. 'Ringing' or other noises in the ears; or deafness.
2. Headache.
3. Nausea, vomiting.

If these occur:

(a) stop the aspirin for 1 day,
(b) then give it in a lower dose.

A large overdose of aspirin is very dangerous. Immediately make the patient vomit if he is conscious. Treat immediately as described in Chapter 34.

Paracetamol

Paracetamol relieves pain and often reduces a fever. However, it is not usually as effective a drug as aspirin. It does not have the anti-inflammatory effects of aspirin. However, it does not cause gastro-intestinal irritation and bleeding as aspirin does.

An overdose of paracetamol is very dangerous. Treat immediately as described in Chapter 34 and transfer the patient urgently to a medical officer for special treatment to try to stop severe liver damage.

Doses of analgesic drugs

Aspirin (300 mg tablets).

- 300–1200 mg (1–4 tabs) each 6 hours if required for pain.
- Use a small dose (1–2 tabs) for a small adult or for mild pain in large adult.
- Use a large dose (3–4 tabs) for a more severe pain in a large adult.

Codeine compound tablets (aspirin 300 mg and codeine 8 mg in each tablet).

- 1–4 tablets each 6 hours if required for pain.
- Use a small dose (1–2 tabs) for a small adult or less severe pain in a large adult.
- Use a large dose (2–3 tabs) for a severe pain in a large adult.

Pethidine (50 mg/ml – 2 ml amps of 100 mg and 1 ml amps of 50 mg)

- 1–2 ml/kg each 6 hours if required for pain.
- Small adult, pain not very severe, 50 mg (1 ml).
- Small adult, severe pain, 75 mg (1.5 ml) (1½ ml).
- Large adult, pain not very severe, 75 mg (1.5 ml) (1½ ml).
- Large adult, severe pain 100 mg (2 ml).

Morphine (10 mg/ml – 1 ml amps of 10 mg).

- 0.2 mg (1/5 mg)/kg each 6 hours if required.
- Small adult 7.5 mg (7½ mg) 0.75 ml (3/4 ml).
- Large adult 10 mg (1 ml).

Lignocaine plain 1% solution (50 ml vial) and

Procaine plain 1% solution (2 ml amp).

- Inject the smallest volume needed into or around the affected area to cause analgesia of the part of the body affected.
- Never inject more than 50 ml at any one time into a patient.

Paracetamol (500 mg tablets).

- 500–1000 mg (1–2 tabs) each 6 hours if required for pain.

IVI Ketamine, IMI Ketamine for general anaesthetic.

IVI Lytic cocktail for general analgesic effect.

IVI Lignocaine for regional anaesthesia.

Do *not* use these three drugs *unless*:
1. you have been trained in their use; *and*
2. you have all the necessary equipment for resuscitation and artificial ventilation available and ready.

8

Notification of Disease and Death

disease control and prevention work and can send you special advice or special help.

The Health Officer may report these things to Health Department Headquarters. Headquarters need to know what diseases occur so that they can send the proper staff, drugs and equipment to help. Headquarters may also help to report certain communicable diseases (the Quarantinable Diseases) to the World Health Organization (WHO).

There are two types of condition which are notified to the Health Officer:

1. Diseases which are monitored and reported regularly at the end of each month.
   (a) Count and record every single case of these diseases (no matter whether an inpatient or an outpatient).
   (b) Send the number of cases of each disease to the Health Officer at the end of each month.

There are three types of notification:

1. Notification of the Provincial or District Health or Medical Officer of:
   (a) the number of cases each month of the diseases which are being monitored;
   (b) events of public health concern.
2. Notification of the coroner and the police of all cases of 'sudden and unnatural' death.
3. Notification of the relatives and friends of the nature, treatment and prognosis of the patient's illness.

> Keep a copy of the list of diseases you must monitor and report in a safe handy place.

---

2. 'Events of Public Health Concern'. If any of these things happen, notify the Health Officer immediately, by the fastest possible method:
   (a) outbreaks or epidemics of known diseases;
   (b) outbreaks or epidemics of unknown diseases;
   (c) single cases of dangerous diseases not usual in the area, e.g. cholera, plague, yellow fever;
   (d) natural disasters (floods, earthquakes, etc.) which may affect people's health;
   (e) unusual events such as diseases or deaths of animals (e.g. fish or rats) which may affect people's health.

Notification of the Health Officer

If certain diseases or conditions occur you must notify these to the Health Officer.

The Health Officer can then help you in your

9

Control and Prevention of Disease — summary of patient management

Figures 9.1 and 9.2 illustrate important points in control and prevention of infectious disease. *Use these five methods for the prevention and control of all (non-infective as well as infectious) diseases.*

See Chapter 11 for details of control and prevention of infectious diseases.

Control and prevention of disease

To control and prevent disease, you need a knowledge of both:
1. the cause of the disease, and
2. the epidemiology of the disease.

You can then choose the most effective means (one or more) to control and/or prevent the disease. The four means for control and prevention of infectious diseases are:
1. Kill the specific agent (an infecting organism) in the body of the original host (clinical case, sub-clinical case or carrier) or reservoir (man, animal, dust, etc.).
2. Block the means of spread from the reservoir to susceptible persons.
3. Increase the resistance of susceptible persons.
4. Prophylactic treatment. Give a drug to stop the infection in probably infected persons before the infection produces clinical disease.

Always give *health education to the patient and to his relatives* about those things which they can do to control and prevent the disease the patient has.

Always use a case of a disease as an opportunity to give *health education to all the community*.

Never forget to use each case of a disease to give *health education to your own health workers* about that disease including its prevention.

The summary of the management of a person with a medical problem

When a patient comes to a health worker with a symptom, the management of this problem may well include some or all of these things:
1. taking a medical history;
2. doing a clinical examination;
3. making a differential diagnosis;
4. doing or ordering tests;
5. making a provisional diagnosis;
6. deciding on the prognosis;
*7. deciding on inpatient or outpatient treatment;
*8. ordering proper nursing care;
*9. giving specific treatment to cure the disease;
*10. giving symptomatic treatment to relieve symptoms;
*11. giving proper explanations and comfort to the patient and to his relatives;
*12. giving health education about the control and prevention of the disease to the patient and to his relatives;
*13. consulting with a medical officer (MO), transferring the patient to MO care or referring the patient to next visiting MO;
14. notifying the Health Officer, the Coroner, the patrol officer, the police, the relatives, etc.;
15. controlling the spread of the disease;
16. preventing the disease occurring in the patient again and also in the community;
*17. discharging the patient and giving final health education;
*18. following up the patient.
(* These 9 things were previously listed as 'treatment' of a patient.)

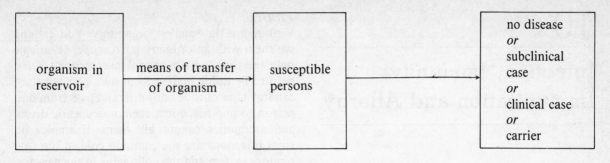

Figure 9.1 Aetiology and epidemiology of disease.

Figure 9.2 Means of control and prevention of disease.

10

Infection, Immunity, Immunisation and Allergy

Infection

The specific agents (organisms) which cause infectious diseases are around people all the time. Why do these specific agents not cause disease in all people all the time?

There are many epidemiological answers. Here are some:

1. The specific agents – only some organisms cause disease.
2. The body – man's body has defences against the organisms that cause disease.
3. Transfer – sometimes the organism has ways of transferring to another person, sometimes it cannot use these ways of transferring.
4. The environment – changes in the environment can change the organism, man's body and the transfer of the organism.

This chapter considers:

(a) the organisms which can cause disease, and
(b) the body's defences against these organisms.

The specific agents which cause infections

The specific agents which cause infections are organisms such as:

viruses   protoza
rickettsiae   worms
bacteria   fungi.
insects (called 'infestations')

Viruses

Viruses are the smallest organisms. You cannot see them with an ordinary microscope. (You can only see them with a special microscope.) They need to be inside body cells to multiply; but they can stay alive outside body cells and pass from one person to another. Most chemotherapeutic drugs and antibiotics cannot kill them. Examples of virus infections are the common cold in the respiratory system and the polio virus in the nervous system.

Rickettsiae

Rickettsiae are organisms which are bigger than viruses, but smaller than bacteria. You can see them, but not easily, with an ordinary microscope. Like viruses, they need to be inside body cells to multiply. Some antibiotics (tetracycline and chloramphenicol) can kill them. An example of rickettsiae is the typhus organism.

Bacteria

Bacteria are small organisms. You can only see them with a microscope. They can live in many places, inside and outside the body. Most bacteria are harmless – some are helpful to us. However, some bacteria can cause disease such as pneumonia in the lungs and leprosy in the skin and nerves. Chemotherapeutic drugs and antibiotics can kill most bacteria.

Protozoa

Protozoa are one-called organisms. They are much bigger than bacteria but usually you can only see them with a microscope. Some protozoa cause disease such as malaria in the blood and amoebic dysentery in the intestine. There are chemotherapeutic drugs which will kill most protozoa.

Fungi

Fungi are simple organisms usually with more than one cell, and are something like plants. Some cause disease such as tinea on the skin and thrush in the mouth. There are chemotherapeutic and antibiotic drugs which can kill most fungi.

Worms

Worms are organisms with many cells. You can usually see them easily without a microscope. Worms are common parasites of man and animals. Many worms have complicated life cycles with different stages in man and other animals. Examples of worm infestations include filariasis in the lymph vessels and roundworm in the intestine. There are chemotherapeutic drugs which can kill most worms.

What determines if these organisms will cause infection and disease or not?

Pathogenicity
Some kinds of organisms *can cause disease* in *most* people they attack. These are called *highly pathogenic*.

Some organisms *can cause disease* in *only a few* of the people they attack. These are called *mildly pathogenic*.

Some organisms *cannot cause disease* in *any* of the people they attack. These are called *non-pathogenic*.

Virulence
The disease caused by organisms can be *mild* (e.g. common cold caused by the cold virus) or *severe* (e.g. meningitis caused by bacteria) or somewhere in between (e.g. influenza caused by influenza virus). Organisms which cause *severe disease* are called *virulent*. Organisms which cause *mild disease* are called *non-virulent*.

The number of organisms
The number of organisms that enter the body can determine if they will cause disease or not. A certain number of organisms must stay alive after entry to cause disease. This number is different for each specific agent. This fact is very important.

The body defences against infection

The body surfaces
The skin and mucous membranes act as a wall which can stop many organisms entering the body. Secretions (or fluids made by the glands) on the body surfaces can contain antibodies which kill the organisms. Secretions can also wash away organisms. Damaged or diseased skin makes it easier for many organisms to enter the body.

The body defence cells
Some cells in the blood and in the tissues can surround and kill and digest many (but not all) organisms.

The body immune system
When organisms enter the body certain cells in the blood and lymph glands start to grow and change.
1. Some cells produce proteins called antibodies which go into the blood and also into the tissues. These antibodies then join themselves to the organisms. This helps the body defence cells to digest the organisms or the body to destroy them in other ways.
2. Other cells produce types of antibody which do not go into the blood and tissues but remain on the surface of the cell which made it. These cells then circulate in the blood and can travel through the capillary walls into the tissues. These cells (called 'immune cells') then attack and destroy the organism themselves. This is called 'cellular immunity'.

If organisms have entered the body and caused an infection before, antibodies and immune cells can still be in the body. These antibodies and immune cells can then attack immediately any new organisms that enter the body. If organisms have not entered the body and caused an infection before, there will be no antibodies and immune cells ready to attack them. It will take a week or more for the necessary antibodies and immune cells to grow and start to attack the organisms.

Examples of infections

Acute infection with bacteria and the inflammatory reaction
This is what *can* happen:
1. The pathogenic organisms must first get onto the surface of the body (skin or mucous membrane).
2. The organisms must overcome the body surface defences. Usually the organisms must find a break in the skin or mucous membrane. However, some organisms can break through unbroken skin or mucous membranes.
3. The organisms must then grow and multiply in the tissues more quickly than the body defence cells, antibodies and immune cells can kill them.
4. If the organisms are not immediately killed, the body usually establishes an inflammatory reaction. The blood vessels in the area dilate (open up more widely) and bring more blood to the area. Defence cells and antibodies then

go through the dilated blood vessel walls into the affected area and attack the organisms.

5. A protein from the blood called fibrin sometimes makes a wall around the area so that the organisms cannot spread to other tissues.
6. The whole body prepares to fight the infection. The body cells in the area release chemicals. These chemicals cause more white blood cells to be made, raise the temperature and make many other changes.
7. If the body defences do not kill the organisms quickly, the organisms can release poisons called toxins. The blood then carries the toxins around the body and they can poison the body in a number of ways. This is called 'toxaemia'. These toxins can cause malaise, raised temperature, fast pulse rate, nausea, vomiting and diarrhoea. Certain toxins can cause clinical disease, e.g. tetanus. (See Chapter 25 page 263)
8. If the body defences do not kill the organisms quickly, the organisms can also destroy tissues in the area of the infection. The dead tissues and blood cells and organisms are called pus.
9. The organisms can spread through the lymph vessels to the lymph nodes and cause inflammation in these places too – lymphangitis in the lymph vessels and lymphadenitis in the lymph nodes.
10. The organisms can be carried around in the blood stream. This is called bacteraemia. The infection can spread to other organs.
11. The organisms can grow and multiply in the blood. This is a very serious and often fatal disease. It is called septicaemia.

Acute infection with viruses and the inflammatory reaction

1. There can be all the symptoms and signs of acute inflammation.
2. There is no pus (e.g. there is only a watery nasal discharge in a viral common cold).
3. There can be a loss of function of the organ that is infected (e.g. viral hepatitis).
4. There can be the general symptoms and signs of toxaemia (e.g. influenza).

Chronic infection and inflammation produced by tuberculosis

1. There are the usual symptoms and signs of chronic inflammation.
2. There is slow destruction of the body tissues.
3. Thick pus (like cheese) is formed.
4. Fibrous tissue tries to make a wall around that area of the body so that the infection cannot spread.
5. Healing is by the contraction and shrinking of the fibrous tissue. This causes scarring.

There are many other types of reaction to infection.

Immunity and immunisation

Immunity is when a person has a resistance to a disease. Sometimes immunity is complete – the immune person can never get the disease again.

More often, the immunity is relative – the body has defences against infection; but, if the body is weakened or if the infecting agent is very strong

Figure 10.1 Diagram to illustrate the classification of the different types of immunity.

or present in large numbers, the immunity can fail and disease can happen.

There are different types of immunity as shown in Figure 10.1.

1. *Inherent* (*inborn*) *immunity* is the immunity a person has without being infected or immunised etc. It varies with race, sex, family, etc.
2. *Acquired immunity* is due to specific antibodies or immune cells which develop in the body after an infection or immunisation. These antibodies or immune cells join onto the attacking organism or toxin and destroy it.
3. *Natural active immunity* follows a natural infection. After the infection some antibodies or immune cells can stay in the blood (or another part of the body) all the time. Also, the body 'remembers' how to make the antibodies immediately the organism tries to attack again.
4. *Natural passive immunity* is only in infants for the first few months of life. The infant gets the antibodies through the placenta or in its mother's milk if the mother has these antibodies. The antibodies do not last in the infant after 3–9 months.
5. *Artificial active immunity* is produced by immunisation (or 'vaccination') with any of the following three things:
   (a) Dead infectious organisms.
   (b) Living infectious organisms which are exactly like the organisms which cause disease, but cannot cause disease themselves (because they are avirulent or nonvirulent organisms).
   (c) A substance like the poison or toxin of an organism but not poisonous itself (called 'toxoid').

   The body makes antibodies or immune cells against all of these three things. These antibodies or immune cells are also effective against the real live organisms or toxins that cause disease. Some of these antibodies and immune cells stay in the blood or other parts of the body after the immunisation. The body also 'remembers' how to make them immediately the disease-producing organism or toxin attacks.
6. *Artificial passive immunity* is produced by giving serum from another person or animal who has antibodies against the disease. This kind of immunity lasts for weeks or months, but after this time there are no antibodies left and there is no immunity.

However, if the antibodies come from a horse or other animal, the human body can have a severe or even fatal reaction to the other proteins in the serum when it is injected. This is even more likely if the serum is used more than once.

Active immunity is always better than passive immunity.

Allergy

Allergy is an inflammatory reaction of part of the body caused by some foreign substance in or on the body. This substance does not normally cause inflammation in normal people. However, some people (who are 'allergic') develop an abnormal immune reaction to these substances. If these people contact the substance again there is an immune reaction between the abnormal antibodies and the substance. In this reaction, histamine and other substances are released. These substances cause the 'allergic' reaction.

Immunity is a helpful reaction of the immune system of the body to a foreign substance. Allergy is a harmful reaction of the immune system of the body to a foreign substance.

There are many types of allergy including:
asthma,
hayfever,
urticaria ('hives'),
oedema (angio-oedema), and
shock.

Allergic reactions can be caused by things which:
touch the skin,
are inhaled (breathed in),
are swallowed, or
are injected.

Treatment includes:
1. adrenaline injections for severe acute reactions (See Chapter 20 page 170);
2. antihistamine drugs either orally, IMI or IVI, e.g. promethazine 25–50 mg (1–2 tabs or 1–2 ml by injection);
3. the usual treatment of any complication;
4. avoiding any further contact with the cause;
5. other special drugs sometimes used by medical officers, including hydrocortisone, prednisolone, etc.

11

Infectious Diseases and Chemotherapy

this causes a temparory increase in the frequency of the disease.

How diseases can be caused

Organisms
The specific agent or cause of a disease is a living organism (which is a parasite). These include:
viruses,
rickettsiae,
bacteria,
fungi,
protozoa,
worms, and
insects.
See Chapter 10 page 34 details of these organisms.

The reservoir of the infection
People who may spread the disease include the following:
1. people who have symptoms and signs of the disease ('cases');
2. people who are incubating the disease;
3. people who have an infection which cannot be seen (no symptoms and signs) (also called 'sub-clinical cases');
4. people who have the disease and are getting better ('convalescent carriers');
5. people who have the disease chronically ('chronic carriers').

Animals, dirt, dust, etc. can also be reservoirs.

The exit of organisms from the reservoir
If the reservoir is a person, the organisms can go out (exit) through:

1. the respiratory tract through the mouth or nose;
2. the gastro-intestinal tract in faeces or vomitus;
3. the urogenital tract by discharges or in urine;
4. the skin and other mucous membranes (eyes, for example) by discharges.

The communicable or infectious period
This is the time during which the organism can be transferred directly or indirectly from an infected person to another person (or from an infected animal to a person).

Infectious diseases

Definitions

Infectious disease
Infectious diseases are also called contagious or communicable diseases, and are diseases caused by harmful organisms which can spread from one person to another.

These harmful organisms can:
1. exit from (or leave) some reservoir of infection (a person, animal or place);
2. transfer to (or spread to) susceptible persons (persons who can get the disease);
3. penetrate (or enter) susceptible persons;
4. have pathogenicity (cause disease by either multiplying or making toxic products in the body).

Endemic disease
A disease is endemic in an area if it happens continuously in the area.

Sporadic disease
A disease has a sporadic incidence when it does not happen continuously in the area.

Epidemic
An epidemic of a disease is when large numbers of people are affected in a short period of time and

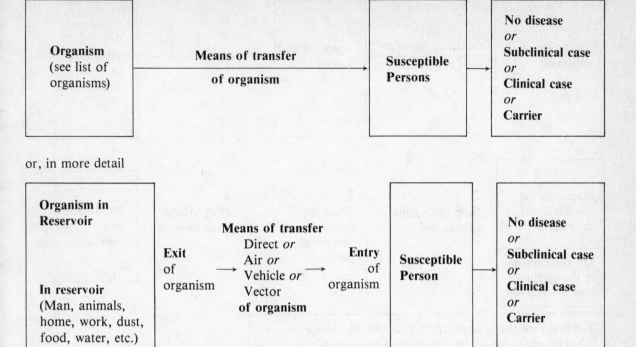

or, in more detail

Figure 11.1 Diagrams showing how disease may be caused.

The means of transfer of organisms

Infection can be spread by:
1. Direct contact (including droplets).
2. Droplets, droplet nuclei and dust in the air which can be inhaled.
3. 'Vehicles', such as:
   fingers,
   food and drink,
   water,
   instruments, and
   blood contaminated injections.
4. 'Vectors' – usually insects.

The entry of the organism (into a susceptible person)

Organisms can enter a person by:
1. inhalation (breathed into the respiratory tract),
2. ingestion (swallowed into the gastro-intestinal tract),
3. inoculation (injected through the mucous membranes or the skin).

The susceptible person

A person has defences against infection (see Chapter 10 page 35):
1. skin and mucous membranes covering the body surfaces,
2. the body defence cells,
3. the body immune system.

If an organism enters the body, the defences usually cause an inflammatory reaction.

The time that passes after a person gets an infection and before the signs and symptoms of the disease start is known as the 'incubation period'.

Means of control and prevention of infectious disease (see Figure 11.2)

1. Kill the organism in the original reservoir (man, animal, dust, etc.).
2. Stop the means of transfer.

Figure 11.2 Diagrams to show the means of spread of infectious disease (upper diagram) and the means of control and prevention of infectious disease.

If the infection is spread by *direct contact*, then:
- avoid exposure to carriers and persons with the disease,
- disinfect discharges,
- improve personal hygiene,
- give barrier nursing to the patient.

If the infection is spread by *droplets* etc. in the air, then:
- cover mouth during coughing and sneezing.
- avoid overcrowded rooms and crowds,
- have good ventilation in all rooms.

If the infection is spread by *vehicles*, then:
- if instruments – improve personal hygiene, disinfection of instruments, give barrier nursing to the patient;
- if other people (fingers) – improve personal hygiene, give barrier nursing to the patient;
- if food – supervise preparation, handling and hygiene of food;
- if water – purify the water;
- if needles or syringes – sterilise syringes and needles properly.

If the infection is spread by *vectors* then:
- control or eradicate the insects.
3. Raise the resistance of susceptible persons.
- Immunise these people — use active immunisation if possible, and passive if no active immunisation is available.
- Improve general health.
4. Prophylactic treatment (or 'chemoprophylaxis'). Give drugs to persons who are probably infected before the organisms cause disease. This is not often possible.
5. Use the occurrence of a case of the disease to give health education on the means of control and prevention of the disease.

Chemotherapy

Chemotherapy is giving a person a chemical which attacks the organisms which cause disease. The chemical is absorbed into the body and kills or stops the growth and multiplication of the organisms which are infecting that person. If possible the chemical will not harm the body of that person.

Chemotherapeutic drugs can sometimes cure an infection alone; but usually other treatment is needed too.

Chemotherapeutic drugs are of three kinds:
1. natural plant products (e.g. quinine, etc.),
2. antibiotics made by bacteria or fungi to kill other bacteria or fungi (e.g. penicillin, tetracycline, chloramphenicol, streptomycin, etc.),
3. chemicals made in the laboratory (e.g. sulphadimidine, INAH, dapsone, chloroquine, metronidazole, diethylcarbamazine, etc.).

A chemotherapeutic drug is usually effective against only one of the groups of pathogenic organisms as shown in Table 11.1.

A chemotherapeutic drug is also usually effective against only some of the members of that group. Table 11.2 shows some examples for antibacterial drugs.

Infecting organisms which are killed or can not grow or multiply in the presence of a chemotherapeutic drug are 'sensitive' to that drug. Organisms which are not killed and can grow and multiply in the presence of a chemotherapeutic drug are 'resistant' to that drug.

Some organisms have always been resistant to certain drugs. Some organisms which were sensitive to a chemotherapeutic drug can develop resistance to that drug. Development of resistance depends on the organism and the drug. Development of resistance can often be stopped by:
1. using the drug in the proper dose for long enough, and,
2. using at least two drugs to which the organism is sensitive at the same time.

Table 11.1 Examples of different types of drug.

Anti-viral drugs	Anti-bacterial drugs	Anti-fungal drugs	Anti-protozoal drugs	Anti-helminthic drugs
Acylovir No anti-viral drugs available in most countries	Penicillin Streptomycin Tetracycline Chloramphenicol Sulphadimidine INAH Thiacetazone Dapsone	Griseofulvin	Quinine Chloroquine Amodiaquine Pyrimethamine Metronidazole	Diethyl-carbamazine Thiabendazole

Table 11.2 Effectiveness of some antibacterial drugs.

	Penicillin	Chloramphenicol	INAH	Dapsone
Pneumococcus (Pneumonia)	effective	effective	not effective	not effective
Salmonella typhi (Typhoid fever)	not effective	effective	not effective	not effective
Mycobacterium tuberculosis (Tuberculosis)	not effective	not effective	very effective	not effective
M. leprae (Leprosy)	not effective	not effective	slightly effective	very effective

Rules for using antibacterial chemotherapeutic drugs

1. Do not give a patient with a fever for which no cause can be found antibacterial chemotherapeutic drugs, unless he becomes very 'sick' (see Chapter 36 page 396)
2. Always use the proper dose of chemotherapeutic drugs – never use less.
3. Always give chemotherapeutic drugs for the full course. For chemotherapeutic drugs used for bacterial infections, this is:
   - mild infections – at least 5 days or for 2–3 days after clinically cured (whichever is longer);
   - severe infections – at least 10 days or 2–3 days after clinically cured (whichever is longer);
   - tuberculosis – at least 18 months;
   - leprosy – at least 5 years.
4. Do not stop antibacterial chemotherapeutic drugs in less than 48 hours because they do not seem to be effective. If the patient is getting worse *add* another drug before the 48 hours are finished. If the drug has no effect after 48 hours, then try another drug. However if the patient gets very sick and looks as if he will die, change to chloramphenicol (see Chapter 12 page 46).

Notes on some antibacterial chemotherapeutic drugs

Sulphonamides

Sulphonamides, (e.g. sulphadimindine) were effective against many bacteria in all parts of the body. Now some bacteria have become resistant to them. Sulphonamides are not used much now (except for urinary tract infection) as other drugs are more effective. The dose of sulphadimidine is 1 g (2 tabs) four times a day for 10 days.

Sulphonamides are also effective for trachoma (see Chapter 31 page 341).

Sulphonamides also have an antimalarial effect. This is a weak effect, but if it is combined with another drug such as pyrimethamine, the effect of both drugs together is powerful. For malaria not sulphadimidine but a similar sulpha-drug (such as sulphadoxine) is used (see Chapter 13 page 56).

Possible side effects include the following:
1. Formation of crystals in the urine if the patient does not drink enough when the drug is taken. Always make sure the patient drinks enough to pass a lot of urine when he takes a sulphonamide.
2. Allergic reactions, such as fever, skin rashes and jaundice.

All side effects are uncommon.

Penicillin

Penicillin is effective against most organisms which cause infections in all parts of the body (except those that cause bowel or urinary tract infections). Organisms which cause bowel or urinary tract infections are usually resistant to penicillin.

A few of those organisms which cause severe infections (including meningitis, septicaemia and pneumonia) are also resistance to pencillin. Some organisms which are sensitive have now developed resistance to penicillin.

Penicillin is given for most infections except bowel and urinary tract infections. If the infection does not improve, tetracycline can be used instead. If the infection is a serious one which threatens life (e.g. meningitis, peritonitis, severe pneumonia, etc.), or an essential body part (e.g. eye, bone or joint, etc.), chloramphenicol is used instead.

Treatment is given for at least 5 days for mild infections and at least 10 days for moderate or severe infections.

The main side effects are allergic reactions including skin rashes, asthma, shock and fever with arthritis. If allergy happens the patient should not be given penicillin again. You must tell him he is allergic to penicillin and that he must never have penicillin again. You must tell him to tell this to any health worker who ever treats him. You must also write it on the outside of both his outpatient and inpatient notes.

Benzyl (*crystalline*) *penicillin*, 1200 mg or 2,000,000 units IVI or IMI each 3 hours is given for infections which threaten life and 600 mg or 1,000,000 units each 6 hours is given for moderate infections.

Procaine benzyl penicillin, 600 mg or 900,000–1,000,000 units daily is given for mild infections or severe or moderate infections which have improved after benzyl (crystalline) penicillin has been given for some days. Give procaine penicillin only by IMI.

Phenoxymethyl penicillin is absorbed after being taken by mouth. It must be taken each 4–6 hours. It is not used much because you cannot know if the patient will remember to take it regularly. It is never used for moderate or severe infections.

Benzathine penicillin is a long acting penicillin which produces low levels of penicillin in the blood for a long time (a little up to 4 weeks). It is used for a 'one dose treatment' for syphilis and once each month for preventing rheumatic fever. The dose is usually 1.8 g or 2,400,000 units.

Ampicillin and amoxycillin are newer penicillins. These are often not available as they are more expensive. They can be given by IVI, IMI or by mouth. They kill most pathogenic organisms in most parts of the body including the urinary and gastro-intestinal tracts. They can be used instead of penicillin and also for urinary tract infections. They have the same side effects as penicillin. In places where these drugs are scare they are used only:

1. instead of tetracycline when a patient is pregnant; (The dose is 250 – 500 mg (1–2 caps) orally four times a day. Larger doses are given by injection for severe infections.)
2. for gonorrhoea instead of the one large dose of procaine penicillin (see Chapter 19 page 132).

Chloramphenicol is a very powerful antibiotic effective against most infecting bacteria in all parts of the body. Chloramphenicol enters all parts of the body. However, chloramphenicol can cause death in a few patients by stopping the making of blood.

It is therefore used only for:

1. severe infection which immediately threatens life (e.g. septicaemia, meningitis, peritonitis, severe pneumonia, etc.);
2. severe infection which threatens an essential body part (e.g. eye, bone or joint, etc.);
3. infection which does not respond to other antibiotics (e.g. pneumonia, urinary tract infections, etc. which has not improved on penicillin, sulphonamides or tetracycline);
4. infection for which no other treatment is available (e.g. typhoid fever).

Penicillin, or, if this is not effective, tetracycline, are almost always effective for the treatment of infections. However, if chloramphenicol is needed for an acute severe infection which is threatening life or a vital body part (and the risk of disease is more than the risk of the drug) then the proper large dose of chloramphenicol should be used, i.e. 100 mg/kg daily or 25 mg/kg every 6 hours. When the patient is apparently cured then the dose of chloramphenicol is reduced to half (½) of the above, i.e. 50 mg/kg daily or 12.5 mg/kg every 6 hours to complete the treatment course. *For adults of ordinary size 1 g (1 bottle of 1g injection or 4 caps) every 6 hours is the usual dose.* When the patient is apparently cured (or when a patient who needs long treatment improves), then, the dose is reduced to 750 mg (3 caps) for large adults (> 50 kg) and 500 mg (2 caps) for small adults (< 50 kg) each 6 hours.

Chloramphenicol is well absorbed from the intestine after it is given by mouth. Chloramphenicol is therefore always given by mouth unless:

1. The patient cannot swallow it because:
   (a) he is unconscious and there is no intragastric tube;
   (b) he is unco-operative.
2. The patient can not absorb it from the bowel, because of:
   (a) shock (little blood will be going to the bowel);
   (b) vomiting;
   (c) severe diarrhoea.
3. The patient is very sick and you cannot be sure that the drugs will be given by mouth because:
   (a) the staff are not dependable enough (staff are usually more dependable with injections than with oral drugs);
   (b) the patient is not dependable (he may refuse it or spit it out or vomit without telling the staff this);
   (c) of the other usual reasons that *very* sick patients are given injections.

Chloramphenicol acts quickly after IV injection.

Chloramphenicol only acts after some delay if given by IM injection. If it is given regularly every 6 hours this delay is not a problem after the first injection, because the effects of the previous dose will still be present. IM chloramphenicol is given if chloramphenicol by mouth is not possible (see above) and IV chloramphenicol is not needed or not possible. If IM chloramphenicol is given, it is best to give an extra injection IV with the first IM dose, it possible. If the IV injection is not possible, give the extra dose by IMI also.

Tetracycline

Tetracycline is effective against most infecting bacteria in all parts of the body; but some bacteria become resistant to it. Therefore it is not used for very severe infections which are threatening life or an essential body part. It is used for:

1. most infections if penicillin does not cure the patient or if it is best not to give injections or it is not possible to give penicillin (e.g. penicillin allergy);
2. gastro-intestinal or urinary tract infection if other treatment (sometimes including sulphonamides) does not cure them.

The dose is 20–40 mg/kg daily. For severe infections give 500 mg (2 caps) four times a day and for less severe infections or after severe infections improve, give 250 mg (1 cap) four times a day by mouth.

Do not use tetracycline and penicillin together.

Do not give tetracycline to:

1. pregnant women,
2. children, or
3. people with kidney (renal) failure.

If penicillin is not effective for these patients, you can give ampicillin or ask a medicial officer to supply a special drug.

Streptomycin

Streptomycin is effective against a number of bacteria including tuberculosis organisms. However, organisms soon develop resistance to streptomycin. Therefore, you must:

1. Use streptomycin only with other drugs. Do not use streptomycin alone.
2. Use streptomycin only for tuberculosis in adults and children (and then only with INAH), or for neonatal infections before tuberculosis infection is possible (and then only with penicillin).

Do not use streptomycin for any other infections.

See Chapter 14 page 71 for dose of streptomycin.

Summary of choice of antibacterial drug

For mild or moderate infection

1. In all places except the gastro-intestinal or urinary tracts – penicillin[1] (tetracycline[2] second choice).
2. In the urinary tract, except sexually transmitted urethritis (gonorrhoea, etc.) – sulphadimidine (tetracycline[2] second choice).
3. In the gastro-intestinal tract – antibacterial drug usually not needed.

For severe bacterial infection which threatens life or a vital body part

1. In all places in adults (but not for newborn babies) – chloramphenicol in the correct *large* dose.
2. For neonatal septicaemia (before tuberculosis infection is possible) – penicillin in large doses and streptomycin (chloramphenicol is second choice; but make sure only the correct *small* dose is given).

For mild or moderate infections which do not respond to penicillin or sulphadimidine

In all places – tetracycline[2].

If the infection is likely to come back many times and the *patient is likely to need long or repeated courses* of antibacterial drugs, then it is very important to *USE tetracycline*; *DO NOT USE chloramphenicol* (unless the infection threatens life or a vital body part).

For moderate infections which do not respond to either penicillin (or sulphadimidine) or tetracycline

First look for causes of failure to respond to treatment.

If you can find no cause then: in all places – chloramphenicol.

---

1. Penicillin. Do not give if the patient is allergic to penicillin.

2 Tetracycline. Do not give if the patient is pregnant or a child or has kidney failure.

44

Use streptomycin in adults for only TU-
BERCULOSIS and ONLY TOGETHER
WITH INAH. Do not use streptomycin in
any other way.

Continue the antibacterial drug for:
1. two to three days after the patient seems cured
   or;
2. mild infections   – 5 days,
   moderate infections – 7 days,
   severe infections   – 10 days,
whichever is longer.

For special infections
None of the above is correct for these special infections:

urethritis   – see Chapter 19 page 132,
tuberculosis   – see Chapter 14 page 71,
leprosy   – see Chapter 15 page 90.

12

Septicaemia

Septicaemia is present when organisms get into the blood stream and multiply in it.

Septicaemia occurs only in special circumstances:

1. Organisms are put straight into the blood stream e.g.:
   • injection of contaminated drugs or blood transfusion (with organisms in them);
   • an operation where an infected area is cut;
   • passage of a urethral catheter especially when there is infection in the urethra;
   • changing or leaving in too long an infected intravenous cannula;
   • doing a burns dressing.
2. The body is in a state of weakened immunity or resistance e.g.:
   • malnutrition;
   • anaemia;
   • after operation or childbirth;
   • if another infection is present in the body;
   • if the patient has cancer or leukaemia, etc.;
   • if the patient is taking prednisolone or similar cortisone-like drug, or anti-cancer drugs.
3. There is a particularly severe or widespread infection in the body e.g.: certain types of pneumonia.
4. The attacking organism is particularly virulent e.g.: certain types of organisms which can cause meningitis and septicaemia.

If a patient in any of these situations suddenly gets worse, always think of septicaemia.

The first group of conditions is of particular importance in the health centre. Septicaemia can follow simple procedures. A very common cause of septicaemia is the passage of a urethral catheter. In all these procedures in Group 1, virulent organisms may be put straight into the blood stream where they start to grow and produce septicaemia.

If septicaemia develops, the patient may have any of the following:

1. Rigor(s).
2. General symptoms and signs of infection which could include:
   • severe malaise and weakness;
   • nausea, vomiting, diarrhoea;
   • being not fully conscious or being psychotic or even fitting;
   • dyspnoea and fast respiration;
   • raised temperature.
3. Fast pulse, low blood pressure but skin warm (due to dilation of blood vessels in the skin) ('warm shock').
4. Fast pulse, low blood pressure, cold, cyanosed, low urine output ('cold shock').
5. Haemorrhages into the skin – petechia (pinpoint haemorrhages) or larger areas of bleeding or bruises.

However, any patient who has an infection and gets worse or any patient who has had any type of procedure carried out on him and then gets very sick should be thought of as having septicaemia.

Management of septicaemia

1. Chloramphenicol (25 mg/kg each 6 hours).
   For an adult of average weight give 2 g immediately then 1 g every six hours.

   Give by IVI if:
   • shock (essential), or
   • IV drip needed for another reason and is running.

If a patient has a condition which makes it likely for him or her to develop septicaemia, and he or she then develops symptoms and signs suggesting septicaemia, immediately manage as follows:

1. chloramphenicol in large doses (usually 1 g each 6 hours);
2. antimalarial drug as indicated usually quinine;
3. IV drip; but only if needed for shock or dehydration, etc.;
4. treatment of any heart failure;
5. treatment of any infected body part in the usual way;
6. consult a Medical Officer if necessary;
7. do not reduce the chloramphenicol dose unless the patient seems to be cured very quickly;
8. continue chloramphenicol for *at least* 10 days.

Give by IMI *if*
• IV drip not needed, or
• IV drip not possible.
and if
• oral drugs are not reliable enough (as very sick), or
• oral drugs are not effective (as shock or not able to swallow or vomiting or severe diarrhoea).

Give orally (4 caps) *only if*
• is not very sick; or after improves (when oral drugs are reliable enough), and
• can swallow, and
• has no vomiting or severe diarrhoea, and
• is not shocked.

2. Antimalarial drug for all patients.
Quinine 10 mg/kg (7.5 ml (7½ ml) for a small adult or 10 ml for a large adult) by IMI in most cases. Give by SLOW IV drip *if* patient:
• is shocked or
• is unconscious, or
• is very sick
and if patient:
• is in or has been in an area where chloroquine resistant malaria occurs, or

• has been given chloroquine and is still sick.
See Malaria Chapter 13 for further treatment.

3. Set up an IV drip; but only if needed i.e. if shock, severe dehydration, unconscious, very sick, not able to take oral fluids and drugs.
Do not give more fluid than is really necessary (or this may cause cerebral oedema, convulsions and death).
When shock – see Chapter 27 page 305.
When dehydration – see Chapter 23 page 228.
When maintenance fluids only needed – give 0.18% sodium chloride in 4.3% dextrose 1 litre each 8 hours.
When drip for IV injections only needed – give 0.18% sodium chloride in 4.3% dextrose, 1 litre each 12 hours.

4. Look for heart failure. Treat if present.
Give intranasal oxygen 2–4 litres/minute.
Give digoxin 0.5 mg (½ mg) or 500 mcg (2 ml) IVI slowly immediately or, if injection not available, 0.5 mg (½ mg) (2 tabs) orally immediately.
Give only maintenance fluids (see 3 above) (do not give 0.9% sodium chloride). Then see Heart Failure (Chapter 27 page 301).

5. Treat any infected part or any other complication in the usual way.

6. Consult a Medical Officer urgently about further management if you are not sure of the diagnosis or treatment or if transfer for surgery is likely.

7. Do not quickly reduce the chloramphenicol dose.
If the patient is apparently cured very quickly, 12.5 mg/kg (12½ mg/kg) each 6 hours could be given i.e.
• 750 mg (3 caps) each 6 hours for a large adult (> 50 kg) and
• 500 mg (2 caps) each 6 hours for a small adult (< 50 kg)
However, *most patients* should continue 1 g (4 caps) each 6 hours.

8. Continue the chloramphenicol for at least 10 days. Many infections will need longer treatment; however use the reduced dose (see 7) *after* clinical improvement and 10 days high dose treatment.

13

Malaria

Definition

Malaria is a disease caused by infection of the red blood cells by a protozoal organism called *Plasmodium* of which there are four types. Infection causes acute and chronic types of fever, anaemia and enlargement of the spleen. Infection also causes, at times, severe disorders of the brain, kidneys, liver and other parts of the body.

Frequency

Malaria is the most common important infectious disease in the world. Malaria affects many of the people living between the latitudes of approximately 60°N and 40°S (see Figure 13.1). Malaria affects between 100 and 150 million people and each year causes over 1 million deaths.

Cause

Malaria is caused by infection with one or more of four protozoal (one-celled microscopic organism) parasites:
1. *Plasmodium falciparum* is the most common in hot, wet climates.
2. *Plasmodium vivax* is the most widespread of the parasites in the world and is more common than *P. falciparum* in places which have cool or dry seasons.

3. *Plasmodium malariae* is not common.
4. *Plasmodium ovale* is very uncommon.

Epidemiology

Man is the only host of the above malaria parasites.

Transmission of these parasites is usually from the blood of an infected person to a female *Anopheles* mosquito and then to susceptible new persons.

Occassionally transmission is by transfusion of blood which has malaria parasites in it from an infected person to a susceptible new person.

See Figure 13.2 for details of the life cycle of the malaria parasite.

The time from when the mosquito ingests the gametocytes until it has infective sporozoites is at least ten days. The gametocytes can develop into sporozoites only if the temperature is above 15°C (60°F).

The incubation period in man (from the bite of an infected mosquito until the start of symptoms and signs of malaria) is usually about two weeks However it is often much longer. It cannot be shorter than eight days.

Transmission of malaria can occur only if the following four conditions are present:
1. There are human gametocyte carriers present in the area.
2. *Anopheles* mosquitoes are present in the area.
3. The temperature and humidity is right for the parasite development in the mosquito.
4. There are susceptible human hosts (usually babies and children in endemic areas).

Partial or incomplete immunity to malaria (mostly due to antibodies) can develop after 4–10 years of continuous exposure to malaria (if the person does not die from chronic malaria or one of the acute attacks of malaria during this time). This means that older children or adults, who have lived continuously for years in places where malaria is present all the time, develop partial immunity. They are often called 'semi-immune'. However, to develop and keep this semi-immunity, a person has to be repeatedly sick with malaria, as well as being likely to die from malaria for 4–10 years (unless treatment for acute attacks is always immediately available).

Figure 13.1 The distribution of malaria.
(Source: *Vaccination Certificate Requirements and Health Advice for International Travel*, Geneva, World Health Organization, 1986)

Areas in which malaria has disappeared, been eradicated, or never existed

Areas with limited risk

Areas where malaria transmission occurs.

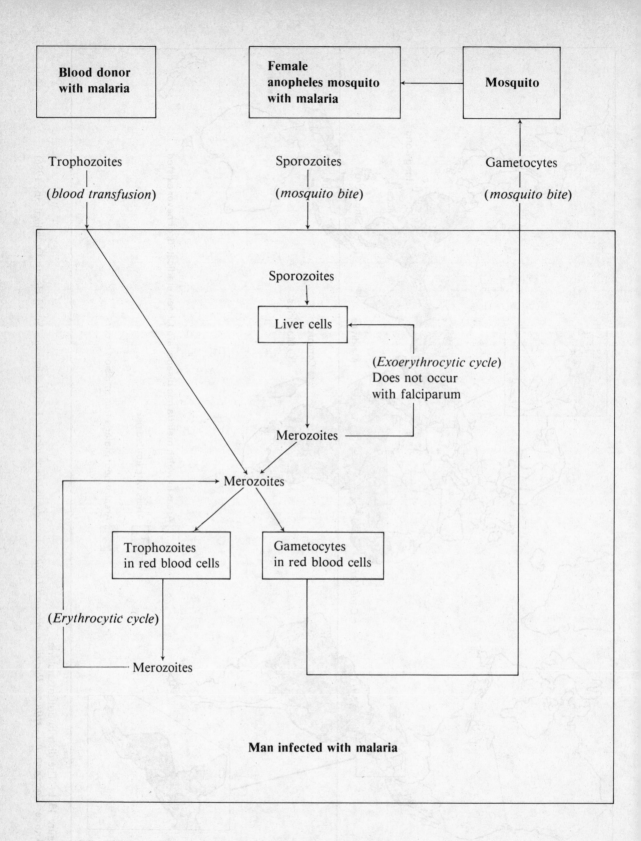

Figure 13.2 Diagram of the life cycle of malaria parasite as it affects man.

Other than these persons who have developed semi-immunity to malaria, all persons of all ages and both sexes are susceptible to malaria.

The persons most commonly affected by malaria are:
1. babies and children in areas where malaria is present all the time;
2. persons of all ages who come to malarial areas;
3. persons of all ages in areas where malaria can occur but where malaria is not present all the time if conditions suitable for transmission of malaria occur (temperature and rainfall change).

Immunity to malaria may be overcome by malaria parasites in the following situations:
1. during pregnancy (especially the last 3 months of pregnancy and especially in the first pregnancy);
2. during another illness;
3. if a person goes for a while with no malaria parasites present in his blood (e.g. the person has been taking anti-malarials and stopped them; the person has been living in a screened house or dormitory; the person has been away from a malarial area, etc.);
4. if a person shifts to a place where there is more malaria or a different type of malaria;
5. if a person is given drugs such as cortisone or prednisolone which stop immunity working properly;
6. possibly if the patient has his spleen removed.

Symptoms and signs, course and complications

Infection with malaria parasites can cause many different symptoms and signs and clinical states. Common clinical states include:
1. An acute attack of vivax (or malariae or ovale) malaria in a non-immune person.
2. An acute attack of falciparum malaria in a non-immune person. One of the seven common complications of acute malaria is likely to develop in non-immune patients with falciparum malaria.
3. Chronic malaria (in the years from the first infection until good semi-immunity has developed).
4. Malaria in semi-immunes.
5. Late complications of malaria.

Acute attack of vivax, malariae or ovale malaria in non-immune people

There may be a few hours to a few days of vague ill health (e.g. feeling cold, aches and pains, nausea, etc.) before any fever and severe disease. Attacks of fever then occur.

At first the patient is cold for ¼–1 hour and the temperature is not raised. The patient then starts to shiver and has a rigor and the temperature rises quickly up to about 40°C. The skin is cold and pale, the pulse fast and the BP often higher than normal. Vomiting, diarrhoea and urinary frequency are common.

Next, a hot stage comes for about an hour. The rigor stops, the patient feels hot, the skin feels hot and dry, the pulse is fast and the BP is often low. Headache, delirium, thirst and vomiting are common.

After this a sweating stage comes. The patient sweats a lot, the temperature falls, the pulse and BP become normal and after an hour or two the patient often goes to sleep. After waking the patient may feel reasonably well.

After about a week the attacks of fever may start to come about each third or fourth day. Until then they occur irregularly.

Jaundice may be seen after attacks of fever.

Anaemia causing pallor gets worse after attacks of fever.

The spleen becomes enlarged and eventually becomes very big.

The liver becomes enlarged but does not become very big.

If treatment is given, there is a good response to treatment within a few hours. Even without treatment the attacks of fever get less frequent. However, relapses occur (because of the liver stage of the parasite) after treatment of an acute attack.

Severe and fatal complications (see page 52) do not usually occur.

Chronic malaria (see page 53) then develops.

Acute attacks of falciparum malaria in non-immune people

The incubation period is usually two weeks. It can be longer; but it can also be as short as eight days.

There may be some hours to a few days of vague ill-health (e.g. feeling cold; headache, backache and pains all over; nausea, vomiting and diarrhoea).

The attack then occurs. The attack may be like other forms of malaria. However, more often the attack does not have the three definite stages.

In an attack the patient may appear to be very sick (as in any febrile illness).

Pains in the head, bones and muscles are severe.

Vomiting and diarrhoea are common.

Mental confusion and delirium are common.

The temperature is usually raised but rigors may not occur. Sometimes the temperature is normal. Most commonly the temperature is raised but it does not go away after an attack and may be continuous.

Sweating is often severe.

Pulse is usually fast.

Blood pressure is often low.

Respiration rate is usually fast.

Anaemia develops quickly.

Jaundice is sometimes present.

The spleen is usually enlarged and tender.

The liver is often enlarged.

If treatment is given there is usually a good response to it after a few hours.

If treatment is not given or if the treatment given is not correct or is not given quickly enough, complications can occur and these include the following:

1. febrile fits (only in children), hyperpyrexia, (complications of fever, see this page);
2. convulsions, unconsciousness, paralysis, psychotic behaviour, etc. (cerebral malaria, see this page);
3. acute anaemia and hypoxaemia ('anoxia'), (see page 53);
4. severe vomiting, diarrhoea and sometimes even dysentery, (gastro-intestinal malaria, see page 53);
5. shock, (see page 53);
6. malarial haemoglobinuria ('Blackwater fever', see page 53);
7. respiratory symptoms and signs (pulmonary malaria, see page 53).

Chronic malaria (see page 53) then develops if the patient does not die from an acute attack or from a complication.

Complications of falciparum malaria

Complications of fever. Febrile fit. Hyperpyrexia

Fever occurs in almost all cases of malaria.

In children, if the temperature rises very quickly, a febrile fit may occur. If the child is given an injection of an antimalarial drug and anticonvulsants and is cooled, the fitting will stop and the child will become fully conscious again. (Occasionally another fit can occur and the child not be fully conscious for an hour or so.) This is different from cerebral malaria (see below).

> Remember that all children who fit must have a lumbar puncture in case they have meningitis (as well as a blood slide taken for malaria parasites and an injection of an antimalarial drug).

Fever alone does not cause fitting in adults. *Adults do not have febrile fits*. All adults who fit must have a lumbar puncture in case they have meningitis (as well as a blood slide taken for malaria parasites, and an injection of an antimalarial drug).

Occasionally, in children and adults, the temperature rises above 40°C and stays there. This is called 'hyper-pyrexia'. This is particularly dangerous if the patient stops sweating and the skin become dry. Cyanosis and mental disturbance may occur. The patient needs urgent cooling or he will become shocked and die.

Cerebral malaria

The malaria parasites may partly block the blood vessels going to the brain and may poison the brain with their toxins and cause an encephalitis (see Chapter 25 page 258). This condition is called cerebral malaria.

Cerebral malaria may cause all sorts of brain and mental symptoms and signs. These include those of depression of the brain functions such as severe headache, drowsiness, paralysis and unconsciousness. They also can include those of irritation of the brain functions such as restlessness, irritability, confusion, abnormal (psychotic) behaviour, twitching and fitting, etc. On examination, the patient is usually febrile, the neck is often stiff, the mental state is often abnormal and any of the above signs may be found.

All patients in a malarious area
- with a severe febrile illness for which no cause can be found, or
- who are unconscious, or
- who have had a fit, or
- with a stiff neck, or
- with an acute psychosis when not known to be psychotic,

must have
1. a lumbar puncture done,
2. a blood smear for malaria parasites made, and
3. full doses of injected antimalarials, preferably quinine.

The loss of consciousness from cerebral malaria may last for some days. Even after this, the patient may still make a full recovery.

Acute anaemia and hypoxia

Acute severe anaemia with hypoxia (symptoms and signs of a low oxygen level in the brain and the rest of the body) occurs especially in those who have a low haemoglobin level (usually below 5 g/dl) who then develop an acute attack of malaria. More red blood cells are destroyed and the anaemia rapidly becomes worse. Poisons from the malaria parasites stop the body cells using properly even what little oxygen is brought by the anaemic blood ('hypoxia' – little oxygen in the tissues). Death can occur quickly from lack of oxygen in the brain and other tissues of the body.

Any patient in a malarious areas who is very pale and develops acute malaria needs urgent treatment for the malaria and an urgent blood transfusion.

Gastro-intestinal malaria

The patient with malaria may develop repeated vomiting, diarrhoea with large volumes of watery stools, or even dysentery. This loss of fluid may lead to dehydration and death.

Any patient in a malarious area who develops gastro-enteritis or dysentery needs a smear for malaria parasites taken, an injection of an antimalarial drug as well as fluids orally or IV.

Shock ('Algid malarial')

The patient with malaria may become shocked with a fast pulse and a low blood pressure. The skin may feel cold but the body temperature, if taken with the thermometer in the rectum, is high. This may occur with or without vomiting and diarrhoea.

Malarial haemoglobinuria ('Blackwater fever')

Malarial haemoglobinuria is very rare. It can occur in persons who have recently moved into the malarious area or have come back to the area or persons who have had irregular antimalarial drugs especially quinine. It can, however, occur in persons without either of these. Due to an abnormal immune reaction, many red blood cells are haemolysed (i.e. broken open and destroyed). Haemoglobin from inside the broken red cells is then free in the blood. This haemoglobin is also passed in the urine which becomes red or brown or black (see Chapter 26 page 294).

The patient may become very anaemic because the red cells are destroyed. Also haemoglobin free in the blood (and not in the RBCs) is very poisonous to the body and especially the kidney. The patient may become shocked and develop kidney failure (when he will pass only a very little urine which is red or brown and has a lot of protein in it). Unless he is given urgent treatment, he will die of the anaemia, the shock or later the kidney failure.

Pulmonary malaria

The respiration rate is usually raised in malaria. In severe cases there may be some respiratory distress. Occasionally, a cough may occur and some abnormal signs may be found in the chest.

Never assume that chest symptoms or signs are due to malaria alone. They always must be treated as due bacterial infections and the patient given antibiotics as well as antimalarials.

Chronic malaria (before immunity is fully developed)

Chronic malaria occurs in persons from the time they are infected with malaria until the time they become semi-immune, i.e. until they develop enough immunity against malaria to overcome most of the malaria parasites and most of the effects of the malaria parasites, most of the time.

This may take 4–10 years. Some people never develop enough immunity and continue to have chronic malaria all their lives.

Symptoms and signs of chronic malaria include:
1. recurrent attacks of acute malaria,
2. anaemia,
3. enlarged spleen,
4. enlarged liver,
5. poor appetite and other gastro-intestinal symptoms and signs,
6. wasting of muscles (abdomen often very enlarged in comparison),
7. reduced resistance to other diseases especially recurrent attacks of bacterial infections and gastro-enteritis.

The above are especially severe in children and often lead to death.

Malaria in persons with immunity ('semi-immunes')

1. Irregular short attacks of malaise, headaches, backache, loss of appetite, fever and sweating occur.
2. Mild anaemia may be present all the time.

Late complications of malaria

After many years a few patients may develop the following:
1. tropical splenomegaly syndrome (see Chapter 21 page 185), or
2. nephrotic syndrome (see Chapter 26 page 287).

Tests

1. Make a blood smear for malaria parasites from all patients with fever or suspected malaria (see Appendix 1, page 60).
2. Do a haemoglobin estimation on anyone who is pale (see Chapter 21 page 191).

Diagnostic features

1. Fever (*all* patients with fever must be treated with antimalarials unless it can be proved that they do not have malaria).
2. Anaemia (*all* patients with anaemia must be treated with antimalarials unless it can be proved that they do not have malaria).
3. Splenomegaly (in non-immunes).

Management

Management may include five things:
1. Give antimalarial drugs (see page 55). Chloroquine for 3 days – if usual case. Quinine for 3 days *then also* pyrimethamine and sulphadoxine once
   • *if* chloroquine resistant malaria proven or possible or
   • *if* a complication especially cerebral malaria or shock.
   Use oral tablets usually.
   Use injection if:
   • unconscious or fitting, or
   • vomiting or severe diarrhoea, or
   • shock.
   See page 55 for which drugs to give by what route.
2. Treat symptoms (see page 57).
3. Treat complications (see page 57).
4. Do not give primaquine also unless in special areas and also the Medical Officer tells you to.
5. Give drugs for prophylaxis only if needed (see page 59).

Note on antimalarial drugs and[1] chloroquine resistant malaria organisms

Commonly used drugs include the following (there are many more):
1. Chloroquine or amodiaquine tablets.
2. Chloroquine injection.
3. Quinine tablets.
4. Quinine injection.

1 For details about chloroquine resistance, see Appendix 2, page 62.

5. Pyrimethamine and sulphadoxine tablets (e.g. 'Fansidar', 'Faludar' or 'Methipox').
6. Pyrimethamine and dapsone tablets (e.g. 'Maloprim').

In many health centre areas the dose of chloroquine usually recommended in textbooks may be too complicated for your staff and your patients to remember.

The doses recommended and the usual number of tablets for a (large) adult are:

10 mg/kg immediately, i.e. 4 tablets immediately;

5 mg/kg 6 hours later, i.e. 2 tablets 6 hours later;

5 mg/kg daily for the following 2 days, i.e. 2 tablets the next 2 days.

That is a total of 25 mg/kg, i.e. 1500 mg, i.e. 10 tablets over 3 days.

In this book a very simple dose is recommended which has been used for many years in Papua New Guinea and has been effective and safe and easy for staff and patients.

Table 13.1   Chloroquine dosage

Size of adult	Dose on Day 1	Dose on Day 2	Dose on Day 3
Small (less than 50 kg)	3 tablets	3 tablets	3 tablets
Large (more than 50 kg)	4 tablets	4 tablets	4 tablets

You, however, will have to follow the rules laid down by the Health Department where you work.

Chloroquine is the best drug to use for malaria. However, in some parts of the world, especially South East Asia and the Pacific and in South America and now also in parts of Africa and India, (see Figure 13.1) some strains of *P. falciparum* have become resistant to chloroquine. These strains of *P. falciparum* are still sensitive to quinine. However, quinine would need to be given for 7–14 days to kill all the parasites. To make the treatment shorter, 3–5 day courses

of quinine followed by one dose of pyrimethamine and sulphadoxine are given for treatment of chloroquine-resistant malaria. Pyrimethamine and dapsone are given for prevention of chloroquine-resistant malaria.

Quinine is a quick acting drug as well as very effective against chloroquine-resistant malaria. Quinine is therefore always used in cases such as cerebral malaria where you have to be sure:
1. the drug will be effective, and
2. action will be quick.

Note on management

All patients with a fever are assumed to have malaria unless it can be proved otherwise. *But always look for other causes*, especially severe infections. Always do a full history and examination and test the urine.

Even if there appears to be another cause of fever, *treat all patients with a fever with a full treatment course of antimalarials unless it can be proved that they do not have malaria*. Treat any other cause as well.

Admit for inpatient treatment if there is a severe attack or a complication.

Treat as an outpatient in a mild attack.

Give antimalarial drugs

Choose drugs according to severity of attack.
• Usual attack. See below.
• Usual attack with vomiting or diarrhoea. See page 56.
• Usual attack but not cured by chloroquine. See page 56.
• Severe attack if patient in or from an area where chloroquine-resistant malaria common. See page 56.
• Patient unconscious or fitting or shocked or very 'sick'. See page 56.

Usual attack. No vomiting. No diarrhoea.
Give oral chloroquine (150 mg base tablets).

Give 10 mg chloroquine/kg body weight daily orally for 3 days.

Table 13.2 Chloroquine dosage

Size of adult	Day 1	Day 2	Day 3
Small (less than 50 kg)	3 tabs	3 tabs	3 tabs
Large (more than 50 kg)	4 tabs	4 tabs	4 tabs

Usual attack but vomiting or diarrhoea

Give IM chloroquine (200 mg in 5 ml amp).

> When possible use oral instead of IM chloroquine.
> Do not give both oral and IM chloroquine at the same time to a patient.

Give 4 mg, i.e. 0.1 ml (1/10 ml) chloroquine/kg patient's body weight (maximum 7.5 ml (7½ ml)) each dose.

The dose if the patient is not able to be weighed is:

- small adult (less than 50 kg) – 4 ml;
- large adult (more than 50 kg) – 5 ml.

After 6 hours if the patient cannot take oral chloroquine repeat the *same* dose of IM chloroquine. However, if patient can take oral drugs, give the first dose of the three daily doses of chloroquine tablets instead (see above). After either the repeat injection or the first oral dose do not give any more chloroquine in the first 24 hours (from when treatment started).

On the second and third days if the patient still cannot take oral chloroquine, then, instead of the once daily dose of tablets, give IM chloroquine twice daily with 12 hours between each dose. Use the *same* IM dose (see above). As soon as possible change to oral chloroquine.

Stop chloroquine after 3 days of treatment.

Usual attack not cured by chloroquine

1. Check that the correct dose of chloroquine was ordered.
2. Check that the chloroquine was ordered for 3 days – once daily if orally or twice daily if injection.
3. Check that *every* dose of the chloroquine was really given.
4. Check that the chloroquine was absorbed (i.e. was not vomited and that the patient did not have diarrhoea).

If the correct dose of chloroquine was not properly given, *then* give the correct dose properly for 3 days.

If the correct dose of chloroquine was properly given, *then* treat as chloroquine-resistant malaria (see below).

Severe attack if patient in or from an area where chloroquine-resistant malaria common

1. Make a (or another) blood smear for malaria parasites.
2. Look carefully for other causes of fever and treat any you find.
3. *If* the blood smear shows trophozoites ('troph' or 'T') or *if* the blood smear result is not immediately available *then* give quinine 10 mg/kg patient's body weight twice daily for 3 days.

Give quinine orally if possible (quinine sulphate 300 mg tablets).

Give quinine by IMI if vomiting or diarrhoea or very sick (quinine dihydrochloride 60 mg/ml (600 mg in 10 ml amps)).

The dose of quinine is:

- small adult (< 50 kg) – 450 mg (1½ tabs or 7.5 ml (7½ ml)) each 12 hours.
- large adult (> 50 kg) – 600 mg (2 tabs or 10 ml) each 12 hours.
- if patient able to be weighed see page 57 for exact dose for injections.

Then, after the 3 days of quinine, give *also* one dose only of pyrimethamine 25 mg and sulphadoxine 500 mg tablets (e.g. 'Fansidar' tablets):

- small adult (< 50 kg) – 2½ tabs,
- large adult (> 50 kg) – 3 tabs.

Patient unconscious or fitting or shocked or very 'sick'

1. Give quinine dihydrochloride (60 mg/ml) (600 mg in 10 ml amp) by IMI or by SLOW IV drip (see page 63), 10 mg/kg twice daily. The drip should run for over four hours.

IMI is usually the best method for giving quinine in a health centre. IV drip is however needed for giving quinine if the patient is shocked. (See Appendix 3 page 63 for method).

If chloroquine has already been given, give no more chloroquine and immediately start the quinine. Do not continue to give chloroquine as well as quinine to a patient.

The dose of quinine is 10 mg/kg patient's body weight each dose. The dose of quinine in ml can be worked out by dividing the patient's weight in kg by 6 (see Table 13.3). If the patient cannot be weighed the dose is:
- small adult (< 50 kg) – 7.5 ml (7½ ml),
- large adult (> 50 kg) – 10 ml.

Table 13.3   Quinine dosage

Patient's weight	Dose in ml
30–39 kg	6.0 ml
40–49 kg	7.5 ml (7½ ml)
50–59 kg	9.0 ml
60–69 kg	10.0 ml
70 kg or more	12.0 ml

The above dose is repeated:
- 6–8 hours after first dose, then
- 24 hours after first dose, then
- twice daily (each 12 hours) after this until the patient can swallow and absorb oral drugs (no shock or vomiting or diarrhoea).

If the patient is very sick and jaundiced or develops side effects of quinine, then reduce the repeat doses of quinine to half (½) of the doses above.

If quinine injection is not available:
1. give chloroquine injections (see page 56) instead,
2. transfer urgently if patient does not quickly improve.

2. See also below for other management at this stage. *This is very important*.
3. When the patient can take oral drugs (see above) change to oral quinine (300 mg tablets):
- small adult (< 50 kg) – 450 mg (1½ tabs) each 12 hours,
- large adult (> 50 kg) – 600 mg (2 tabs) each 12 hours.
4. After three days of oral quinine stop quinine and give *also* one of the following:
   (a) pyrimethamine 25 mg and sulphadoxine 400 mg tablets ('Fansidar' tablets) one dose only:
   small adult (< 50 kg) – 2½ tablets,
   large adult (> 50 kg) – 3 tablets;
   or if no 'Fansidar' available,
   (b) chloroquine tablets for three days (see page 55; but only if chloroquine-resistant malaria is not likely, *or*
   (c) continue quinine tablets for 10–14 days.

A three day course of quinine must ALWAYS be followed by one of the above even if the patient seems to be cured by three days of quinine.

Treat the symptoms

Rest
   Pain – aspirin 600–1200 mg (2–4 tabs) 4th hourly if needed.
   Fever – aspirin and sponge or wrap in wet sheet and fan.
   Vomiting many times – chlorpromazine 0.5 mg (½ mg)/kg IMI once (dose in ml is patient's weight in kg divided by 2 with maximum dose 25 mg (1 ml)). Do not give if systolic blood pressure < 80.

Treat any complications

Cerebral malaria
Give quinine by IMI or by *slow* IV drip (see above and Appendix 3 page 63) immediately.
   Do lumbar puncture *always*.
   Treat for meningitis also if CSF is not clear or is bloody or is not obtained (failed LP) (see Chapter 25 page 256).
   Paraldehyde 0.2 ml/kg (1/5 ml/kg) (5–10 ml) IMI immediately if convulsions. (Then see Convulsions, Chapter 25 page 266.)

Care of unconscious patient (see Chapter 25 page 264).

If not improved in 24 hours do a repeat lumbar puncture. If CSF still clear continue treatment. If CSF not clear or is bloody or is not obtained (failed LP) treat for meningitis also.

When unconsciousness lasts more than 24 hours transfer to medical officer care.

Acute severe anaemia

If Hb less than 5 g/dl and malaria (fever), transfer urgently (emergency) for blood transfusion.

Give IM antimalarials first if vomiting of oral antimalarial drugs is likely during transfer.

Gastro-enteritis or dysentery

IV fluids as for dehydration (see Chapter 23 page 224).

Give IM chloroquine or IM quinine.

Shock

Give quinine by slow IV drip (see Appendix 3 page 63).

IV fluids in another drip as for shock (see Chapter 27 page 307).

Blackwater fever

Do *not* give quinine. Give instead IM chloroquine.

Immediate treatment for shock or acute kidney failure if present. Transfer urgently (emergency) to Medical Officer care.

Very high fever

Up to 40°C:
- Aspirin 600–1200 mg (2–4 tablets) 4th hourly if needed.
- Sponge or wrap in wet sheet. Fan.

Above 40°C:
- Emergency – as above and wrap in a wet sheet, repeatedly wet the sheet and fan vigorously.
- IMI chlorpromazine 0.5 mg (½ mg)/kg (maximum 25 mg or 1 ml).
- Watch carefully for shock and treat if it occurs (see Chapter 27 page 305).
- When improved and treatment stopped, watch carefully for rise in temperature again which needs treatment again.

Give IMI, not oral, antimalarials.

Tropical splenomegaly syndrome

See Chapter 21 page 185.

IF   the patient is very sick or unconscious
THEN   treat this patient with quinine (not chloroquine) by IMI or by slow IV drip. This is especially important.

IF   the patient is in or is from an area where chloroquine-resistant malaria occurs, OR
IF   the patient has not responded to chloroquine already given.

IF   the patient is very ill or shocked and has some history or some signs that suggest he may have an acute severe bacterial infection
THEN   treat for septicaemia too (see Chapter 12).

Transfer to Medical Officer care

This is required only *if* complications occur *and* if is not possible to treat the complications properly in the health centre, e.g.:
1. cerebral malaria with unconsciousness which has lasted more than 1 day;
2. acute anaemia (Hb less than 5 g/dl and fever);
3. shock which cannot be corrected;
4. Blackwater fever.

Prevention and control

Eradication is not possible in most areas.

Kill malaria parasites

Killing all the malarial parasites in the bodies of all the original hosts (by giving antimalarial drugs to all of the population) is not possible in most areas.

In some areas, primaquine is given as well as the usual treatment drugs, to eradicate the infection from persons with malaria. Primaquine was also given in some areas where chloroquine-resistant malaria was just starting to occur but no spraying was being done try to stop the spread of chloroquine-resistant malaria.

Stop transmission

Stop mosquitoes from transmitting the infection from an infected person to another person. This is the main method used in malaria control.

All indoor surfaces of dwellings should be regularly sprayed with DDT or another residual insecticide. *Anopheles* mosquitoes bite at night when most people are indoors or near a house. After feeding, the mosquito likes to rest on a wall (which should be covered with DDT). Before there is time for the malaria to develop in the mosquito, the DDT will kill mosquito. The aim of spraying is to kill all *Anopheles* mosquitoes which have bitten human beings in their houses. (The aim of spraying is *not* to kill *all* mosquitoes.)

Raise the resistance of susceptible persons

This is not yet possible; but immunisation is the main hope for the control of this disease.

Prophylactic treatment

Regular prophylactic antimalarial drugs will stop the development of malaria parasites in the blood (trophozoites). They will therefore prevent clinical malaria. But they will also prevent the development of semi-immunity to malaria. And after a variable period of time (often about a year) they will cause the loss of any existing semi-immunity to malaria.

Prophylactic antimalarial drugs are therefore given only to certain groups of people.

1. People who
   - have no immunity to malaria, *and*
   - have come to a malarious area,
   and who
   - do not need to develop semi-immunity to malaria (e.g. they will not live in the malarious area for the rest of their lives or for many years), *or*
   - do not wish to suffer the ill-health needed to develop semi-immunity to malaria i.e. chronic malaria with repeated acute attacks of malaria for 4–10 years (see page 53); although the danger and severity of this ill-health can be greatly reduced by quick correct treatment of any acute attack which occurs.

This group will include:
(a) adults from areas where malaria does not occur,
(b) adults from areas where the same kind of malaria is not present all the time,
(c) children under 6 years; but only in *some* countries (after the age of 6 the children can clearly complain of the symptoms of malaria and be given quick drug treatment of the acute attack and are then allowed to develop chronic malaria and semi-immunity).

2. People who do have some immunity to malaria but this immunity is reduced for a while due to another condition.
   This group will include:
   (a) women when they are pregnant.
   (b) people sick from another illness e.g. pneumonia (stop antimalarials as soon as the pneumonia is cured) or anaemia (stop antimalarials as soon as haemoglobin is 10 g/dl).

3. People who cannot develop normal immunity to malaria. This group will include:
   (a) patients with Tropical Splenomegaly Syndrome,
   (b) possibly people who have had their spleens removed.

Chloroquine (300 mg) (2 tablets) each week is used for adults in most areas.

In some countries in areas where 10–20% of falciparum parasites are resistant to chloroquine, it has been made a policy to give pyrimethamine 12.5 mg and dapsone 100 mg combined in one tablet (e.g. 'Maloprim') one tablet each week. However, before you give this drug, check that it is policy to do so in your area. Also check whether it is safe for you to give it to women who are, or may be, pregnant. This drug also may not always prevent attacks of vivax malaria.

Appendix 1 Malaria blood smear

You should take a blood smear for examination for malaria parasites ('MPs') from all patients who have a fever. Even though you usually cannot examine the slide in the health centre you should still take one. At the end of the month you should send all the slides to the Malaria Control Office. This will help them tell how much malaria and what kind of malaria is occuring in the area.

Method of making malaria blood films

Both thick and thin blood films are used to detect and identify malaria parasites. These are usually made on the same frosted ended slide. See Chapter 6 page 22 for details.

1. For best results make a spreader. Break off the corners of a glass slide making sure that the edge of the slide is smooth. It must not be chipped or rough because this will spoil the thin blood film.

edge smooth -
not chipped or rough

2. Imagine that the non-frosted area of a standard clean slide is composed of three equal parts.

3a. Put one large or preferably three small drops of blood in the middle of the part nearest the frosted end.
3b. Put one small drop of blood at the beginning of the next part.

4. Bring the edge of a second slide to contact the surface of the blood slide just in front of the one drop of blood – push this spreader slide backwards until it just touches the drop of blood, which will then spread along its edge.

5. Hold at an angle of 45° and spread the drop of blood by pushing the spreader forward. (See Chapter 6 page 23 for details.)

6. With the corner of the spreader slide, spread the 3 drops to form a circular thick film about 1 cm in diameter. Spread the blood evenly. If you can just see the print of a newspaper through it, the smear is the right thickness.

IF YOU CAN READ THE TYPE. THEN THE BLOOD FILM IS TOO THIN

IF YOU CAN ___ THE TYPE. THE BL___ TOO THICK

IF YOU CAN JUST SEE THE TYPE. THE BLOOD FILM IS CORRECT

7. Leave the slide flat so that the thick film will dry evenly. Use a pencil to write the slide number on the frosted end of the slide.

Interpretation of reports of malaria smears

A report of 'negative' means that after the examination of 100 high power fields under the microscope, no malaria parasites were seen. Therefore it is very unlikely that the patient's illness is caused by malaria.

If malaria parasites are found, the number of parasites per field is counted and recorded like this:

1. If the number of parasites in an average field is higher than 20 (e.g. 43) only one field is counted and the total number of parasites reported (e.g. 43/1).
2. If the number of parasites present in an average field is between 3 and 19, (e.g. 14) then ten fields are counted, and the total number of parasites reported (e.g. 140/10).
3. If the number of parasites present in an average field is less than 3 (e.g. 1 or 2) in most fields, then 100 fields are counted and the total number reported (e.g. 120/100).

If mixed infections are found, then each species is reported separately.

Trophozoites and *P. falciparum* gametocytes are reported separately.

The presence of trophozoites or gametocytes shows infection with malaria parasites. But only trophozoites harm humans. Trophozoites indicate the patient's illness may be caused by malaria. Gametocytes do not harm humans. The presence of gametocytes in the blood does *not* suggest that the patient's illness may be caused by malaria. Chloroquine treatment may cure a patient of falciparum malaria and trophozoites will disappear from his blood within one week. However, as chloroquine does not kill *P. falciparum* gametocytes, the smear may show gametocytes for another 3–4 months although the patient is cured. The gametocytes are however infectious for mosquitoes.

Trophozoites ('Troph' or 'T') present in a slide mean the patient may be sick with malaria.

Gametocytes ('G') do not mean the patient may be sick with malaria (but the patient can pass on the disease to mosquitoes).

A more accurate method of estimating parasite density is to estimate the number of parasites present in 1 cmm of blood. When examining the film, the laboratory worker counts 200 white cells and all the parasites present in the fields which contained the 200 white cells. He then multiplies the number of parasites by 40 (as there are about 8000 white cells per cmm) to give the number of parasites per cmm. Again mixed infections are reported separately, and trophozoites and *P. falciparum* gametocytes are reported separately.

Another method of recording parasite density is as follows:

- Less than 10 parasites in 100 fields.   +
- More than 10 parasites but less than 100 parasites in 100 fields.   + +
- More than 100 parasites in 100 fields but less than 10 parasites in 1 field.   + + +
- More than 10 parasites in one field. + + + +

Again, mixed infections are reported separately and trophozoites and *P. falciparum* gametocytes are reported separately.

Appendix 2 Chloroquine resistant malaria

In some parts of the world, especially in South East Asia, the Pacific, South America and now also in parts of India and Africa (See Figure 13.1 page 49), some malaria parasites have become resistant to treatment with chloroquine and the related drug, amodiaquine. This has happened with only some *P. falciparum* parasites. A full treatment course of chloroquine does not 'cure' the patient as it previously did, i.e. make the patient clinically well *and* clear the blood of all the asexual parasites (trophozoites in the RBCs).

Resistance against chloroquine is divided into three types depending on the results of blood slides taken after a proper three day treatment course of chloroquine. The first day of treatment is called day 0. For exact details of the tests see the WHO publications. A simplified explanation is as follows.

S Sensitivity *P. falciparum* trophozoites are cleared from the blood within 7 days and do not later appear (unless reinfection). (In fully sensitive parasites the trophozoites have usually all gone within 2 days.)

R_1 Resistance *P. falciparum* trophozoites disappear from the blood slides within seven days as in S; (however they are *not* all killed); trophozoites reappear in the blood slides before 4 weeks have gone.

R_2 Resistance The number of *P. falciparum* trophozoites in the blood slides is reduced but the blood is not cleared of trophozoites within 7 days; also the number of trophozoites rises again before 4 weeks have gone.

R_3 Resistance The number of *P. falciparum* trophozoites in the blood smears is not significantly reduced by treatment. (It may even rise.) Trophozoites therefore are still present after 7 days.

The definitions are further explained in the following graphs.

These tests are difficult to do in areas where malaria is common as most patients will be infected with malaria again before four weeks have gone. However, the time from the bite of an infected mosquito until an attack of that malaria infection (with a significant number of malaria parasites (trophozoites) in the blood slide) is usually (10–) 14 days. Therefore, any trophozoites in the blood after 7 days and before 14 days (from the first day of the chloroquine treatment course) are almost certainly because of chloroquine resistant malaria in the body.

Before deciding that a patient has chloroquine resistant malaria
1. Make sure it is falciparum and not one of the other types of malaria which have a persistent liver cycle and are not 'cured' by chloroquine.
2. Make sure that the patient did swallow and did absorb the chloroquine (i.e. did not have vomiting and/or diarrhoea).

Appendix 3 Method of giving quinine by slow IV drip

Give quinine by a slow IV drip *only if*:
1. It has been possible to get a drip running immediately (before 15 minutes have passed). (An immediate IMI is better than a late IV drip.)
2. The staff are able to keep the drip running.
3. The staff will not let the drip run in quickly. (A rapid IVI of quinine will cause sudden death.)

If not, it is better to give the quinine by IMI.
Give quinine by IMI *when*:
1. IV drip was not started immediately (before 15 minutes have passed).
2. The staff are not capable of keeping the drip running.
3. You are not certain that the staff will not let the drip run quickly.

IM quinine is not as effective as IV quinine especially if the patient is shocked. Also it may cause an injection abscess.

Method of giving quinine by slow IV drip

Use 10 ml/kg patient's body weight of 4.3% dextrose in 0.18% sodium chloride solution to dilute the quinine. Let the fluid run out of a flask of dextrose saline until the required amount is left (e.g. 500 ml for an adult).

Add the dose of quinine to the solution by injecting the quinine into the flask.
Mix well.
Run the drip *slowly over four (4) hours*.
• Order the number of drops per minute.
• Mark on the IV flask the level for each hour.
• Then, every hour check that the fluid has fallen to the level of this mark, but *no more*.

14

Tuberculosis

Definition, cause, pathology and epidemiology

Tuberculosis is a disease which effects the lungs and other parts of man; and, sometimes, other animals. It is usually a chronic disease; but sometimes it can be acute.

Tuberculosis is caused by an infection by a bacterial bacillus called *Mycobacterium tuberculosis*. When the *M. tuberculosis* bacillus is stained in the laboratory and then covered with acid, it keeps the colour of the stain. (Most other organisms lose their colour.) *M. tuberculosis* is therefore called an acid fast bacillus. This is shortened to AFB. (*M. leprae* is also an AFB. See Chapter 15 page 76).

Tuberculosis is very common in developing and tropical countries especially where there is poor general health, nutrition, housing and public health services and especially in urban areas.

Tuberculosis is nearly always spread by persons with tuberculosis of the lungs who are not being treated. These people cough out tuberculosis organisms in droplets and droplet nuclei into the air. These droplets or droplet nuclei are then inhaled into the respiratory tract of another person. The *M. tuberculosis* organisms then start to grow, if the person does not have some immunity to the organism.

Some immunity against infection with tuberculosis organisms can be given by previous infection with tuberculosis or by deliberate immunisation using similar organisms (e.g. BCG).

If the organisms grow, they cause a small area of bronchopneumonia. The organisms then spread to the lymph nodes in the chest. They are then carried by the lymph into the blood. Then the blood spreads the organisms to the whole body. In the 1–2 months while it is happening, the body is slowly developing immunity to the organisms. When this immunity has properly developed usually the body then kills the organisms and the infection heals. This is called '*primary tuberculosis*'. A few organisms may remain alive (in the lungs or any other part of the body to which they spread) for many years or the rest of the person's life. But these organisms are usually surrounded by scar tissue and are not able to cause disease.

'*Post primary tuberculosis*' happens if the organisms start to grow again and escape from their surrounding scar tissue. This can happen at any of the places they spread to in primary tuberculosis. It happens most commonly in the lungs; but it can also happen in lymph glands, meninges, bones and joints, kidneys, etc.

Sometimes in primary or post primary tuberculosis, when the organisms are in the blood and spread to many or all organs of the body, they continue to grow and multiply in all these places and cause '*miliary tuberculosis*'. Figure 14.1 shows the stages of infection with tuberculosis organisms.

Symptoms and signs

Symptoms and signs of tuberculosis are caused by:
1. disease of the organ infected by the *M. tuberculosis* organisms – destruction of the organ and the formation of pus in it; and
2. toxins made by the *M. tuberculosis* organisms– causing general symptoms and signs of infection.

The symptoms and signs of primary tuberculosis, post-primary tuberculosis and miliary tuberculosis are outlined in this section.

Primary tuberculosis

The body's defence system usually wins the fight before any organ is badly damaged. Usually there

Figure 14.1 Diagram showing the stages of infection with tuberculosis organisms.

is only a mild febrile illness, the cause of which is not found out by the health worker.

Post-primary tuberculosis

Pulmonary tuberculosis
Symptoms include the following:
1. Chronic cough, almost always. The cough stays and does not go away even after treatment with antibiotics. *Anyone who has a cough for more than 4 weeks must be examined for tuberculosis.* Often a cough is the only symptom or sign of tuberculosis.
2. Sputum, usually – usually made of pus.
3. Haemoptysis, sometimes – it can be large or small.
4. Pain in the chest, usually of pleuritic type; but this is not common.
5. Shortness of breath, sometimes. This comes early in the disease if the disease is severe (e.g. miliary tuberculosis) or there is a large pleural effusion; otherwise it only comes after many years when most of the lungs are destroyed.
6. Fever, sweating etc. especially at night. (i.e. general symptoms of infection) – not very common.
7. Loss of weight – only if acute severe disease or late disease.

Signs include the following:
1. Sometimes mild fever; usually only in severe or late disease.
2. Sometimes wasting and weight loss; usually only in acute severe or late disease.
3. Sometimes anaemia; usually only in acute severe or late disease.
4. Sometimes abnormalities on chest examination; but often not. If abnormalities in the lung are present, they are most likely to be those of upper lobe disease or of pleural effusion.

Patients with tuberculosis can also get ordinary pneumonia or acute bronchitis. When you ask how long they have had a cough, they often say for only as long as their acute chest infection. They think the previous chronic cough was normal. Therefore always ask all patients with acute chest infections if they *also* had a chronic cough before the start of this present infection. Send sputum from such patients for AFB tests.

Pneumonia or other chest infection which is unusual or not 'typical' in anyway, may be caused by tuberculosis. Suspect pneumonia of being caused by tuberculosis if *any* of the following are true:
1. it is in an upper lobe of the lung;
2. the signs in the chest are much worse than you expect because the patient does not seem very 'sick';
3. the pneumonia does not get better as quickly as it should with proper treatment; or
4. the patient had a chronic cough before the start of the pneumonia.

Send sputum from such patients for AFB tests. If the patient is still not cured after two weeks of proper treatment send three more sputum slides for AFB tests.

Everyone who has had a cough for more than four weeks *must* have three samples of sputum sent for AFB (TB) tests even if the person has no other symptoms or signs (see exception later).

Lymph node (gland) tuberculosis
Usually children or young adults are affected; but anyone can be affected.

Usually neck nodes are affected; but nodes in other areas can be affected (see Figure 14.2).

Usually the only symptom is a lump which does not go away, but gets bigger.

Usually the only sign is enlarged firm lymph nodes which are matted (or joined) together and which are not tender or red or hot. Sometimes there may be a sinus discharging pus over the nodes.

Any chronic enlargement of cervical lymph nodes with no obvious cause (e.g. infection in the ENT or head) which does not improve after antibiotics for 3 weeks, must be biopsied to look for tuberculosis (especially if the tuberculin test is positive.

Kidney tuberculosis
Symptoms are those of an urinary tract infection or blood in the urine.

Signs are often not present; but there may be

kidney tenderness or epididymitis (inflammation of the tubules at the back of the testis).

Tests usually show pus or blood or protein in the urine.

Treatment with sulphadimidine and then tetracycline or chloramphenicol does not cure the patient. Refer or non-urgently transfer such patients to a medical officer for definite diagnosis and treatment.

> Any patient with a urinary tract infection which does not improve after proper treatment, must be transferred to a medical officer for diagnosis and treatment.

Vertebral tuberculosis (see also Chapter 29 page 324)

Symptoms and signs include the following.

The patient has back pain and stiffness which lasts for months, which never improves but instead becomes steadily worse.

When you examine the back it is stiff (i.e. it will not bend normally). When you feel (or gently hit with the side of your hand) all along the spine, you find a tender part.

If no treatment is given the infected bones of the spine collapse and a lump or deformity occurs in the line of the spinal bones (see Figure 14.3).

If treatment is not quickly given, weakness or paralysis or loss of sensation in the legs and not being able to pass urine may occur (because of pressure on the spinal cord).

Figure 14.3 Tuberculosis of the spine. Note the deformity of the spine (often called a 'gibbus'). Tuberculosis of the spine is often called 'Potts Disease'. This patient needs urgent transfer for treatment before she becomes paraplegic.

Figure 14.2 Tuberculous cervical lymphadenitis. The gland must be biopsied.

Suspect vertebral tuberculosis if there is chronic increasing backache with tenderness and stiffness.

Transfer such patients for X-ray and definite diagnosis.

> Any patient who has chronic backache which is becoming worse and who has a stiff spine with a tender part, must be transferred for examination for spinal tuberculosis.

Tuberculous arthritis (see also Chapter 29 page 323)

The hip or knee joints are most often affected, but any joint can be affected.

Children or young adults are most often affected, but anyone can be affected.

Symptoms are usually chronic continuous pain and stiffness of the joint or a limp which slowly becomes worse.

Signs include:
1. *chronic arthritis which slowly becomes worse* (swelling, tenderness, warmth, pain on moving joint, limited movement of joint, not able to use joint properly, etc.);
2. *wasting of muscles, usually severe*, which move the joint is typical;
3. nearby lymph nodes are usually enlarged;
4. a sinus discharging pus may be present over the joint late in the disease.

Any chronic arthritis which becomes progressively worse over months should be suspected of being tuberculous arthritis.

Transfer all such patients for definite diagnosis.

> Any chronic arthritis (i.e. with inflammation of the joint) which becomes progressively worse over months, should be suspected of being tuberculous arthritis. Tuberculosis is even more likely if only one joint is involved, and especially if the tuberculin test is positive. Such cases should be referred or transferred for tests.

Meningeal tuberculosis (see also Chapter 25 page 259)

Most often the patient is a child, but the patient can be any age.

Symptoms and signs are the same as for acute bacterial meningitis (see Chapter 25 page 256) but the disease is less acute.

The history is usually much longer (i.e. more than a few days). A contact may have tuberculosis or a chronic cough not yet diagnosed as tuberculosis – check the family.

At first the patient is usually not as sick and febrile as you would expect for bacterial meningitis. Also, the patient may be wasted and have signs and symptoms of tuberculosis elsewhere. The patient does not improve as he should on proper meningitis treatment. (See Chapter 25 page 257.)

The CSF is sometimes yellow or forms a web after standing; but it can appear normal to naked eye examination.

> Transfer urgently
> (1) all cases with the above this history, examination and tests
> (2) all cases of meningitis or encephalitis or cerebral malaria which do not improve after 2 days of proper treatment,
> for definite diagnosis and special drug treatment as meningeal tuberculosis is likely.

Abdominal (peritoneal, intestinal or lymph node) tuberculosis

Symptoms include: swelling of the abdomen, usually; bowel colic, sometimes; general symptoms of infection, e.g. weight loss, fever, malaise often.

Signs include: abdominal ascites, usually; masses or tenderness sometimes; general signs of infection, e.g. fever, weight loss, anaemia, sometimes.

> Suspect abdominal tuberculosis in a patient with ascites if:
> • no oedema of the back or legs, or
> • no response to treatment with diuretics, or
> • abdominal masses or tenderness are also present, or
> • general signs of infection are present.

Transfer all suspected cases for definite diagnosis.

Miliary tuberculosis

The patient may have a family or contact history of tuberculosis or a past history of a chronic cough or another condition which suggests tuberculosis.

Symptoms are usually not specific but are severe – malaise, fever, sweating, weakness, nausea, vomiting, diarrhoea, cough, shortness of breath, headache, etc.

Signs are usually not specific but are severe – not fully conscious, fever, fast pulse, dyspnoea, weight loss, anaemia, etc.

Antibiotics and antimalarials do not help the patient who quickly becomes worse.

Transfer such cases urgently if they do not improve with proper treatment for septicaemia (see Chapter 12) and chloroquine-resistant malaria (see Chapter 13 page 54) within 48 hours.

Tests

Sputum tests for AFB

This is how to do the sputum test for AFB:
Saliva from the mouth is *no use* for this test. *Sputum* coughed up *from inside the chest* and spat out is *essential*.

Give the patient a container (such as a bottle or plastic bag), or if one of these is not available, something such as a banana leaf. Ask the patient to stand either outside in the open air or facing an open window. Ask the patient to breathe deeply three times, then to cover his mouth and then to cough deeply when he feels ready to cough. When he coughs deeply to produce sputum, tell him to spit the sputum into the container holding it close to his mouth.

Now look to see if the specimen is suitable for examination.

A proper specimen is thick with solid pieces of pus or yellowish material and 2–5 ml in volume.

If the sputum is not suitable ask the patient to repeat the process until a good specimen is obtained. At times it is necessary to give physiotherapy (hit the patient on the back when he coughs or make him bend or lie down with the head lower than the chest and hit his back while he coughs) to get a proper specimen.

This first specimen, which you collect when you first see the patient at the health centre, is called specimen 'A'.

Tell the patient to collect another specimen of sputum in the same way at home immediately when he wakes the next morning and then return with it. This is called specimen 'B'.

When the patient comes back the next day with the specimen 'B', collect the third specimen at the health centre. This is called specimen 'C'. To make a smear from the sputum specimen, take a clean slide and mark it on the rough end with the patient's name, address, etc. With an applicator stick (or any kind of stick), lift out one or two thick yellow solid pieces of sputum. Then spread this sputum around the other two-thirds of the slide thickly and evenly.

Allow the slide to dry in the air (for about 15 minutes). Make sure it is protected from flies and insects. After it is dry, 'fix' it by passing it 3 times through the flame of a spirit lamp (or over any non-smoky flame, e.g. over a hurricane lamp if a spirit lamp is not available), until it is just hot enough to be uncomfortable if held on the back of the other hand. Make sure the patient's sputum and name are facing upwards. Place the slide into a slide box, or protect it with another slide tied to it but separated from it by broken applicator or match sticks. It must be kept away from cockroaches or other insects. Burn the specimen containers and applicator sticks.

The sputum smear will show AFB in almost all cases if the patient has pulmonary tuberculosis causing symptoms. In some early cases, before a bronchus is broken open by the disease, the sputum will be negative. The most common causes of slides being negative, when, in fact the patient does have pulmonary tuberculosis, are:
1. saliva and not sputum was put on the slide,
2. errors were made in the laboratory.

In places where tuberculosis is common any patient who has a cough which has lasted for more than 4 weeks or who has any other symptoms or signs suggesting pulmonary tuberculosis, should have his sputum tested for AFB three times.

Take one specimen of sputum *immediately* (Specimen A). Ask the patient to cough up a second specimen early the next morning (Specimen

B). Collect a third specimen the day the patient brings back specimen B (Specimen C).

From each sample, make a smear of the sputum, fix it by heating it, and send it to the laboratory with a request for tests for AFB.

If a patient has negative slides for AFB and you still strongly suspect pulmonary tuberculosis, repeat the slides ('A', 'B' and 'C').

If the patient has these repeated slides negative for AFB and you still strongly suspect tuberculosis, discuss the case with the Health or Medical Officer to see if non-urgent transfer for chest X-ray is needed.

In places where tuberculosis is not common and chronic bronchitis (COLD) is very common,[1] if a patient has a true chronic cough treat with procaine pencillin for 1 week. If the patient is then cured, discharge him.

If he is not cured treat with tetracycline for 1 week, and if he is then cured, discharge him.

If he is still not cured *and* he is over 40 years old *and* has never been where tuberculosis is common *and*:

- has never lived in the same house as a person from an area where tuberculosis is common, *and*
- has never had contact with a tuberculosis patient, *and*
- has no other symptoms or signs of tuberculosis, *then* discharge with PD of chronic bronchitis (COLD).

All other cases continue the tetracycline for 2–4 weeks and send sputum smears for AFB.

Gastric aspirate examination for AFB

This is done for children or adults who are not able to produce sputum.

Three (3) fasting morning specimens are collected.

This test is not as accurate as sputum (false negative and false positive results can occur).

---

1 These rules will probably not apply in your area, unless there are particular environmental conditions. Unless your Health Department tells you that these rules can apply in your place, cross them out of this book.

Tuberculin test (also called 'Mantoux' Test)

Purified Protein Derivative of tuberculosis organisms 'PPD (TR23)' can be injected intradermally (into the skin). If the body's defence cells have learned to fight tuberculosis organisms, there will be an acute inflammatory reaction in the skin at the site of the injection within a couple of days.

Give PPD by *intradermal* injection only.

At 72 (or up to 96) hours, measure and write down on the patient's chart the diameter in mm of the swelling (not the redness).

0–9 mm negative
10+ mm positive

If the reaction is negative there is no immunity to tuberculosis organisms and, as long as the PPD was active and the test was done properly, infection with tuberculosis organisms is unlikely (but still possible).

A positive reaction means that there is some 'immunity' against tuberculosis organisms: tuberculosis organisms have been in the body in the past or are there at present.

But, remember that:

1. The tuberculin test may be negative when the patient does have active tuberculosis disease. Times when this occurs include:
   (a) when the tuberculosis infection is very severe, e.g. miliary tuberculosis or tuberculous meningitis;
   (b) when another illness is present (such as measles or chickenpox);
   (c) when the patient has malnutrition;
   (d) when the patient is taking certain drugs (especially prednisolone or cortisone-like drugs);
   (e) when the PPD was not reliable, or the test was not done properly.
2. The positive tuberculin test does *not* mean that the patient is sick with tuberculosis disease. It means only that tuberculosis organisms are or were alive in his body. Do *not* diagnose tuberculosis disease just because the tuberculin test is positive.

BCG immunisation which causes an ulcer in a few days (instead of the usual few weeks) has the same meaning as a positive tuberculin test, and is called an accelerated BCG reaction.

Lymph node biopsy

Lymph nodes near the body surface i.e. just under the skin and can be easily held between the finger and thumb – the biopsy can be done at the health centre.

Deep lymph nodes – refer or transfer to a medical officer for biopsy.

Chest X-ray

A chest X-ray is not possible at a health centre and is almost never necessary for diagnosis.

A normal chest X-ray makes pulmonary tuberculosis unlikely.

An abnormal chest X-ray means further tests (mainly sputum for AFB) are needed to see if the abnormality on the X-ray is caused by tuberculosis or another disease.

Diagnostic features

1. Every cough which has lasted for more than 4 weeks.
2. A chronic cough is especially suspicious when there is also – sputum, or haemoptysis, or chest pain, or fever or weight loss.
3. Swollen lymph glands in the neck with no obvious cause (especially no ENT or scalp infection) which do not go away after treatment with antibiotics.
4. Tuberculin test usually (but not always) positive. The positive tuberculin test diagnoses only infection (past or present), *not* disease.

Treatment

The two most important things in the treatment of the patient are:
1. Give *at least* two antituberculosis drugs.
2. Give these drugs *regularly* for *at least* the shortest amount of time that is needed for them to cure the disease. For the drugs usually available this means *at least* 12 months or even better 18 months.[2]

Treatment is divided into two parts:
1. short-term intensive chemotherapy for 8 weeks (2 months) with 3 drugs (INAH and streptomycin and thiacetazone) (called 'A' treatment);
2. maintenance treatment for 16 more months with any 2 of the above 3 drugs:
   either fully supervised outpatient treatment twice weekly with streptomycin and high-dose INAH (called 'B' treatment),
   or unsupervised home treatment daily with INAH and thiacetazone tablets being taken by the patient himself each day (called 'C' treatment).

Do not start treatment unless:
1. sputum is positive for AFB; *or*
2. lymph gland (or other) biopsy is positive for tuberculosis; *or*
3. patient has suspected severe tuberculosis and would die before test results could be obtained or transfer was possible (diagnosis *must* later be confirmed in these cases);) *or*
4. tuberculosis has been diagnosed by a medical officer in another way.

Always do a full medical history and physical examination and test the urine first.

Diagnose and treat any other conditions present especially anaemia and other bacterial chest infections.

Treatment of the patient only is not the proper management of the problem caused by the diagnosis of a case of tuberculosis. Remember the other things needed in the management of the patient. (See box on page 72)

Here is a very effective fairly cheap regimen for management of patients with tuberculosis. This regimen is at present used in Papua New Guinea. If there is a different policy in your area, change the necessary details. However, the basic plan in all effective management policies will be the same as in this regimen.

---

2 A new drug called rifampicin is now available which, if used together with INAH can cure tuberculosis in 9 months. Another drug called pyrazinamide is also available, which, if used together with rifampicin and INAH, can cure tuberculosis in 6 months. However these drugs are still very expensive and do have serious side effects and the use of them is not yet possible in health centres in most developing countries. The use of these drugs will not be described. The use of one of the older but very effective and cheap regimens is described.

> Management includes 4 things:
> 1. Register patient. Fill in index and treatment cards. Arrange treatment and patient follow-up. Arrange contact tracing. Give health education.
> 2. Treat with *at least* 2 drugs *regularly* for *at least* 18 months.
>   (a) Give INAH and streptomycin and thiacetazone daily for 8 weeks ('A' treatment).
>   (b) Then give *either*
>   • streptomycin and high dose INAH twice weekly ('B' treatment) for 16 months, *or*
>   • INAH and thiacetazone daily ('C' treatment) for 16 months.
> 3. Check that the infection is controlled by the drugs. Send sputum for AFB (Specimen 'P') every 3 months.
> 4. Transfer to medical officer care if needed.

Register the patient. Arrange treatment and follow-up. Arrange contact tracing. Start health education.

1. Confirm the diagnosis (if the diagnosis was made by another health worker).
2. Register the patient in the register book and give him a number from the register.
3. Fill in his details on the index card. Put the card in the index card file.
4. Fill in the details of the treatment plan on the treatment card. Send the treatment card to the treatment centre.
5. Start patient and family education.
6. Arrange contact education and examination.
7. Arrange for sputum smears for AFB every 3 months (e.g. 1st week of January, April, July and September) if sputum positive.
8. Check treatment attendances and smear results on the treatment charts every 3 months (e.g. 1st week of February, May, August and November). Write results on index cards.
9. Notify the Health Department of the patient in the monthly report. (*Every* month fill in TB report form from the index card file.)

Give INAH, streptomycin, thiacetazone

Give the patient education about the need for regular treatment for 18 months.

Tell him to notify the treatment centre if he intends to move or go on holiday.

Defaulter action

If the patient does not attend for one week the treatment centre worker must *visit* him weekly until he attends regularly. If the patient still does not attend for three weeks, the treatment centre worker must tell the supervisor.

The supervisor must then *visit* the patient regularly until he attends.

If the patient will not attend for three months or you cannot find him, tell the Health Department Medical Officer.

Give short term intensive treatment for 8 weeks ('A' treatment)

Give 3 drugs every day for 8 weeks.

Adults weighing more than 40 kg:

1. isoniazid or INAH 300 mg daily
2. thiacetazone 150 mg daily
} one combined INAH and thiacetazone tablet daily

3. streptomycin –
   • 1 g (2 ml) IMI daily if less than 40 years old
   • 0.75 g (1.5 ml) (1½ ml) IMI daily if more than 40 years old.

Adults weighing less than 40 kg:

1. INAH 150 mg (1½ tabs) daily
2. thiacetazone 75 mg daily
} ½ of one combined INAH and thiacetazone tablet daily

3. streptomycin 0.75 g (1.5 ml) (1½ ml) daily.

This can be given as an inpatient or outpatient depending on:
1. the medical condition of the patient;
2. the nearest treatment centre being close enough for daily attendance;
3. the treatment centre worker being experienced enough to observe the patient on initial therapy and educate him;
4. what the patient and his family want.

Watch carefully for drug toxicity, especially rash, dizziness, fever, jaundice. If toxicity occurs, stop treatment and urgently transfer the patient to a Medical Officer.

Before discharge to OPD treatment, give the patient education about drug side-effects. Tell him to come immediately to the health centre if he develops itch, rash, blisters, dizziness, fever, nausea, jaundice, etc.

Then continue maintenance therapy for 16 months more

Either 'B' or 'C' maintenance therapy may be given.

You should decide the type of maintenance therapy as early as possible during initial therapy so that you can carefully instruct the patient about it while he is still being seen daily.

Fully supervised maintenance treatment ('B' treatment)

1. Streptomycin 1 g (2 ml) IM twice weekly (Mon. and Thurs.)
2. INAH high dose according to patient's weight, swallowed in the presence of the health worker twice weekly (Mon. and Thurs.).

Patient's weight	Dose INAH
20–25 kg	300 mg (3 tablets)
26–30 kg	400 mg (4 tablets)
31–35 kg	450 mg (4½ tablets)
36–40 kg	500 mg (5 tablets)
41–45 kg	600 mg (6 tablets)
46–55 kg	700 mg (7 tablets)
56–61 kg	800 mg (8 tablets)
61–65 kg	900 mg (9 tablets)
66–75 kg	1000 mg (10 tablets)

3. Pyridoxine 25 mg (1 tab) twice weekly (Mon. and Thurs.)

Give 'B' treatment if:
1. thiacetazone toxicity during initial treatment,
2. treatment centre is close enough for twice weekly attendance,
3. need for carefully supervised taking of treatment (patient not dependable or 'C' treatment not successful),
4. this is what the patient wants.

Home Maintenance Treatment ('C' treatment)

Adults weighing more than 40 kg:

1. isoniazid or INAH 300 mg daily
2. thiacetazone 150 mg daily

} one combined INAH AND thiacetazone tablet daily.

Adults weighing less than 40 kg:

1. INAH 150 mg (1½ tabs) daily
2. thiacetazone 75 mg daily

} ½ of one combined INAH and thiacetazone tablet daily.

The patient attends the treatment centre once every 4 weeks on the 'C' collection day (marked on the calendar distributed by TB Control) to collect a supply of (usually) 28 tablets to take one daily at home.

Give 'C' treatment if:
1. there is no treatment centre near the patient's home or work;
2. patient has a travelling job such as truck driving or shift work;
3. a patient showed during 'A' treatment that he understood and could be trusted to take treatment at home;
4. this is what the patient wants.

Progress sputum examination for AFB

Send one sputum slide (Specimen 'P') every 3 months (e.g. the first week of every January, April, July and October) if the patient was originally sputum positive.

Note on ethambutol

Ethambutol can be used by medical officers in some special cases of tuberculosis. If the patient has had or is likely to have a reaction to thiacetazone, the medical officer may give an 'Alternative "A"' regimen ('AA' regimen) of INAH and streptomycin and ethambutol (instead of the usual 'A' regimen of INAH and streptomycin and thiacetazone).

Ethambutol is an effective safe drug. But, if a dose higher than the proper dose is given, it can cause blindness.

The dose is 15 mg/kg daily or 50 mg/kg twice weekly.

Transfer

Transfer to Medical Officer care any of the following:

1. patients who are strongly suspected of having tuberculosis; but you cannot prove the diagnosis at the health centre;
2. patients who develop serious drug reactions (urgent);
3. patients with complications, especially significant haemoptysis (urgent);
4. patients with suspected drug resistant infection, i.e. patients who continue to have positive sputum for AFB after 6 months supervised regular treatment which you know has been given and taken (non-urgent).

Note on health education and contact tracing

The patient

Teach the patient about the disease and the need for regular treatment for 18 months. Make the patient memorise the month and the year he should finish treatment (if all goes well).

Tell him if he does not take treatment the disease will destroy his lungs and infect others. Tell him if he takes regular treatment for 18 months he will be cured and he will not infect others.

Tell him to come to the treatment centre immediately if he gets itch, rash, blisters, nausea, fever, jaundice, etc.

Tell him to tell the treatment centre if he intends to move to another place or go on holiday.

Ask if he has any worries or questions, and answer them.

Family, other contacts and community education

All contacts (family, those who live in the same house, friends, workmates, schoolmates, etc.) should be seen.

Educate them about the symptoms of the disease and tell them that drugs cure it and tell them to come back if symptoms develop.

Question and examine them for cough, enlarged lymph glands and wasting, etc. Any who have chronic cough or other symptoms or signs should have sputum tested for AFB, and biopsy of any enlarged lymph nodes.

If tuberculin testing or X-rays are available, do these especially in children who cannot produce sputum. Give any child contact under 7 years who has a positive tuberculin test but is otherwise well prophylactic INAH for 1 year. Give newborn (and probably all young children) who are close household contacts of infectious sputum positive pulmonary tuberculosis patients prophylactic INAH, even if the tuberculin test is negative (especially if the patient is the mother). (*Make sure that the child does not have tuberculosis as then the child needs at least 2 drugs, i.e. INAH and streptomycin.*)

Give BCG to other children and to adults who have a negative tuberculin test.

Educate everyone to come to the Health Centre if symptoms develop.

Explain to all the family and contacts how tuberculosis can be treated and how they can help the patient and *make sure* he or she gets regular treatment.

Control and prevention

Get rid of the reservoir of infection

Persons with pulmonary tuberculosis spread the disease by coughing.

Almost as soon as a patient starts on antituberculosis drugs, he becomes non-infectious.

If all pulmonary cases of tuberculosis could be found and kept on treatment, the disease could no longer spread.

Therefore, every time you see any patient for any reason, ask if he has a cough. If it has been present for more than 4 weeks, send sputum for tests for AFB.

Once a case is found, it is important to examine all the patient's contacts to find who gave him the disease and to whom he has given the disease, before they spread it further (see above).

Stop the means of spread of the organisms

Measures to stop droplet spread help. Educate people to cover the mouth when coughing. Encourage housing which is not overcrowded (especially where people sleep).

Raise the resistance of susceptible persons

The resistance of the general population can be raised by general public health measures (malaria control, prevention of malnutrition, treatment of anaemia, etc.).

The resistance of individual persons can be greatly increased by BCG immunisation given before tuberculosis infection usually happens. In places where infection happens all the time and where it is not known how long the effect of BCG lasts, give BCG:

1. at birth or as soon as possible after;
2. at 7 years or the first year at school;
3. at 13 years or the last year at school;
4. to adults who have not had BCG before;
5. to contacts with a negative tuberculin test and no evidence of disease (if you give prophylactic INAH, give BCG after INAH completed).

Check all patients for BCG scars. If the correct number of BCG scars is not present, give BCG.

Prophylatic treatment

You should give prophylactic treatment to contacts of infectious patients who have been infected. This is to kill the few organisms in the infected contact before the organisms multiply and produce clinical *disease*. In practice this is usually done only for children under 7 years with *M. tuberculosis* infection shown by a positive tuberculin test. It is also given to newborn children (and probably best given also to all children under the age of 3) who are household contacts of sputum positive tuberculosis patients (especially if this person is the mother), even if the tuberculin test is negative. These children are given INAH for a year. Do not give INAH alone if there is any evidence of tuberculosis *disease* (as well as tuberculosis *infection*); give at least 2 drugs instead. After a course of INAH prophylaxis is finished, then give BCG.

15

Leprosy

Definition, cause, pathology

Leprosy is a chronic bacterial infection of man. It is common in parts of the world where living and public health standards are not good. The infection causes chronic inflammation of and destruction of the skin and the peripheral nerves. Sometimes it can also cause inflammation and destruction of the eyes, the mucous membrane of the upper respiratory tract, the muscles, the bones, the testes and other organs.

Leprosy is caused by an infection with *Mycobacterium leprae*, a bacterial bacillus. If you stain the *M. leprae* bacillus in the laboratory and then cover it with acid, it keeps the colour of the stain. (Most other organisms lose their colour.) *M. leprae* is therefore called an acid fast bacillus. This is shortened to AFB. (*M. tuberculosis* is also an AFB, see Chapter 14.)

M. leprae grows very slowly inside body cells. It likes to grow in skin and in nerve cells more than in other cells. It also likes to grow in cool areas of the body more than in warm areas of the body. It therefore grows best in cool areas of the skin and in nerves which are near the surface of the body. However, if there is not much body defence against the organism, *M. leprae* can grow in all organs of the body.

The body defends itself against *M. leprae*. It does this by its immune cells. (The body also makes antibodies against *M. leprae*; but these do not kill the organism or stop it growing.)

In most people, *the body has very powerful cellular immunity*. This destroys all the *M. leprae* organisms before any damage is done to the body. The infected person does not get the disease.

If the body has bad cellular immunity (or none), the *M. leprae* organisms grow and multiply and spread through all parts of the body and cause disease. This is called '*lepromatous leprosy*'.

If the body has good cellular immunity but not enough to kill all the M. leprae *organisms*, the body fights the organisms and keeps them in 1–3 places in the skin and/or in 1–3 of the nerves. But, the skin and nerves can be severely damaged in the fight. This is called '*tuberculoid leprosy*'.

There are also *people with intermediate cellular immunity, which is neither good nor bad*. They can get disease with features of both lepromatous and tuberculoid leprosy. The organisms grow and multiply, but the cellular immunity stops them spreading to all of the body. Disease occurs in many parts of the skin and many nerves. This is called '*borderline leprosy*'.

Table 15.1 shows the relationship between cellular immunity and the outcome of *M. leprae* infection.

Epidemiology

Organisms can only spread from patients with lepromatous and borderline leprosy. The organisms spread only from their upper respiratory tract secretions and lepromatous ulcers and ulcerated ENL lesions.

Spread is by direct or indirect contact; but probably mainly droplets from the respiratory tract.

Organisms spread to the respiratory mucous membrane or the skin of another person.

The incubation period is usually 2–4 years; but it can be shorter or very much longer at times.

All persons are susceptible; but children and males more commonly get the disease. However, most people (99%) infected with *M. leprae* organisms overcome the organisms and get no leprosy disease.

The world distribution of leprosy is shown in Figure 15.1 on page 78.

Table 15.1 *This table shows how the body's resistance (cellular immunity) to M. leprae organisms determines what happens after the body is infected with M. leprae.*

Body resistance to organism	None	Between none and good	Good but not quite normal	Normal
Number of M. leprae which grow in skin	Many	Many; but not as many as lepromatous; more than tuberculoid	Some but not many	None
Where M. leprae grow	Everywhere in all organs	In skin – in many areas / In nerves – in many areas	In skin – in 1–3 areas / In nerves – in 1–3 areas	Nowhere
Name of disease	Lepromatous (L) / (LL)	Borderline (B) / (BL) (BB)	Tuberculoid (T) / (BT) (TT)	No leprosy
Number of people in the population	Very few	A few	A few	Most
	Of the few (1%) of people infected with M. leprae who develop leprosy only 10–20% of these few (1%) develop this lepromatous type of leprosy	Of the few (1%) of the people infected with M. leprae who develop leprosy, most of these few (1%) develop this tuberculoid or borderline type of leprosy		Most of the people infected with M. leprae (99%) do not develop leprosy disease

Symptoms and signs

Leprosy causes:

1. Skin patches or infiltrations (see below).
2. Nerve enlargement and/or tenderness and/or loss of function (motor and/or sensory) (see page 81).
3. Anaesthesia (loss of sensation) of areas supplied by affected nerves. Injuries, burns, ulcers and destruction occur in anaesthetic areas.
   The parts affected are the hands and feet and eyes (see page 83).
4. Weakness, wasting, paralysis of muscles supplied by affected nerves. Deformities of affected areas can then occur.
   The parts affected are the hands and feet and eyes (see page 84).
5. Changes in other organs (only in lepromatous leprosy) – the eyes, upper respiratory tract, bones, muscles, joints, testes, etc. (see page 85).
6. 'Reactions' (see page 86).

Skin patches or infiltration

Look at all the skin of the body. Remove as many clothes as possible. Ask the patient to stand in good even natural light or sloping sunlight.

Look very carefully at the face. Examine especially the ears, eyebrows, forehead, cheeks and

Figure 15.1 The distribution of leprosy.
(Source: WHO Technical Report Series No. 716, 1985 (Report of a WHO Study Group on Epidemiology of Leprosy in Relation to Control))

nose for infiltration and nodules.

Look first for all lesions present. Find out their type (see below), number, size, if they are all the same, and if they are symmetrical (same number on both sides) or not symmetrical.

Next look at the individual lesions and find out what type they are. Find out if they are flat or raised, if the edges are definite or not definite, the appearance of the centre, the appearance of the surface, the colour, and if the lesion is anaesthetic.

Figure 15.2 Close up view of an early tuberculoid type skin lesion.

Figure 15.3 A typical large tuberculoid type skin lesion of the arm.

Figure 15.4 Well advanced lepromatous leprosy.

If: the lesions are 1–3 patches of any size, that are not all the same and are not symmetrical, *and*

if: the individual lesions are raised with a distinct edge, healing in the centre, dry, pale, without hair, and anaesthetic,

then: the patient has *tuberculoid type skin lesions*. (See Figures 15.2 and 15.3).

If: the skin lesions are very many (too many to count), small, all the same and symmetrical, *and*

if: the individual lesions are flat, without a clear, edge the same all over, shiny (red, not pale) and not anaesthetic,

then: the patient has *lepromatous type skin lesions* (*see Figure 15.4*).

If: there are no individual lesions and all the skin is affected, so that the skin of the whole body is thick with deep lines, folds and nodules, which are shiny and perhaps anaesthetic at the ends of the limbs,

then: the patient has *late lepromatous type skin changes*. See Figures 15.5, 15.6 and 15.7.

Figure 15.5 Late lepromatous leprosy.

Figure 15.6 Lepromatous leprosy with nodules on the ear. Nodules are more easily seen on the ear than other places. You can see nodules on the ear even more easily if you examine the patient from behind.

Figure 15.7 Late lepromatous leprosy. Swelling of all the skin of the body is often more easiy seen in the swelling of the fingers and hands, as in this patient.

If: the patient has many patches (but which still can be counted) and which are various sizes and which may or may not be symmetrical, *and*

if: the individual patches are different (some looking like tuberculoid patches and some looking like large lepromatous patches)

then: the patient has *borderline type skin changes* (see Figures 15.8 and 15.9).

Sometimes in borderline type skin changes the patches merge into normal skin and this normal skin merges into other patches. It is then difficult to see which is normal and which is abnormal skin, and the skin looks like a relief map in an atlas. These changes are characteristic of borderline leprosy.

Test any skin patches for loss of sensation (anaesthesia) with cotton wool or a pin (see Figure 15.10). First touch some normal skin with a piece of cotton wool when the patient has his eyes open. Ask the patient to put a finger on the same place as you touched. Then ask the patient to close his eyes. Touch normal skin again. Ask the patient to put a finger on the place you touched. Do this several times on normal skin with the patient's eyes closed until you are sure that he understands what to do. Then touch the skin in places where there may be loss of sensation as well as places where there is normal skin. If the patient does not put his finger on places you touch, then he feels nothing in these areas. He has anaesthesia in these

Figure 15.8   Borderline leprosy.

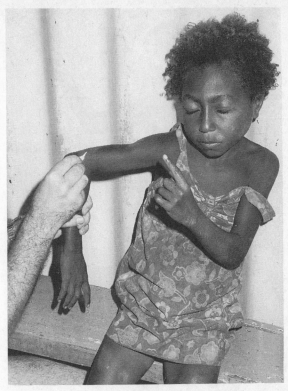

Figure 15.10   Testing for anaesthesia of a patch in the skin. (See text for description.) Compare with testing for anaesthesia in hands and feet. (See Figure 15.15.)

areas. Repeat this several times on places which appear to be anaesthetic. Check the opposite side of his body in the same places.

Nerve damage – enlargement and/or tenderness and/or loss of function

The important nerves most commonly affected by leprosy which can be palpated (felt) are the ulnar, median, radial, lateral popliteal and posterior tibial (see Figure 15.11).

Feel for enlargement or tenderness of the
- ulnar nerves at inside of elbows (Figure 15.12),
- posterior tibial nerves behind the inside of the ankle joints (Figure 15.13),
- lateral popliteal nerves at the outside of the knees (Figure 15.14).

Nerves in the skin near a patch may be enlarged.

Nerves going to the face and the eye may be affected; but these cannot be felt easily.

Figure 15.9   Borderline leprosy.

median

facial

ulnar

radial

lateral
popliteal

posterior
tibial

Figure 15.11 The position of nerves commonly
affected in leprosy and which can be felt to be
abnormal – enlarged or tender. The method of
examining the three most important areas are shown in
Figures 15.12, 15.13 and 15.14.

Figure 15.13 Method of palpating for tenderness
and/or enlargement of the posterior tibial nerve.

Figure 15.14 Method of palpation for tenderness
and/or enlargement of the lateral popliteal nerves.

Figure 15.12 Method of palpating for enlargement
and/or tenderness of the ulnar nerve.

Anaesthesia of areas supplied by affected nerves (hands, feet and eyes)

Ulnar nerve damage causes anaesthesia in the little finger and half of the next finger.

Median nerve damage causes anaesthesia in the rest of the hand.

Lateral popliteal nerve damage causes anaesthesia in the outside part of the leg.

Posterior tibial nerve damage causes anaesthesia underneath the foot.

Damage to the nerve going to the eye causes anaesthesia the cornea of the eye.

1. Test the hands feet and eyes for anaesthesia, (see Figure 15.15 and below).
2. Look and feel for burns, blisters, cuts, ulcers, swellings, hot areas, etc. on the hands and feet. These can be present in anaesthetic areas without patient noticing (see Figure 15.16).

Figure 15.16 Blister from burn due to loss of sensation.

Figure 15.17 Hand destroyed because of loss of sensation and lack of special care of the anaesthetic hand. The patient had trauma including burns, cuts, blisters, etc., as the patient has in Figure 15.16, but they did not hurt and as he did not know how to look after his hand, this is what happened.

Figure 15.18 Photograph of plantar ulcers (i.e. ulcers on the sole of the foot). These ulcers were caused by injuries (such as cuts and bruises) which the patient did not worry about or care for because there was no pain. If the patient had cared for his feet properly (see page 92), he need not have got these ulcers. If the ulcers had been treated properly they would have healed. The dressings used by the health worker for this patient were useless. For proper treatment of plantar ulcers see page 93. Note that these ulcers are NOT caused by the leprosy organisms in the ulcer. These ulcers are caused by nerve damage with loss of sensation under the foot.

Figure 15.15 Testing for anaesthesia in the hands and feet. Note the difference from testing for anaesthesia in a skin patch (see Figure 15.10). Gently but firmly touch the palms of the hands and soles of the feet with the tip of a pencil or a piece of wire. With his eyes closed, the patient must put a finger close to the place you have touched. If he puts his finger more than 2 cm away from the place you touched, he has lost enough sensation for him to severely damage this part of his body without knowing it.

3. Look for severe destruction of the hands or
   feet which can be caused by the anaesthesia and
   injuries which the patient does not notice because there is no pain (see Figures 15.17 and
   15.18).

Test for anaesthesia in the eye by getting the
patient to look upwards and towards his nose and
then touch the cornea with a small piece of cotton
wool from the side of his face. If the patient still
has sensation, the eye will blink.

Weakness, wasting or paralysis of muscles supplied by affected nerves

(hands, feet and eyes)

Ulnar damage causes a claw hand, affecting
mostly ring and little fingers. The patient cannot
straighten or bend these fingers properly (see
Figure 15.19).

Median damage causes claw hand of the
other fingers which the patient cannot bend or
straighten properly, and paralysis of thumb so
that the patient cannot pinch or lift it away from
the palm of the hand (see Figure 15.20).

Radial damage causes wrist drop or the wrist
cannot bend backwards (see Figure 15.21).

Lateral popliteal damage causes foot drop or
the foot cannot bend up at the ankle (see Figure
15.22).

Posterior tibial damage causes paralysis of
small muscles of the foot, and claw toes.

Facial damage causes paralysis of eyelid – the

Figure 15.20   Testing for weakness of one of the
muscles supplied by the median nerve.

Figure 15.21   Testing for weakness of muscles
supplied by radial nerve.

Figure 15.19   Testing for weakness of one of the
muscles supplied by the ulnar nerve.

Figure 15.22   Testing for weakness of muscles
supplied by the lateral popliteal nerve.

patient cannot close his eye properly (lagopthalmos) (see Figure 15.23).

A quick test for paralysis of hand muscles is as follows (see also Figure 15.24):

1. Ask the patient to hold his hand like the hand on the left of Figure 15.24 (wrist up, fingers straight but bent to 90° where they join the palm, and thumb across the palm).
2. Look for clawing of little and ring fingers (both of patient's hands) from ulnar weakness.
3. Look for clawing of other fingers (patient's left hand) for median weakness.
4. Look for wrist drop (not present) from radial weakness.
5. Check if the thumb cannot go across the palm (not present) from median weakness.

Later effects

Fixed deformities occur later in the disease if treatment is not successful. The joints become stiff in the position in which they are paralysed and cannot be straightened even with another hand helping.

Damage of other organs only in lepromatous leprosy

Nose – swollen mucous membrane causes blocked up nose which can bleed. Later, the bone collapses and the nose becomes flat.

Figure 15.23 Bilateral lagopthalmos. The patient is trying to close both eyes. The eyes turn upwards, but the eyelids will not close.

Figure 15.24 A quick test for paralysis of the hand (see text).

Bones of hands and feet – these become weak and easily crushed, and the fingers and toes, etc. become shorter.

Testes – these become smaller, and sterility and gynaecomastia (swollen breasts) develop.

Eyes – iritis with loss of vision can occur (see Chapter 31 page 343).

'Reactions'

There are two types of reaction. It is not important to remember which one is which; however it is important to recognise that a reaction is occurring.

Type I reaction occurs in borderline leprosy and affects the nerves and the parts of the skin that are already affected by leprosy. The edges of the skin patches may become swollen, painful and tender. More seriously, the affected nerves may become swollen, painful and tender. There may be a sudden loss of sensation. There may be sudden paralysis.

Figure 15.25 Leprosy reaction with ENL. ENL are inflamed tender nodules, most common on the front of the legs and the backs of the arms and on the face.

Type II reactions occur in lepromatous leprosy. Small, painful lumps called erythema nodosum leprosum (ENL), may develop in the skin so this reaction is often called an ENL reaction. There may be also acute inflammation of any of the organs involved in lepromatous leprosy. Especially important are acute iritis (painful red eye with some loss of sight), acute orchitis (painful swelling of a testis or both testes) or painful swelling of nerves with sudden loss of sensation or paralysis.

If a reaction occurs there may also be general symptoms and signs of inflammation – fever, fast pulse etc.

Classification of types of leprosy

Lepromatous, tuberculoid and borderline leprosy are the three main types of leprosy.

But leprosy can be divided into six types:
1. indeterminate,
2. tuberculoid,
3. borderline,
4. lepromatous,
5. neural, and
6. clinically dapsone resistant leprosy.

Indeterminate leprosy

Indeterminate leprosy may occur soon after the leprosy organisms have entered the body and started to grow, but before it has been decided if the body's defences or the organisms will win the fight.

One (or a few) flat (or slightly raised), indistinct, slightly pale, sometimes slightly anaesthetic patch in the skin may be found. Skin smears (see page 87) may show a few AFB, but may be negative.

Unless the smear is positive for AFB, do not diagnose indeterminate leprosy. Either biopsy the lesion (see page 90) (*but* do *not* biopsy a lesion on the face), or see the patient each 6–12 weeks until either the lesion goes away, or the lesion is obviously leprosy, or the lesion is examined by a medical officer. Many people with a diagnosis of 'indeterminate leprosy' do not have leprosy at all.

Tuberculoid, borderline and lepromatous leprosy

See Table 15.2.

Neural leprosy

Some cases only involve nerves and have no skin lesions.

Some cases may have had skin lesions which healed, and only nerve changes remain.

These are both called 'neural' leprosy, or, if many nerves are involved, 'polyneuritic' leprosy.

Dapsone resistant leprosy

See page 96.

Tests

Skin smear for BI and MI

Do a skin smear in all cases of suspected leprosy – especially lepromatous or borderline leprosy.

How to make a skin smear

Take smears from the ear lobes, the eyebrows and any suspicious skin lesions. Pinch the skin firmly between your thumb and forefinger so that it cannot bleed. With a sharp scalpel, make a slit in the skin 2–3 mm deep and 5 mm long. Then scrape the tissues from the bottom of the wound with the point of the scalpel blade. Use the material on the scalpel blade to make the slide. Warm the slide over a flame until it is just too hot to hold on the back of the hand.

Pack the slide where no insects can reach it, and send it to the laboratory with a request form asking for examination for AFB, including both BI and MI (see Figure 15.26).

Bacillary Index (BI) tells how many *M. leprae* organisms there are in the slide. The Bacillary Index is high (e.g. BI 6+) in lepromatous cases. Some bacilli may be seen in borderline cases (e.g. BI 1–4+). No bacilli are seen in tuberculoid cases (BI negative or 0). If originally high, the BI takes years to become negative, even during successful treatment.

Morphological index (MI) tells the percentage of the *M. leprae* organisms that are seen which are morphologically normal (or solid staining or in one piece). The morphological index therefore shows what percentage of organisms are alive. Before treatment MI may be up to 60%. (It is never much more than 60% and never 100%.) MI should fall to 0% after 6 months of successful treatment. The MI should stay at 0% if treatment is effective.

Repeat the smear (for MI and BI) each 3 months (e.g. 1st week of each January, April, July and October), if the original smear was positive.

Diagram 1.

Pick up a fold of skin and squeeze it tightly between thumb and first finger.

Diagram 2.

A small slit is made in the skin fold. (Use a sterile scalpel - keep squeezing the skin tightly so it cannot bleed.)

Diagram 3.

The base of the skin slit is scraped with the tip of the scalpel. (Keep squeezing the skin fold to prevent bleeding.)

Diagram 4.

Place the smear from the patient onto a properly labelled glass slide.

Diagram 5.

	1	2	3
NAME or number DATE			
	4	5	6

e.g. 1. right ear
2. left ear
3. right eyebrow
4. left eyebrow
5. whatever site
6. whatever site

This is how to label and place the patient's smears on the slide. Use a diamond pencil or sticking plaster to label. Do NOT use pencils or paper labels which can rub off. The arrow is to show where you start numbering the smears. Place the smears ON THE SAME SIDE of the glass as the LABELLING. On the requisition slip - use the same numbering as shown in the diagram. Give the actual site from which each smear came.

match sticks

rubber band

Slides can be packed in pairs like this. The smears must face inwards.

Figure 15.26   Diagrams 1–6 show how to make skin smears for AFB (see text).

Table 15.2 Main features of the main three types of leprosy

	Type of leprosy			
	Tuberculoid (TT) Type	Borderline (BB) Group	Lepromatous – early (LL) Type	Lepromatous – late (LL) Type
1. Skin				
(a) lesions				
– type	patches	patches	patches	the patches join; all the skin is affected
– number	1–3	many – but can be counted	many – cannot be counted	
– size	small or large	vary	small	
– all the same	no	no	yes	
– symmetrical (i.e. same both sides)	no	sometimes	yes	
(b) individual lesions				
– flat or raised	raised at edge	some flat; some raised	flat	the skin is all thickened with folds and nodules
– edge distinct or indistinct	distinct	some distinct; some indistinct	indistinct	
– appearance of centre	healing and scarring	some healing; some not	all the same	
– appearance of surface	no sweating; no hair	some normal; some not sweating; no hair	sweating; hair	
– colour	pale at edge	some pale; some shiny	shiny (red) not pale	shiny (red) not pale
– anaesthesia	anaesthetic	some anaesthetic but not complete	no anaesthesia	anaesthesia
2. Nerves				
Cutaneous (skin) (sensory)	only nerves going to a patch	nerves going to patches	hands and feet both sides	much of arms and legs both sides
Peripheral and cranial number	1–3	many	none or all	all
Symmetrical (i.e. same both sides)	no	sometimes	yes	yes
swollen	yes (very)	yes	only a little	yes
tender	no	no; yes if in reaction	no; yes if in reaction	no; yes if in reaction

Table 15.2 Continued

	Type of leprosy			
	Tuberculoid (TT) Type	Borderline (BB) Group	Lepromatous – early (LL) Type	Lepromatous – late (LL) Type
3. Anaesthesia of area supplied by affected nerves	yes (usually)	yes	no	yes
4. Paralysis and wasting of muscles supplied by affected nerves	yes (usually)	yes	no	yes
5. Other organs affected				
(a) mucous membranes of URT	no	not marked	yes	yes
(b) bones	no	not marked	yes	yes
(c) muscles	no	not marked	yes	yes
(d) testes	no	not marked	yes	yes
(e) general symptoms and signs	no	not marked	yes, especially if reaction	yes, especially if reaction
6. Reactions	no	yes (Type 1)	yes (Type 2)	yes (Type 2)

Skin biopsy

Do a skin biopsy if the diagnosis of tuberculoid or borderline leprosy is not certain.

Take a skin biopsy from the edge of the patch. The bigger the biopsy the better the report can be; but an oval piece of skin about 1 cm in length is enough. Infiltrate the area with local anaesthetic. Mark a narrow oval of skin 1 cm in length to be cut out. With a sharp scalpel cut along the mark you have made, down to the *fat* under the skin. Lift the biopsy up by the fat underneath the skin *very carefully* (with the smallest forceps you have), and cut through the fat to remove the skin biopsy. Do not squeeze the skin with the forceps because this will make it difficult to examine under the microscope. Drop the biopsy into 20–30 ml fixative solution or formal-saline. Stitch up the skin. For best results, ask your laboratory to send you Ridleys FMA for fixative solution. Leave the biopsy in this solution for 2 hours; then rinse it with water and put it in 70% alcohol. If you do not have this special fixative, use formalin and leave the specimen in the formalin.

Course and complications

Indeterminate leprosy cures itself without treatment in 3 out of 4 cases. Treatment will cure the other types.

Tuberculoid leprosy will often cure itself without treatment. But before this happens, severe nerve damage can occur. Treatment will kill the infection and soon stop more nerve damage occurring.

Lepromatous leprosy never cures itself but becomes worse. Reactions are common. Many organs are damaged. Treatment can cure the infection. After some years of regular correct treatment, reactions become less common and then stop.

Without treatment, borderline leprosy will later become like either tuberculoid or lepromatous leprosy. Meanwhile severe nerve damage occurs. Treatment can cure the infection and after some years the reactions will stop.

When the infection is stopped and the *M. leprae* all killed, damaged nerves and other organs cannot recover. But, further damage can be stopped by proper treatment. Proper treatment before much damage occurs is the most important thing.

Treatment

The most important things in the treatment of the patient are:
1. Give dapsone[1] *regularly for at least five years* to patients with tuberculoid leprosy and *regularly for life* to patients with lepromatous or borderline leprosy.
2. Give a second drug e.g. clofazimine with the dapsone at the start treatment to patients with lepromatous or borderline leprosy.
3. Give the patient education about:
   (a) the need for regular treatment for many years or for life,
   (b) the care of hands/feet/eyes if these are anaesthetic, and
   (c) the need for quick and proper treatment of reactions, for when reactions later occur.

Do not start treatment unless:
1. the diagnosis is certain because of typical symptoms and signs, or
2. the diagnosis was not certain but is now confirmed by a test (skin smear or biopsy).

If the diagnosis is not certain:
1. do a skin smear for AFB if you suspect lepromatous or borderline leprosy;
2. do a skin biopsy if you suspect tuberculoid or borderline leprosy;
3. if a biopsy is not possible, then, review the patient each 6–12 weeks instead;
4. wait for the results before starting treatment.

Always do a full medical history and physical examination and test the urine. Diagnose and treat any other conditions you find, especially anaemia or tuberculosis.

---

1 A new drug called rifampicin is now available which will kill most of the *M. leprae* organisms in the body very quickly. This will make the patient non infectious more quickly. But as it does not quickly kill *all* the *M. leprae* organisms in the body, it does not *cure* the patient quickly. Rifampicin is given together with dapsone. After rifampicin is given together with dapsone to patients with lepromatous or borderline leprosy, the patient must continue to take dapsone for life. Rifampicin is very expensive and it has serious side effects. The use of it is not possible in most developing countries at present. There are also other drugs which are effective against *M. leprae* organisms.

Treatment of the patient only is not the proper management of a case of leprosy. Remember the other things needed in the management of the patient. (See box below.)

Details of an effective and cheap regimen for management of patients with leprosy. This regimen is used in Papua New Guinea. If there is a different policy in your area, change the necessary details. The basic plan in all effective management policies will be the same as this regimen.

Management includes 9 things:
1. Register patient. Fill in index and treatment cards. Arrange treatment and patient follow-up. Arrange contact tracing.
2. Give dapsone and, if necessary, clofazimine.
3. Treat reactions quickly and effectively.
4. Educate about the care of anaesthetic hands/feet/eyes and the use of footwear.
5. Physiotherapy for weak, paralysed or deformed hands/feet/eyes.
6. Plaster of paris casts, footwear, etc. for plantar ulcers.
7. Arrange surgery if necessary.
8. Check that the infection is controlled by drugs.
9. Transfer to Medical Officer care if necessary.

Do all necessary administrative procedures

1. Confirm the diagnosis (if the diagnosis was made by another health worker).
2. Register the patient in the register book and give him a number from the register.
3. Fill in details on the index card. Put the card in the index card file.
4. Fill in details of the treatment plan on the treatment card. Send the card to the treatment centre with the patient.
5. Start patient education and family education.
6. Arrange contact education and examination.
7. Arrange for a skin smear for BI and MI of AFB immediately, and then (if positive) every 3 months (e.g. 1st week of January, April, July, September) until MI = 0: then every year.

8. Check smear results and attendances on the treatment charts every 3 months (e.g. 1st week of February, May, August, November). Write the results on the index cards.
9. Notify the Health Department in the monthly report. (The Leprosy Report form is filled in from the index file every month.)

Give antileprosy drugs

Give education to the patient about the importance of regular treatment for many years or for life if he has lepromatous leprosy.

Commence short-term intensive ('A') treatment.

Give dapsone 100 mg (2 tabs) every day for 12 weeks to *all* patients.

Give clofazimine 100 mg (1 cap) every day for 12 weeks to *all* borderline and lepromatous cases (i.e. all cases with smears positive for AFB). (It is not necessary to give clofazimine to tuberculoid cases.)

Patients should be admitted as inpatients for the first month, for education and for observation for drug side effects (fever, skin rash and/or jaundice).

After 12 weeks give *either*:

Dapsone fully-supervised twice weekly outpatient ('B') treatment – 300 mg dapsone (6 tabs) twice weekly taken by the patient at the treatment centre each Monday and Thursday, *or*:

Dapsone home ('C') treatment – 100 mg dapsone (2 tabs) taken every day by the patient at home. The patient collects 56 tablets from the treatment centre each 4 weeks and takes 2 tabs every day.

Continue dapsone – until it is stopped by the medical officer (5 years after the last sign of activity for tuberculoid patients but never for lepromatous patients).

Visit – all patients who do not come for treatment (see the rules for 'defaulter action'). The treatment centre worker visits if the patient misses one week of treatment. The OIC of the supervising centre visits if the patient misses one month of treatment.

Notify the OIC of the Leprosy Control Unit at the Provincial or District Health Office if the patient does not have his treatment for three months.

Treat any reaction

Give health education to the patient about the symptoms and signs of reaction. Tell him that he should immediately report to the health worker if he gets any of these symptoms or signs: lumps in the skin; swelling of skin patches; nerve pain; sudden paralysis; sudden loss of sensation; painful eyes; any loss of sight; painful and swollen testis.

Treat reactions as follows:

1. Treat anything which may have caused the reaction (e.g. illness, accident, anxiety, etc.).
2. Make the patient rest in bed if possible. Support any affected part in a sling or a well padded splint.
3. Continue the full dose of dapsone; 100 mg (2 tabs) everyday.
4. Aspirin 900–1200 mg (3–4 tabs) four times a day until reaction stops, or for 3 weeks.
5. Chloroquine:
   450 mg (3 tabs) every day for 1 week, then
   300 mg (2 tabs) every day for 1 week, then
   150 mg (1 tab) every day for 1 week.
6. If the reaction is a Type 2 reaction (that is, reaction with ENL) and if the reaction does not quickly improve with the above treatment give clofazimine:
   • 300 mg daily (1 cap three times a day) until it stops, then
   • 200 mg daily (1 cap twice a day) for 1 month, then
   • 100 mg daily (1 cap once a day) for 1 month, then
   • 100 mg (1 cap) three times a week for 1 month then stop treatment.
   Do not give clofazimine for a Type 1 reaction (i.e. reaction without ENL).
7. Transfer any cases as recommended on page 96.

If the patient has anaesthetic hands or feet or eyes, give education about their care and supply protective footwear

Give a copy of a suitable booklet in the patient's own language for him to read.

Special care for anaesthetic hands includes:
1. Soak in water every day.
2. Precautions to stop burns.
3. Precautions to stop injuries.

4. Every night and morning look at both sides of the hands for burns or injuries, and feel for hot areas.
5. Wash, dress and splint any burn or injury.
6. Get medical treatment if the burn or injury does not improve quickly (dressings, splint, antibiotics, etc.).

Special care for anaesthetic feet includes:
1. Soak in water every day.
2. Always wear footwear to stop injuries or burns from the outside.
3. No running, jumping, long steps, long walks, etc. to prevent injuries to the foot from the inside.
4. Every night and morning: look for lumps, wounds or ulcers; feel for hot areas; feel for deep tenderness.
5. Wash and dress any injury and do not use the foot until it is better, (i.e. go to bed or use a crutch or stick).
6. Ask for medical treatment if the injury does not improve quickly (usually a plaster of Paris (POP) cast is necessary).

Special care for anaesthetic eyes includes:
1. Look at the eye every night and morning.
2. If the eye becomes red, ask for medical help (i.e. to remove any foreign body (not felt by the patient) to treat any infection to treat any reaction if necessary).

If the patient has weakness or paralysis or deformity of hands, feet or eyes, start physiotherapy

1. Any recent paralysis is probably caused by a reaction. Transfer the patient for special drugs, special plasters and special exercises.
2. Any foot drop which has started in the last 6 months is also treated as a reaction. Transfer for treatment with special plasters and special drugs.
3. In other cases, ask the patient to do the special exercises.

Treat any plantar ulcer with a plaster of Paris (POP) cast and footwear

> These ulcers are not caused by leprosy organisms in the ulcerated areas. These ulcers do not happen without a definite cause. These ulcers are always caused by an injury or pressure on part of the foot.

Because of anaesthesia, the patient does not feel the cause of injury. So he does nothing about this cause. The injury becomes worse and worse. Even when he does know of the injury he continues to walk on the foot. This makes the damage worse and stops healing. (A person with normal sensation would have too much pain to walk.)

Abnormal positions of parts of the feet due to muscle weakness or deformity cause a lot of pressure on some areas of the foot. This can damage the skin and other tissues in this area, and ulcers then form.

Secondary bacterial infection usually occurs and makes the ulcer worse.

Note that the ulcer is *not* caused by leprosy organisms or bacterial infection but *is* caused by anaesthesia and injury.

It is important that you tell the patient how to prevent ulcers. Treatment for ulcers includes the following:

If there is secondary bacterial infection

(i.e. if the foot is hot, red, swollen, etc. or pus is discharged from the ulcer).

1. Rest the foot:
   - Rest in bed with the foot higher than the rest of the bed.
   - Use crutches to walk (to toilet, etc.).
   - The foot must *not* be put on the ground.
   This is the most important part of the treatment.
2. Antibiotics – give penicillin at first; give tetracycline if penicillin is not effective.
3. Use dressings with Eusol.
4. Cut away any thick dead skin. Do not cut any living tissue (which will bleed).
   Do not cut out bone from inside the ulcer. Remove *loose* pieces of bone with forceps.

Prepare suitable footwear (before POP applied)

1. If the foot is not deformed, get a sandal or shoe of the patient's size. Get a soft rubber insole and stick it inside the sandal or shoe.
2. If the patient's foot is deformed, take a POP cast of the foot. Send the cast to the leprosy shoe workshop. They will make a suitable shoe with an insole shaped to fit the patient's foot and send it back to you.

When infection is controlled

1. Apply a below knee POP cast (see Figure 15.27).
2. When the cast is dry apply a wooden rocker or walking iron to the POP (see Figure 15.28).
3. The patient can then walk on the POP.

Figure 15.27 A below-knee plaster of Paris cast fitted with a 'home made' walking rocker made out of scrap wood and an old car tyre. The whole job was done by an orderly, and although it was not perfect, the ulcer was completely healed in 6 weeks.

the width of the plaster of Paris cast

a little less than the length of the foot.

Figure 15.28 Diagram of a simple rocker: (A) from underneath; (B) from the side. The main part or platform is made from 3 or 5 ply or a piece of wood such as the top of a packing case. The rockers are made of 2 pieces of wood nailed on across the whole width of the platform. Underneath these, rubber cut from an old car tyre is nailed on. Apply the below-knee POP one day and do not let the patient walk on it. The next day make the botton of the cast flat with POP and then plaster the rocker on with a POP bandage. Do not allow the patient to walk on it until the next day.

4. The patient may be kept in the health centre or discharged and checked every week, to make sure the POP is not damaged.
5. Remove the POP (and apply a new one) if there is pain under the POP or any other suspicion of pressure.
6. After 6 weeks remove the POP cast. In most cases the ulcer will be healed. If it is not healed remove any dead hard skin, treat any infection, and then re-apply a POP cast.

After removing the POP cast (when the ulcer is healed)

1. Immediately tell the patient to put his new shoes on.
2. The patient must *always* wear these shoes. He must never walk anywhere without these shoes.
3. Allow the patient to walk only a little the first day and then a little more every day. After 3–6 weeks he can walk normal distances.
4. Get new shoes for the patient before the old ones wear out. Do not allow anyone to repair the shoes with nails or wire. These could damage the patient's foot.

Surgery

If physiotherapy is not successful, surgery may help. Cases which surgery may help include patients with:
1. completely wasted hand muscles;
2. foot drop for more than 6 months;
3. lagopthalmos for more than 6 months.

Check that the *infection* is controlled by drugs

Look for signs of drug resistance.
Do smears for BI and MI every 3 months on borderline or lepromatous patients.
Do clinical examination at least every 12 months.

Patients likely to develop dapsone resistant leprosy include:
1. patients who have lepromatous leprosy,
2. patients who have had dapsone for many years,
3. patients who have had only dapsone (and no other antileprosy drug),
4. patients who have had only small doses of dapsone,
5. patients who have had irregular dapsone, either because they were unreliable or because it was reduced during repeated reactions.

Signs of dapsone resistant leprosy include:
1. A mixture of old and new lesions.
   There may be the wrinkled ears and resolving nodules etc. of treated leprosy.
   There are *also* new lesions, especially nodules.
2. Some of the new lesions may not be typical.
   Nodules are often in unusual places, e.g. on the eyes, abdomen, front of elbows, etc.
   Lesions may not be symmetrical.
   Some lesions may be large and raised.
3. The new lesions will have a high BI and MI when the rest of the body and old lesions have a much lower or negative BI and MI.
4. The MI of the new lesions will not fall to 0 after 6 months of daily supervised high dose dapsone treatment (100 mg daily).

Make sure the nodules are not just one of the following:
1. ENL nodules. These are usually tender and come and go over a few weeks.
2. Recurrence of leprosy because the patient has stopped taking his drugs.

Figure 15.29 Dapsone resistant leprosy (DRL). A close-up photograph of new nodules in a patient, who also has signs of old treated lepromatous leprosy. The nodules are on the front of an elbow. The other elbow was not affected. The lesions are raised and some have a sunken central part. The lesions had a BI of 5 and an MI of 50% whereas the smear from the ears had a BI of 1 and an MI of 0.

Patients with suspected dapsone resistance should be treated with supervised dapsone 100 mg daily or 300 mg twice weekly.

If they do not greatly improve in 3–6 months and the MI does not fall to 0 (the BI will not change in 6 months) they must be transferred to medical officer care for special tests and treatment.

Do not give patients with suspected dapsone resistant leprosy clofazimine. (They must be treated with *2 new* antileprosy drugs together.)

Control and prevention

Kill the organism in the body of the original host or reservoir

Discover and treat all the infectious (lepromatous and borderline) cases. When they start treatment, leprosy patients become non-infectious almost immediately and cannot spread the disease.

How to find cases of leprosy:

1. Contact education and examination.
   You should see all contacts (family, those who live in the same house, friends, workmates, schoolmates, etc.) and educate them about the symptoms of leprosy and tell them it can be cured. You should then examine and test them all. You should tell them to come to the health centre if symptoms develop later. All contacts of lepromatous patients should be examined every year for 5 years.
2. You should educate and examine special groups during other health examinations – especially school children.
3. You should educate the general public.
4. You should arrange surveys in areas of known or suspected high prevalence of leprosy. (Whole population surveys are not usually as useful as using your available resources or (1) and (2).)

Stop the means of spread of the organism

This is not possible and is not worth trying.

Isolation of cases is not possible and should not be tried.

Improvement in housing and living standards and general public health will do far more to stop the spread of leprosy than any special rules for leprosy patients (if the patients take their antileprosy drugs).

Raise the resistance of susceptible persons

1. The resistance to leprosy of the general population is raised by: better nutrition, better housing, the treatment of other diseases, and general public health methods.
2. The resistance of individual persons in some groups of people in some countries is raised by BCG immunisation.
3. It is hoped that specific immunisation against leprosy will soon be developed and be available.

Prophylactic treatment

This is not given (except in very unusual circumstances in infants).

Transfer

Transfer to Medical Officer care the following cases:

1. All *new* cases who before treatment is started, have:
   - (a) reaction and/or
   - (b) tender nerves.
2. All cases with a *reaction* which
   - (a) involves vital body parts (especially the nerves or eyes), or
   - (b) is severe, or
   - (c) does not stop with treatment.

   These include patients who have:
   - tender nerves,
   - acute paralysis or loss of sensation,
   - acute orchitis (painful, swollen testis),
   - iritis (eye red or painful, or sight becoming worse),
   - severe general signs and symptoms,
   - reaction which does not stop after 3 weeks of treatment, or
   - reaction which returns after reaction treatment has stopped.
3. Any *new* patient who may have *drug resistant organisms* – These include:
   - (a) A patient who is not clinically improving or whose smear is not improving (MI does not fall to 0 and then stay at 0) after 6–12 months of proper supervised treatment.
   - (b) A patient whose infection or smear gets worse after early improvement after 6–12 months of proper supervised treatment.
4. Any *old* patient on dapsone treatment alone (or on and off dapsone) who may have *dapsone resistant leprosy*. These may include those who have *both*:
   - positive smears (MI more than 0 at any time or BI still positive after 5 years), or
   - clinical signs of dapsone resistant disease, or
   - smear signs of dapsone resistant disease (new nodules with high BI and MI while other places in the body have negative or low BI);

   and also do not improve after supervised dapsone treatment every day for 6 months (clinical signs do not improve and MI does not become 0).

   Do not start these patients on clofazimine before transfer.

Refer to visiting Medical Officer:
1. any case with complications especially paralysis or deformity, for advice and assessment for surgery,
2. any case in 'Transfer' 3 or 4 (see above) if a medical officer visits.

16

Some Common Infectious Diseases

Figure 16.1 A close-up photograph of the measles skin rash. The rash is often very hard to see on a dark skin.

This chapter covers some acute specific infectious diseases which cause fever and occur everywhere

Measles (morbilli)

Measles is a common, very infectious disease. It usually affects children but can affect adults. It is endemic, but small epidemics occur. The cause is the measles virus.

Spread is from the respiratory tract of an infectious patient by direct contract or by droplets.

The incubation period is of medium length (1–2 weeks).

The pattern of the disease is as follows.

1. At first the symptoms and signs of a quite severe viral-type upper respiratory tract infection (URTI) and conjunctivitis with fever develop. This lasts for about a week.
2. Then Koplik spots appear in the mouth. The Koplik spots are like white grains of salt on the red mucous membrane, usually on the inner side of the cheek. If you see Koplik spots, the disease is not a usual URTI, but measles.
3. After about 4 days, the typical measles rash comes (See Figure 16.1). There are many slightly red and raised patches of various sizes on the skin. These start on the face and shoulders and then spread to the rest of the body. The other symptoms improve as the rash appears.
4. Secondary bacterial infection of the respiratory tract often occurs, especially otitis media and pneumonia. This usually happens when the rash is improving.

Treatment of measles itself is symptomatic only – rest, aspirin, and antimalarials (if in a malarious area).

Treatment of secondary bacterial complications is with antibiotics.

If otitis media occurs see Chapter 20 page 157. If pneumonia occurs see Chapter 20 page 164. If gastroenteritis occurs see Chapter 23 page 220.

> If the patient is a child see a textbook on children's diseases.

Immunisation is possible with a live virus vaccine.

German measles (rubella)

Rubella is not a commonly diagnosed disease. It usually affects children and young adults.

It is endemic but small epidemics occur. The cause is the rubella virus.

Spread is by direct contact or by droplets from the respiratory tract of adult patients, or by any discharge from an infant with congenital infection.

The incubation period is of medium length (2–3 weeks).

The patient is infectious from 1 week before the rash appears until 4 days after it appears.

The symptoms and signs are usually mild – mild fever, etc. then a rash like mild measles and enlarged lymph nodes behind the neck.

Treatment is symptomatic only.

The disease is important only because pregnant women infected in the first 4 months of pregnancy may have deformed babies.

Patients with rubella should not be allowed to come into any type of direct or indirect contact with pregnant women. Infectious patients include normal child or adult patients and babies born with the disease.

Young girls should try to have the disease before the age when they may become pregnant.

Immunisation is possible with a live virus vaccine.

Chicken pox (varicella)

Chickenpox is a common infectious disease. It usually affects children, but can also affect adults. The cause is the chickenpox virus.

It is endemic, but small epidemics occur. Spread is by direct contact and by droplets from the respiratory tract of infectious patients (but not from the crusts of the sores). The incubation period is of medium length (2–3 weeks). The patient is infectious from the day before the rash appears until 1 week after it appears.

The disease causes:

1. Mild general symptoms and signs of infection (fever, malaise, etc.).
2. A typical rash (see Figure 16.2):
   • macules, papules, vesicles, pustules and crusts (see Figure 32.2),
   • mostly on the trunk and face,
   • with new lesions appearing from time to time (so that at any one time in any one place there are lesions at different stages).

In adults a severe chickenpox virus pneumonia sometimes occurs.

Treatment is symptomatic only, with aspirin and calamine lotion and antimalarials (if in a malarious area). If the skin lesions become

Figure 16.2 Photographs of a patient affected by chickenpox at about the end of the first week. Note that the lesions are at different stages.

infected by bacteria, give antibiotics by injection or by mouth and skin preparations (see Chapter 32 page 350).

If pneumonia occurs see Chapter 20 page 165.

> If the patient is a child, see a textbook on children's diseases

Herpes zoster

Herpes zoster (shingles) is caused by a re-infection with the chickenpox virus in someone who has had chickenpox before.

A rash like the chickenpox rash appears (see Figure 16.2 and Figure 16.4) *but*
- it is in the area of skin supplied by only one nerve (see Figure 16.3),
- it is usually on only one side of the body,
- it stops exatly at the midline of the body,
- it usually appears on the trunk or the face,
- there is severe pain in the affected area often before the rash appears, as well as during the rash, and sometimes for months or years after the rash goes.

Management is as for chickenpox, but powerful drugs, including pethidine, may be needed to

control pain at first. If the eye is affected, put chloramphenicol ointment into the eye every 3 hours, keep the eye covered and transfer the patient urgently to medical officer care.

Other viral diseases with skin rash

The diseases described so far have:
1. fever and other generalised symptoms and signs of infection,
2. skin rash – which is typical of the disease, and
3. other complications.

There are many other viral diseases which are similar, except that the rash is not typical of only one disease. These viral infections cannot therefore be identified by most health workers, but this does not matter.

If the patient is not very 'sick', treat only the patient's symptoms and give antimalarials (if in a malarious area – see Chapter 36 page 397).

If the patient is very 'sick' treat him for septicaemia and malaria (see Chapter 12). If he does not improve, transfer him to medical officer care. If complications such as encephalitis occur, transfer the patient to medical officer care.

Figure 16.4 Herpes zoster of the right side of the face. Note that the lesions stop exactly at the midline. Note that the eye is affected and the patient therefore needs urgent treatment and transfer to medical officer care.

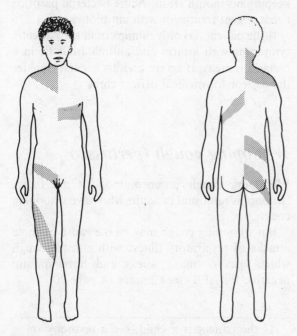

Figure 16.3 Diagram to show some of the possible distributions of the herpes zoster rash.

Mumps

Mumps is a common disease which usually affects children. It is not very infectious, so not all children get it. Many adults are therefore not immune to mumps and so it can also affect adults. The cause is the mumps virus.

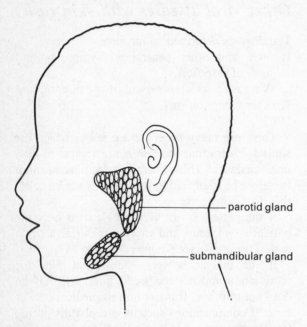

Figure 16.5 Diagram to show the anatomical position of the parotid and submandibular salivary glands.

Figure 16.6 Mumps. The child on the left has parotitis with swelling in front of and below his left ear – in the position of the parotid gland (see Figure 16.5).

Spread is from an infected patient from the respiratory tract and mouth by direct contact and by droplets. The incubation period is of medium length (2–3 weeks). The patient is infectious from a week before the salivary gland swelling appears until all the swelling goes. One attack gives immunity against mumps for life.

The disease causes the following:
1. mild general symptoms and signs of infection,
2. painful, tender swelling of one parotid gland, which lasts for about a week (see Figures 16.5 and 16.6),
3. often painful, tender swelling of the other parotid gland as the first one improves.

Complications include:
1. acute orchitis (painful tender swelling of one or both of the testes) – common in adults;
2. acute pancreatitis with upper abdominal pain and vomiting;
3. viral meningitis and/or encephalitis (see Chapter 25 page 260).

Make sure the patient does not have acute bacterial parotitis. This is an acute severe inflammation of the parotid gland with severe pain, severe tenderness and a lot of swelling as well as fever. It usually occurs in someone who is already sick and not drinking much and not keeping his mouth clean. Acute bacterial parotitis needs urgent treatment with antibiotics.

If the patient has only mumps treat the patient's symptoms with aspirin and antimalarials (if in a malarious area). If severe orchitis occurs, transfer the patient for medical officer care.

Whooping cough (pertussis)

Whooping cough is uncommon in adults. A 'whoop' is not usual in adults who have whooping cough.

But whooping cough may be the cause of some attacks of respiratory illness with chronic cough which last for many weeks and have sputum negative for AFB (see Chapter 14 page 70).

If the patient is a child, see a textbook on children's diseases

100

17

Acute Infectious Diseases with Limited Distribution

This chapter is about some acute specific diseases which cause fever but which occur only in certain parts of the world:

1. Bacterial infections
   - Relapsing fever
   - Leptospirosis
   - Bartonellosis
   - Plague

2. Rickettsial infections
   - Typhus fevers

3. Virus infections
   - Dengue fever
   - Sandfly fever
   - Yellow fever
   - Viral infections spread by insects from infected animals or men which are related to dengue fever and yellow fever and can cause 'Haemorrhagic fever'.
   - Viral infections spread by direct contact from infected people (and possibly infected rats) which can cause 'Haemorrhagic fever'.

Find out which of these diseases occur in your area. If any of these diseases do not occur in your area, do not learn about those diseases.

See Chapter 36, page 395 for diagnosis and management of a patient who has a fever and you are not sure of the cause of the fever.

Relapsing fever

Relapsing fever is an acute bacterial infection which causes repeated attacks of acute severe fever and damage to the blood, blood vessels, liver, spleen, eyes, nervous system and heart.

There are two types of relapsing fever. One type is caused by a bacterium which normally lives in small animals and is spread by ticks. This is called endemic tick-borne relapsing fever. The other type is due to a bacterium which normally lives in man and is spread by lice. This is called a epidemic louse-borne relapsing fever. The two diseases are clinically similar but the epidemic louse-borne type is the more severe.

Endemic tick-borne relapsing fever

There are many areas where this disease occurs. Find out if it occurs in your area.

The bacteria which cause endemic relapsing fever normally live in small animals (such as rats and bats). Ticks bite these animals to suck their blood, and bacteria are carried from an infected animal to another animal by the ticks. These ticks like to live in the cracks of walls and floors of houses. During the night these ticks come out and bite animals and people (to suck their blood). The ticks can pass on the bacteria to any person they bite. The infected tick also passes on the bacteria to its offspring through its eggs. An infected woman can pass on the disease to her child through her placenta. Figure 17.1 shows the means of spread.

The symptoms and signs of the infection include:

1. A high fever with chills, headache and body pains; often nausea and vomiting; often liver

Figure 17.1 Diagram showing the means of spread of endemic tick-borne relapsing fever.

enlargement and, in severe cases jaundice. After 4–5 days the temperature goes down and the patient stays well for 4–5 days or longer.
2. Then a relapse occurs with the same signs though usually they are less severe.
3. This cycle of a fever for 4–5 days and then being reasonably well for 4–5 days may happen up to 10 times.

Complications occur. These include:
1. meningitis with CSF which is clear to naked eye examination (see Chapter 25 page 260);
2. encephalitis (with unconsciousness or fitting) (see Chapter 25 page 260);
3. iritis (see Chapter 31 page 343) and loss of sight.

Apart from loss of sight, relapsing fever can look exactly like malaria; it is not possible to tell if the patient's condition is caused by malaria unless his blood slide is examined.

Like malaria, people who do not die from the relapsing fever, should become immune to it. The people most affected by relapsing fever are therefore (1) new-comers to the area, (2) infants and children, (3) pregnant women.

If women are infected during pregnancy they usually have a miscarriage, stillbirth or premature labour; but, if the baby is born alive, it can be born infected and will soon have the symptoms and signs of relapsing fever.

Differential diagnosis
This includes malaria and all the causes of fever (see Chapter 13 and Chapter 36 page 395).

If the patient is in or from an area where malaria occurs it is not possible to tell without tests if his fever is caused by relapsing fever or malaria. Always take a blood slide (See Figure 17.2). If possible have the slide examined immediately. If the bacteria (*Spirochaetes* or *Borrelia*) are seen and no malaria parasites are seen the patient has relapsing fever. If malaria parasites (plasmodia) are seen but no bacteria are seen the patient has malaria. If it is not possible to have the slide examined immediately you must treat the patient for both conditions.

If the patient has jaundice see Chapter 24 page 248

Treatment
Penicillin, tetracycline and chloramphenicol all kill the bacteria of relapsing fever. However some of the bacteria are becoming resistant to penicillin.

When antibiotics kill many bacteria quickly, the toxins from the dead bacteria often cause a severe reaction. This reaction can include a high fever, fast breathing and cough, fast pulse and low blood pressure, encephalitis, shock or heart failure and death. Do three things to avoid this reaction.
1. Keep the patient in bed for the first 2 days of treatment.
2. Keep everything needed for treatment of the reaction ready (see Chapter 12 and Chapter 37).
3. Give only a small dose of antibiotic at first.

Start treatment with procaine penicillin 200 mg or 600,000 units (2 ml) IMI. Give the same dose for the next four days; or on the second day

A

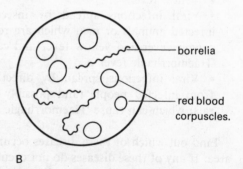

B

Figure 17.2 Always take a thick and thin blood slide (A) from every patient with any illness and in a area where malaria and relapsing fever occur. Ask for examinations for both malaria and relapsing fever parasites. The appearance of relapsing fever parasites (*Borrelia*) under the microscope is show in B. They are seen between the red cells; malaria parasites are seen in the red cells.

change to oral tetracycline and give 250 mg (1 cap) four times a day for a week. However do not give tetracycline to pregnant women or children.

Always treat with antimalarials too (see Chapter 13 page 55) unless you are certain (from good blood slide results) that the patient does not have malaria.

Control and prevention
The only effective way is to stop the spread of the organism by getting rid of the ticks.
1. Treat the home with gamma BHC regularly. This is expensive.
2. Make better houses with no cracks in the walls, floors, ceilings in which the ticks can live.

Epidemic louse-borne relapsing fever

See page 101, Relapsing Fever, first.

Cause and epidemiology
The type of bacterium which causes epidemic louse-borne relapsing fever is a parasite of men and lice only. The lice do not pass on the disease to their offspring (see Figure 17.3). This disease starts when an infected person or an infested louse brings the disease to a group of people who are infested with lice. People have lice because they do not wash themselves or their clothes properly. Epidemic louse-borne relapsing fever is normally less common than the endemic type; but large epidemics can occur.

Figure 17.3 Diagram showing the means of spread of epidemic louse-borne relapsing fever.

The *symptoms and* signs are similar to the symptoms and signs of the endemic type (see page 101) though there are some differences:
1. The attacks are often more severe with fever and bleeding nose at first, hepatitis with jaundice, enlarged spleen, bleeding, meningitis and encephalitis, and then shock or heart failure as the attack ends.

2. The attacks last longer (up to 10 days) and there may be less time between attacks; but there are usually fewer attacks.
3. Half the people affected may die if they are not treated.

Treatment is the same as for the endemic type (see page 102).

Control and prevention
1. All cases must be treated; but there will still be infected lice.
2. The main means of control is therefore to stop the means of spread. All lice both on patients and other people should be killed. People should take precautions not to get lice from other people (see above).
3. Immunisation is not possible.
4. Prophylactic treatment is not needed if precautions about lice are taken.

Leptospirosis

Leptospirosis occurs in most parts of the world. It is a bacterial infection of the whole body but affects mostly the liver and kidneys.

Leptospirosis is normally an infection of rats, pigs and dogs and the organisms are excreted in the urine of these animals. Leptospirosis in man is therefore common (1) where rats are common; (2) if there is rat urine in water which people use and (3) when people live and work with animals.

Infection with the bacteria can cause the following:
1. fever of unknown cause (this may be mild or severe);
2. hepatitis with jaundice, tender liver and bile in the urine;
3. kidney damage with a lot of protein in the urine;
4. meningitis;
5. heart failure or shock.

If a white blood cell count is done, it is high. The disease can last about 3–4 weeks. For differential diagnosis see Table 17.1 page 110.

Antibiotics improve the patient if given early in the disease. Treatment of the other conditions (see above) caused by the infection is also needed.

Bartonellosis

Bartonellosis is a bacterial infection of the red blood cells and the inside of blood vessels. It is carried by sandflies. It occurs only in parts of South America.

The acute stage is caused by the bacteria breaking many red blood cells open (haemolysis). The symptoms and signs are: high fever, pains all over the body, vomiting and diarrhoea, enlargement of liver and spleen, anaemia and often unconsciousness and death.

If the patient does not die, he then improves for a month or so. Then many small red lumps full of blood come up on the skin. These are most common on the head and toward the ends of the arms and legs. These lumps go away after 2–3 months.

Treatment is by antibiotics. Chloramphenicol is best as secondary infections, which may be sensitive to only chloramphenicol, often occur. Other treatment and often blood transfusion are usually needed also. A severely affected patient usually needs transfer for Medical Officer care after antibiotics and treatment of the patient's other conditions are started. (See Chapter 12 page 46.)

People who live in the area where bartonellosis occurs, and do not die from the infection, become immune. It is mostly new-comers to the area and children who are severely affected.

Prevention is by spraying the areas where sandflies breed with insecticide and the use of repellents and protective clothing.

Plague

Plague is an acute infection with bacteria (*Yersinia pestis*) which causes:
1. inflammation of lymph nodes,
2. septicaemia, and
3. pneumonia.

Plague occurs in parts of North and South America, Africa and Asia (see Figure 17.4).

In most of these places plague is endemic and is a disease passed from one bush animal to another, often rats, by infected fleas. The infected bush animals often do no die.

If infected fleas from bush animals infect village or town rats, these newly infected rats often die and the fleas then look for a new host and may find man. Man can also be infected when hunting among infected bush animals.

After a bite from an infected flea the person develops bubonic plague – fever, severe sickness and swelling of the lymph nodes (called a bubo) near the flea bite. He then develops septicaemia. He may also develop pneumonia and cough up many of the plague bacteria. These plague bacteria can be breathed in by other people and these people then develop a severe plague pneumonia and usually die quickly. One patient with pneumonic plague can cause an epidemic. An epidemic can also be caused by infected fleas passing from one person to another.

The clinical features are therefore as follows.

Bubonic plague
Usually fever with rigors and severe generalised symptoms and signs of infection occur.

Swelling of the lymph nodes near the flea bite, called a bubo, also occurs. The bubo may become very tender. The swelling is often the size of an egg. If the patient lives, after a week or so the bubo bursts through the skin and pus comes out.

Usually the patient gets worse with severe toxaemia, bleeding into many parts of the body, septicaemia, sometimes pneumonia and death in 1 – 2 weeks.

Septicaemic plague
The patient becomes so ill so quickly with the septicaemia that he dies in coma and shock within 3 – 5 days, before the bubo can become very big.

Pneumonic plague
This may appear in a patient who has bubonic plague or in a person who has inhaled plague bacteria coughed out by a patient.

The onset is acute with fever, rigors and marked toxaemia. There is severe shortness of breath and a cough. At first the sputum is watery but it soon becomes bloodstained. Often the clinical signs in the chest are not marked.

The patient dies in 1–2 days.

Minor plague
An occasional patient (usually during an epidemic) who has bubonic plague is not very sick and the bubo bursts and discharges pus. The patient can walk around; but his pus may infect others.

Figure 17.4 The distribution of plague.
Source: *Weekly Epidemiological Record*, Vol. 55, p. 244 (1980)

probable plague area

known focus

Diagnosis can be confirmed by the examination of:
1. fluid aspirated from a bubo,
2. 10 ml of venous blood, and
3. sputum.

Take these samples and immediately start treatment. Do not wait for any results if you strongly suspect plague. Treatment can be with chloramphenicol, tetracycline or streptomycin. As streptomycin should not be used in a health centre except for tuberculosis and as the patient is usually very sick, treat with choramphenicol as in Chapter 12. It is most important to give immediate treatment to try to save the patient's life and also to try to stop spread of the disease.

As soon as the disease is suspected start control methods immediately.
1. Take the necessary tests from the patient.
2. Start the patient on treatment.
3. Start all contacts including yourself on prophylactic treatment (usually tetracycline 250 mg (1 cap) four times a day for a week).
4. Notify the health or medical officer who will immediately confirm the diagnosis and take over control procedures.
5. Kill all fleas on the patient and staff and contacts.
6. Apply insecticides (e.g. 10% DDT powder) to places where rats run.
7. Kill rats.

If you do these things you may save many lives.

Plague is a Quarantinable Disease and the Government will notify its occurrence to the World Health Organization and neighbouring countries.

Typhus fever

Typhus fevers occur only in special areas or in special conditions. Only one type is likely to occur in your area although the epidemic type can occur anywhere if the conditions are right (see page 107). Find out if typhus occurs in your area; and if so, what type.

The typhus fevers are acute infectious diseases caused by rickettsiae (see Chapter 10 page 34). These organisms are carried to people by infected insects. These rickettsiae cause inflammation of the inside of blood vessels going to all parts of the body. The damage to blood vessels and toxins produced by the organisms cause the symptoms and signs of typhus.

The onset is usually sudden with fever and a rigor; the fever usually lasts for about 2 weeks.

Pains and weakness in the muscles are marked.

Headache is severe. Mental disturbance and deafness can occur. In severe cases encephalitis and unconsciousness follow.

The face is usually flushed and the conjunctivae are red.

A rash comes by about the fifth day. At first the rash is like measles and is of pink macules which go pale when pressed. However, unlike measles, it starts near the axillae and spreads mainly to the trunk. Later on it does not go away when it is pressed, as bleeding occurs into that part of the skin.

In the second week, especially in older people, the condition may get worse and often leads to death.
• The spleen becomes enlarged.
• The pulse becomes faster and the blood pressure lower.
• The encephalitis gets worse.
• Blood vessels can block and cause death of parts of the skin or the fingers or the toes etc.
• Bleeding can occur.
• Kidney failure can occur.
• Heart failure or shock can occur.

After the second week, those who have not died, usually improve slowly.

Treatment is usually very effective – as long as it is given soon enough.
1. Give tetracycline or chloramphenicol. Tetracycline is used if the diagnosis is certain.
   • Give the antibiotic as soon as possible before the serious effects of the disease occur which the antibiotic cannot cure.
   • Give a large dose for the first dose i.e. tetracycline 1 g (4 caps) or chloramphenicol 2 g (8 caps)
   • After the first dose give the normal dose for any severe infection i.e. tetracycline 500 mg (2 caps) each 6 hours or chloramphenicol 1 g (4 caps) each 6 hours.
2. Give good nursing care and the usual treatment of any of the complications which have already occurred.

Control and prevention depend on the type of typhus which is present (see below). There are four main groups or types of typhus.

Epidemic louse-borne typhus

Epidemic typhus is carried from person to person by the human body louse (see Figure 17.5). This disease occurs in places where a lot of people are crowded together and people do not wash themselves and their clothes properly. Suspect epidemic typhus if an illness that could be typhus occurs in a group of people e.g. refugees.

Figure 17.5 Diagram showing the spread of epidemic louse-borne typhus.

Treatment is as described for typhus fever.

Report any case or cases of suspected epidemic typhus to the Medical Officer and health officer as the diagnosis needs to be confirmed by tests and control measures started to stop an epidemic.

Control of epidemic louse-borne typhus is best done by killing all lice on patients and on all other people. This is done by better personal hygiene and an insecticide, usually DDT.

1. Wash the patient. Put clean clothes on the patient. Then treat the patient, the clothes and the bedclothes with 10% DDT powder.
2. Sterilise the patient's clothes by heat. If a steriliser is not available use a hot iron. If ironing is not possible treat the clothes with 10% DDT powder and leave them for 2 weeks before they are worn again.
3. Get staff to apply DDT powder to their own clothes.
4. Treat the whole population with DDT. Special blowers are available which can blow about 60 g of 10% DDT powder into a person's clothes without their undressing. This should be repeated 1 week later.

A typhus vaccine exists to raise the resistance of people to the disease. However the vaccine is usually not available where epidemic typhus occurs. The dose for adults is 1 ml by sub-

cutaneous injection repeated after 2–4 weeks. Booster doses are needed each year to keep up the immunity but are often given each 3 months during an epidemic.

Endemic flea-borne murine typhus

Endemic flea-borne typhus is carried to people from fleas which have fed on infected rats (see Figure 17.6).

Figure 17.6 Diagram to show the spread of endemic flea-borne murine typhus.

Endemic flea-borne typhus is a much milder disease than epidemic louse-borne typhus and death rarely occurs. It is usually a short-lived 'fever of unknown cause'. Treatment is as described above.

Control is by control of rats and fleas. DDT is often put where rats are known to run. Typhus vaccine can be used in special circumstances.

Sporadic tick-borne typhus

Tick-borne typhus is normally a disease of small animals and ticks. Occasionally an infected tick may bite a person. Infected ticks may be brought into a house by dogs which do not themselves suffer from the disease (see Figure 17.7).

Figure 17.7 Diagram to show the spread of sporadic tick-borne typhus.

The disease is usually mild. However at the place where the tick bit the person, a black ulcer (called an eschar) usually appears and the nearby lymph nodes are usually enlarged.

However in America a severe form of typhus

called Rocky Mountain Spotted Fever is carried by ticks.

Treatment is as described for fever typhus (see above).

Control and prevention is the avoidance of bites from ticks. Do not allow dogs to sleep on beds.

Sporadic mite-borne scrub typhus

Mite-borne scrub typhus is normally a disease of small animals and mites in jungle areas of Asia and the Pacific. People are affected if they are bitten by infected mites (see Figure 17.8).

Figure 17.8 Diagram to show the spread of mite-borne scrub typhus.

The disease can be quite severe and cause death. Also a black ulcer (eschar) can form the mite bite. Nearby lymph nodes become enlarged. Numerous eschars can be present and many lymph nodes enlarged if many infected mites bit the person.

Prevention is by keeping away from areas known to have infected mites or by people wearing protective clothing and repellents if they have to go to that area.

If an area where people must live becomes affected, then the bush has to be cleared, small animals killed and the area treated with insecticide.

Dengue fever

Dengue occurs in most parts of the world. A number of viruses can cause this disease. Dengue viruses are spread by mosquitoes. Dengue usually occurs in small epidemics.

At first there is mild upper respiratory tract and conjuctival inflammation. Soon after there are complaints of severe headache, pain on moving eyes, backache and joint pains. The patient may not be able to eat or sleep.

On examination there is fever, conjunctival inflammation, tender eyes, rash on the skin (often like measles, though often more red in colour and starting on the arms), small vesicles on the palate, and enlarged non-tender lymph glands.

In some cases, after 2–3 days the patient improves for 1–2 days; but the disease returns again and lasts for about 7–10 days in all.

In some epidemics in some countries, especially in children, bleeding and shock can occur. Dengue is therefore one of the causes of 'haemorrhagic fever' (see page 110). There is no improvement when antimalarials or antibiotics are given.

Unless a blood slide can be examined for malaria and is negative, all cases of dengue in malarial areas must be treated with antimalarials (see Chapter 13 page 55) as well as rest and other symptomatic treatment. However do not give aspirin which could make any bleeding worse. Use paracetamol instead. If the patient is very ill, treat for septicaemia (see Chapter 12 page 46). If bleeding or shock occurs, treat as in Chapter 27 page 305.

The means of control and prevention is to kill mosquitoes, especially around houses and prevent mosquitoes breeding.

Sandfly fever

Sandfly fever is a virus infection which is similar to dengue fever. The differences are:
- It is spread by sandflies.
- The illness lasts for a shorter time – usually only 3 days.
- There is usually no skin rash.
- Although unpleasant, no deaths occur.

Yellow fever

Yellow fever occurs only in western and central Africa and the north part of South America. It may spread to other tropical areas (see Figure 17.9).

Yellow fever is an acute viral infection which can cause:
1. fever.
2. liver damage with jaundice (hepatitis),
3. kidney damage with protein in the urine and sometimes kidney failure, and
4. bleeding into all parts of the body.

The yellow fever virus is usually passed between monkeys and mosquitoes. A person can be

Figure 17.9 The distribution of yellow fever.
(Source: *Vaccination Certificate Requirements and Health Advice for International Travel*, Geneva, World Health Organization, 1986)

Jungle   Urban

Figure 17.10   Diagram to show how yellow fever virus spreads.

infected if he is bitten by an infected mosquito in the jungle (jungle yellow fever). If an infected monkey, mosquito or person comes to a town, the disease can then be passed between people and mosquitoes in the town (urban yellow fever). (See Figure 17.10)

People who live in an area where yellow fever is common and do not die from an attack usually become immune or suffer only mild attacks. Severe attacks occur when people from other areas go to an infected area or the disease spreads to a new area.

A typical severe attack is as follows:

1. At first there are severe general symptoms and signs of a viral type infection, similar to dengue fever – fever; pains in the head, eyes, back and joints; red watery eyes; nausea, vomiting etc. The pulse is usually slow, not fast.
2. After a few days the temperature falls and the patient may improve.
3. After some hours or a day or so, however, the patient may get much worse. He or she develops a high fever (although the pulse is still slow), jaundice and a tender liver and bile in the urine (hepatitis), a lot of protein in urine and also bleeding into the skin and from the nose, mouth, lungs, intestine, etc.

4. Death occurs from liver or kidney failure or bleeding. If these can be successfully treated and the patient lives for about 12 days, the patient usually recovers.

Yellow fever is one cause of 'haemorrhagic fever'.

The differential diagnosis includes malaria, septicaemia, relapsing fever, leptospirosis and viral hepatitis. If laboratory tests are available these would help (see Table 17.1).

For treatment of yellow fever in a health centre, see page 111.

Other viral fevers similar to dengue or yellow fever including 'haemorrhagic fevers'

There are a large number of viral diseases which can cause symptoms and signs similar to dengue or yellow fever.

These diseases can cause fever often with a slow pulse (which should make you suspect some unusual or viral disease), generalised aching and pains all over the body, rash, liver damage (hepatitis), kidney damage (proteinuria or kidney

Table 17.1   *Table to show the differential diagnosis of some causes of a fever with jaundice if you have laboratory tests to help. Remember that pneumonia is also a very common cause of fever and jaundice; but there are also signs in the chest.*

Causes of Jaundice and Fever	Proteinuria	WBC total	Blood slide
Yellow Fever	A lot	Low	Negative
Malaria	Little or none	Low or normal	Plasmodia
Relapsing Fever	Some	High	Borrelia
Septicaemia	Little or none	Variable – often high	Negative
Leptospirosis	A lot	High	Negative
Viral Hepatitis	Little or none	Low or normal	Negative

failure), bleeding, shock and other conditions.

Fortunately most are usually mild like sandfly fever and Kyasanur Forest Disease. Some (e.g. dengue) can be moderately severe and can sometimes cause a 'haemorrhagic fever'. Others, such as yellow fever, Kyasanur Forest Disease, Lassa Fever, Marburg Disease and Ebola Fever can be severe; and if severe, often cause a 'haemorrhagic fever'.

One group of the viruses is carried to man by insects (especially mosquitoes and ticks) usually from infected animals but sometimes from infected people. These diseases include dengue, sandfly fever, Kyasanur Forest Disease and yellow fever.

Another group of these viruses are spread from man to man by body fluids or body secretions during close personal contact. They may also be spread to man from rats living in a person's house. These diseases include Lassa Fever, Marburg Disease and Ebola Fever.

Diagnosis of these diseases is not possible (unless a known epidemic of one of them is occurring) without special laboratory tests not available at a health centre. The medical officer must be notified so that he can make arrangements for these tests to be done. Unless a definite diagnosis is made, the best treatment control and prevention measures cannot be carried out.

There is no specific cure for any of these diseases. However if the patient can be kept alive until his body can make enough antibodies to kill the virus, he will probably recover. In a severe case medical officer care in a hospital will be needed to do this.

However there are a number of other diseases which can cause similar symptoms and signs. Try to make sure the patient does not have one of these. Treat for these diseases if they are treatable and cannot be ruled out. These diseases include the following:
1. malaria,
2. septicaemia,
3. relapsing fever,
4. leptospirosis,
5. typhus, and
6. acute severe viral hepatitis.

Management in a health centre of a severe acute disease which causes fever, especially if there is also haemorrhage, of unknown cause therefore includes the following:

1. Do *not* transfer the patient unless the Health Officer tells you to do so as epidemics can be caused by transfer.
2. Immediately notify the medical officer and the health officer.
3. Barrier nurse the patient.
   • Staff must take care not to get blood, urine, saliva, etc. onto themselves.
   • Staff should wear gloves and gowns.
   • Staff should put insecticide (e.g. 10% DDT powder) on their clothes if the case is possibly epidemic typhus.
   • Treat the patient and his clothes and his bedclothes with 10% DDT powder.
4. Treat for septicaemia. (See Chapter 12.)
5. Treat for falciparum malaria. (See Chapter 12 and Chapter 13 page 55)
6. Treat for hepatitis if it occurs. (See Chapter 24.)
7. Treat for kidney failure if it occurs. (See Chapter 25.)
   However, unless kidney failure does occur, make sure you give the patient enough fluid to give a good urine output (2 litres/day).
8. Treat shock if it occurs. (See Chapters 12 and 27.)
9. Do not give aspirin which may make bleeding worse.
10. Treat bleeding if it occurs. (See Chapter 27 page 307)
11. Nurse the patient under a mosquito net (and, if possible, in a room which has insect screens on the door and windows).
12. Have the patient's room and the whole health centre sprayed with a residual insecticide.
13. Destroy any breeding places for mosquitoes around the health centre.
14. Treat the patient's room with gamma BHC if ticks occur in the area.
15. Try to kill any rats by poison or other means. Also put insecticide along known rat runs.
16. Take 20 ml of blood and keep it in the refrigerator at 4°C for special laboratory tests. Take and keep blood and urine for the usual laboratory test (see Chapter 6 page 24). If the patient dies, get permission to take at least a piece of liver for examination (a piece aspirated (sucked back into a syringe) through a very thick needle put into the liver through the skin, is better than none).

18

Some Subacute and Chronic Infectious Diseases with Limited Distribution

This chapter is about the following diseases:
1. Bacterial infections
   - Typhoid fever
   - Brucellosis
2. Protozoal infections
   - Leishmaniasis
   - Trypanosomiasis
3. Worm infections
   - Schistosomiasis

Typhoid fever

Typhoid fever is an acute or subacute disease caused by the typhoid bacteria. At first it causes malaise, fever, abdominal pain and constipation. Later, it causes diarrhoea, rash, enlargement of the spleen and very severe toxaemia. This stage may be complicated by intestinal haemorrhage or perforation. Sometimes, mild cases may cause only a non-specific illness and fever.

Cause, epidemiology, pathology

Typhoid fever is caused by infection with typhoid bacteria (*Salmonella typhi*). The reservoir is persons infected by the typhoid bacteria.

The faeces or urine of infected people may contaminate food or the water supply. This may occur if they handle food, or if they do not use a toilet. It may also occur if the water supply is not safe from contamination by excreta or is not treated. Sometimes flies carry the bacteria from faeces to food.

The bacteria multiply in the bowel and then spread through the whole body. They grow best in the lymph glands, spleen, gall bladder and parts of the wall of the intestines.

The stools of the patient are often infectious for weeks or months; and the patient may become a carrier for life.

An attack of the infection usually produces considerable immunity.

Symptoms and signs, course and complications

For the first week the patient has the general symptoms and signs of infection with some special features. He has malaise, headache, pains all over and fever. He may have a cough and nose-bleeds. He usually has mild abdominal pain and constipation. On examination, the patient has fever but the pulse may be slower than expected. Nothing else special is found.

During the second week the patient becomes worse. General symptoms and signs may be severe. Abdominal pain becomes more severe and diarrhoea occurs. On examination the patient may not be fully conscious. The fever and slow pulse are still present. There may be signs of bronchitis in the chest. The abdomen is usually distended and may be tender especially in the right iliac fossa. The spleen is enlarged. A rash made up of red spots, each of which lasts for a day or so, may be seen, especially on the abdomen.

During the third week, the general and abdominal symptoms and signs become worse. The patient may become unconscious and die.

During this third week two complications may also occur.
1. The bowel may perforate (get a hole in it through to the peritoneal cavity). There is a sudden abdominal pain and rapid worsening of the patient's condition and the symptoms and signs of general peritonitis develop.
2. Haemorrhage may occur from the intestinal wall into the intestine. The patient may pass blood from the rectum; or simply become pale and shocked (and later pass blood).

If the patient does not die he or she usually starts to recover quickly after the fourth week. However, in some cases, after about two weeks, there is a return of the symptoms and signs, though usually not as severe as before.

A much milder disease often occurs. Sometimes it may be only a fever with perhaps a mild gastro-intestinal upset, or some of the other symptoms or signs of the more severe disease.

Tests

None are available at the health centre.

The white cell count is usually not raised unless a complication has developed when it may be high.

Blood and stool cultures may grow the typhoid organism.

Diagnostic features

Generalised symptoms and signs of infection (often 'PUO', 'sick', and no response to anti-malarials, see Chapter 36 page 396).
Slow pulse.
Constipation at first, then diarrhoea
Abdominal distension and tenderness.
Persistence of temperature, after treatment with antimalarials, without any focal signs.

Differential diagnosis

All other causes of fever (see Chapter 36 page 395).
Other causes of gastro-enteritis have to be differentiated from typhoid (Chapter 23 page 220). Other causes of septicaemia (Chapter 12 page 46).

Treatment

Transfer the patient to medical officer care, if this is possible.

Dispose of faeces carefully. Disinfect the bedpan and other articles used by the patient, and carefully wash your hands after caring for the patient.

Give chloramphenicol 1 g (4 caps orally or 1 bottle by injection) each 6 hours. When the fever stops reduce the dose to 500 mg (2 caps) four times a day. However, continue the chloram-phenicol for 2 weeks. (See Chapter 11 page 43)

Treat as for other cases of gastro-enteritis. (See Chapter 23 page 220)

Treat any complication in the usual way.

Transfer

Transfer these cases:
1. All diagnosed cases (in case a blood transfusion or operation is needed).
2. The diagnosis cannot be made and the patient is very 'sick'.
3. A complication occurs especially perforation or haemorrhage.

Control and prevention

1. Kill the organism in the body of the host (reservior) (patients and carriers).
   If typhoid fever is uncommon in the area, investigation is needed to find out where the infection came from. A carrier is usually responsible. A Medical Officer may be able to treat such a carrier. However, *if typhoid is common in an area*, a search would not be made for the source of infection.
2. Stop the means of spread of the organism.
   Patients and carriers should not be allowed to handle food for others.
   Proper disposal of faeces is essential.
   Safe water supply is essential.
   Careful nursing of cases which are infectious is important. Staff must wash their hands carefully after caring for a patient.
3. Raise the resistance of susceptible persons.

There is an immunisation called typhoid vaccine and another called TAB vaccine which will make it less likely for an immunised person to get typhoid. This is only given to a person who is especially at risk of getting typhoid. This is not a highly effective immunisation. The adult dose by sub-cutaneous injection is 0.5 ml (½ ml) repeated 7–28 days later and if possible 6 months later. A booster injection is needed each 3 years to keep up the immunity it produces.

Brucellosis

Brucellosis is due to an infection with the *Brucella* bacteria. The infection is normally one of cattle, goats and pigs and it can cause abortions in these animals. The bacteria can spread to people who live with or work with infected animals or who drink unpasteurised milk from infected animals. The *Brucella* bacteria live mainly in the lymph tissues; but can affect joints and other parts of the body.

At first there can be a fever with severe pains and malaise which lasts for a few weeks. After this the patient usually slowly improves.

However, the fever may come back many times every week or every few weeks. The spleen sometimes becomes enlarged and sometimes very enlarged. Pain in a joint, especially the hip, is common and chronic osteomyelitis of the spine sometimes occurs. Weight loss is common. Depression is common.

In most people this prolonged infection is usually overcome by the body itself after a year or so; but in a few, the infection continues.

Diagnosis can be made only by special blood tests (serology) not possible in a health centre.

Treatment is by a long course of a high dose of tetracycline.

Refer or transfer suspected cases to a medical officer for diagnosis and treatment.

Leishmaniasis

Leishmaniasis is a group of diseases caused by an infection with protozoal organisms called *Leishmania*.

There are three types of leishmaniasis.
1. Skin leishmaniasis also called 'Oriental sore'.
2. Skin and mucous membranes leishmaniasis which occurs only in South America and is called 'Espundia'.
3. Skin, blood, bone-marrow, spleen, liver and lymph node leishmaniasis called visceral leishmaniasis or 'kala azar'.

Figure 18.1 Diagram to show the means of spread of leishmaniasis.

The reservoir of infection includes not only infected people but also infected dogs and many other animals.

The organisms are spread to man by the bite of a sandfly which has been infected from an infected man or infected animal (see Figure 18.1).

Control and prevention of leishmaniasis follow the usual rules.
1. Kill the parasite in the original host or reservoir.
   Find and treat patients with the disease.
   Find and kill any dogs or other animals with the disease.
2. Stop the means of spread.
   Sandflies breed in places like animal houses, rubbish dumps, anthills, crumbling stonework etc. They do not usually fly more than a few hundred yards from where they breed. The following may therefore be effective:
   (a) Move houses away from places where sandflies breed.
   (b) Kill sandflies with regular spraying of insecticide where they breed.
   (c) Protect people from sandflies by clothing, repellents and fine sleeping nets sprayed with insecticide.
3. Raise the resistance of possible new hosts.
   This can be done for only skin leishmaniasis. A sore can be started by injecting material into the skin of an area where a scar will not matter. This will stop sores starting in other areas such as the face where a scar would matter.

Skin leishmaniasis (Old world cutaneous leishmaniasis or Oriental sore)

Skin leishmaniasis occurs in many old world countries; that is Africa, the Mediterranean, the Middle East and Asia (see Figure 18.2)

Children are most often affected as most adults have been infected and have become immune.

The incubation period is from weeks to months.

At first a small reddish itchy lump appears in the skin where the patient was bitten by the sandfly. A crust forms on top of the lump. The lesion gets bigger and usually becomes a rounded ulcer. The ulcer has thick raised edges and a discharge of blood and pus, which dries to form a dark crust (see Figure 18.3). Small new lumps may start around the edge of the ulcer. These lumps then get

Figure 18.2 The distribution of skin leishmaniasis (Oriental sore), and skin and mucous membrane leishmaniasis (New World cutaneous leishmaniasis).
(Source: WHO Technical Report Series No 701, 1984 (Report of a WHO Expert Committee on Leishmaniases))

Figure 18.3 A typical skin lesion of skin leishmaniasis.

bigger and ulcerate. Eventually, as these join, a large ulcer up to 10 cm in diameter may be formed. Sometimes the lesion stays as a large lumpy mass. The ulcer is not painful. The ulcer usually lasts for about a year and then heals leaving a thin scar.

Sometimes there may be more than one lesion if the patient was bitten in several places. Sometimes new lesions form on the skin between the first lesion and the nearby lymph glands.

The patient does not have a fever or feel ill because of the infection.

The diagnosis can be confirmed by aspirating some fluid through a fine needle from the edge of the ulcer and examination of this fluid under the microscrope for the leishmania organisms.

Treatment includes the following:

1. Eusol dressings two or three times a day until the crust is gone and the ulcer is clean.
2. If there is a lot of secondary bacterial infection, give antibiotics such as penicillin or tetracycline.

3. Then keep the ulcer clean and dry under a dressing and it will probably heal in a few weeks.
4. Treat with drugs as for kala azar (see page 118) if the ulcer does not heal after the above treatment, or if the ulcer is on the face, or if there are a number of large ulcers.

Epidemiology. Control. Prevention. (See page 114)

Skin and mucous membrane leishmaniasis (New world cutaneous leishmaniasis)

In Central and South America special types of cutaneous leishmaniasis are found (see Figure 18.2) The worst type is called 'Espundia' in Brazil.

In Espundia, the first lesion may be many on the face, ears, elbows or knees (see skin leishmaniasis, page 114). Either then, or months or years later, lesions appear in the mucous membrane of the nose and mouth. The nasal mucous membrane swells up and then ulcerates. The ulcer may slowly destroy all the tissues of the nose and then the mouth, lips and throat.

The diagnosis can be confirmed as for skin (cutaneous) leishmaniasis (see this page).

Treatment with special and dangerous drugs is needed. Unless you have been specially trained in the use of the drugs, transfer the patient to a medical officer for treatment.
Epidemiology. Control. Prevention. See page 114.

Visceral leishmaniasis (kala azar)

Visceral leishmaniasis occurs in many countries (see Figure 18.4).

A person is infected by the bite of an infected sandfly. The leishmania organisms spread to the bone marrow where they damage the cells that make new blood. The organisms spread also to the lymph nodes, liver and spleen which are damaged and become larger than normal.

In the Mediterranean region children and visitors are the ones mostly affected. In other areas, adults are affected too.

The illness starts with a fever. This is usually not severe at first and the patient continues his normal life. Sometimes however, the fever is severe. The

Figure 18.4 The distribution of visceral leishmaniasis. (Shaded zones are endemic areas, spots indicate sporadic cases.) (Source: WHO Technical Report Series No. 701, 1984 (Report of a WHO Expert Committee on Leishmaniases))

fever may be worse in the afternoon and again at night.

The spleen soon becomes enlarged; and often becomes very enlarged (see Figure 18.5).

The liver becomes enlarged but not very enlarged.

The lymph nodes may become enlarged.

The patient becomes anaemic.

The patient may have repeated attacks of diarrhoea.

The patient becomes thin and wasted and often has a darkening of the colour of the face, hands and feet.

Dermal (skin) leishmaniasis may occur – often after treatment and when the patient is getting better (as the skin is then the place the organisms find it easiest to live). There are pale or reddish thickened areas of the skin on any part of the body. Lumps may form – especially on the face. (See Figure 18.6.)

Figure 18.6 A patient with dermal leishmaniasis. Do not confuse this condition with leprosy. (Source: W. Peters and H. M. Gilles, *A colour atlas of tropical medicine and parasitology*, London, Wolfe Medical Publications 1981) (Dr D. M. Minter)

Figure 18.5 A patient with visceral leishmaniasis. Note the features of the disease listed above.

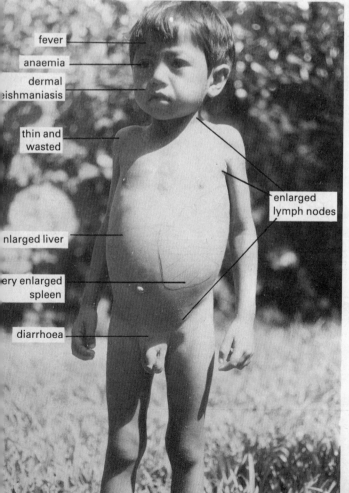

fever
anaemia
dermal leishmaniasis
thin and wasted
enlarged lymph nodes
nlarged liver
ery enlarged spleen
diarrhoea

The diagnosis can be confirmed in the laboratory by finding the leishmania organisms in the blood or in a biopsy. When no laboratory is available the formaldehyde gel test can be used. Put 1 ml of the patient's serum in a test tube. Add one drop of 40% (commercial) formaldehyde (formalin). If the patient has kala azar the serum (1) becomes solid (so that if you tip the tube upside down the serum does not run out) *and* (2) the serum does not stay clear (but goes a milky or dirty colour). Both (1) and (2) are needed for the test to be positive. The test is not positive until a few months after the patient has been infected.

Treatment is different in different parts of the world as the sensitivity of the organisms to drugs varies. Treatment is also by drugs with dangerous side effects. Unless you have been specially trained in the use of the best drugs for your area, transfer the patient for diagnosis and treatment to a medical officer.

Epidemiology. Control. Prevention. See page 114.

African trypanosomiasis (Sleeping sickness)

African trypanosomiasis occurs only in Central West and East Africa (see Figure 18.7).

Figure 18.7 The distribution of African trypanosomiasis. It is caused by two subspecies of *Trypanosoma brucei*. The dots show where *T. b. rhodesiense* is endemic and the open areas show where *T. b. gambiense* is highly endemic.
(Source: D. H. Molyneux and R. W. Ashford, *The biology of* Trypanosoma *and* Leishmania *Parasites of Man and Domestic Animals*, London, Taylor and Francis, 1983.)

Figure 18.8 A trypanosome magnified many times.

Figure 18.9 The appearance of a tsetse fly. The actual size is about 15 mm in length.

African trypanosomiasis is an infection caused by a protozoal parasite called a trypanosome. There are two kinds of trypanosomes which affect man. If a trypanosome is in blood or other fresh fluids examined under the microscope, it can be seen to swim with its tail (see Figure 18.8).

Animals including cattle and large game are affected as well as man.

The trypanosomes are carried from infected man or animals by the tsetse fly (see Figures 18.9 and 18.10). There are two kinds of fly which carry the disease and they have different breeding, living and biting habits.

The trypanosomes cause a chronic disease which causes death. At first a sore forms at the bite. Then a fever occurs when the blood, lymph glands and other organs of the body are affected. Later the nervous system is damaged and this nervous system damage is the usual cause of death. One type of trypanosome causes all of these things in a few months. The other type of trypanosome may take about a year to cause death.

Figure 18.10 Diagram to show the trypanosomes can be spread.

African trypanosomiasis occurs only in people who go into a tsetse fly infected area.

The bite of a tsetse fly is painful; but the pain soon goes. However if trypanosomes were injected by the fly, then 1–3 weeks later a reddish non-painful lump comes up at that place. It can form into an ulcer if it is scratched. The lesion goes away itself in 2–3 weeks. Sometimes the person does not notice the lesion.

The trypanosomes however then go into the blood and cause any of the following.
1. Fever with weakness, headache, etc. The fever may be there for a few days and then be gone for a few days over many months. However the fever can be severe and present all the time. Everyone who has a fever in an area where trypanosomiasis occurs must be investigated for trypanosomiasis. Wet and also stained thick blood films must be examined for trypanosomes before any other diagnosis is

made. The examination should be repeated at least 3 times if the patient does not get better.
2. Lymph node enlargement. Any nodes may be enlarged but those at the back of the neck are the ones most commonly affected. The nodes are smooth, firm, painless and not stuck to the skin or other structures.
   If in an area where trypanosomiasis occurs, aspirate fluid from the node with a fine needle and have it examined for trypanosomes.
3. Skin rashes may occur, especially irregular ring-like reddish patches which do not last for very long.
4. Enlargement of the spleen.
5. Enlargement of the liver.
6. Bone marrow damage with anaemia.
7. Heart damage with a fast pulse even when the fever is not present and later sometimes heart failure.
8. Kidney damage with proteinuria.

After some weeks or months the nervous system is affected. Signs of meningitis, encephalitis and organic psychosis then occur. (See Chapters 25 and 35.) The patient often has headache, abnormal behaviour, sleeps during the day but not at night, shakes, becomes paralysed and passes into a coma and dies. Examination of the CSF shows an increase in the protein and in the cells. However, when there are no nervous system signs, a lumbar puncture should not be done just to see if the nervous system is involved. A lumbar puncture may cause infection of the nervous system from other parts of the body unless the patient is already on treatment.

If the patient is from or is in an area where trypanosomiasis occurs, then trypanosomiasis must be thought of and tests done for it in all cases of:
  fever
  lymph-node enlargement,
  anaemia,
  wasting,
  sleepiness,
  meningitis,
  encephalitis,
  psychosis, and
  unconsciousness.

In any of these conditions, if another cause for the condition is not found and if the condition

Figure 18.11 The distribution of Chagas' disease. (Source: Pan American Health Organization.)

does not get better on the proper treatment for the diagnosis you made, then transfer the patient to a medical officer for the special tests to diagnose trypanomiasis.

Treatment for the disease is effective if given early enough – best before the nervous system is affected. But the treatment has many serious side effects. If you suspect or diagnose a case of trypanosomiasis then transfer the patient to medical officer care at a hospital unless you have been specially trained to use the special drugs that are best in your area.

Control and prevention will depend on the advice of experts who will work out the best methods of your area. The usual methods are:

1. Kill the parasite in the body of the original host or reservoir. This is done only during an epidemic when mass treatment may be given.
2. Stop the means of spread.

   There are two ways to make it difficult for the fly to live in a place. One is to take people away from the area and also chase animals away from the area – the fly then has nothing to feed on. Another way is to put a large number of people into the area and clean the land for agriculture – the fly then has nowhere to live.
3. Raise the resistance of people.

   This is not yet possible.
4. Prophylactic treatment.

   Six monthly injections of a drug can be used: but only in some areas for some people.

American trypanosomiasis (Chagas' disease)

American trypanosomiasis occurs only in Central and South America (see Figure 18.11). The disease is caused by a protozoal parasite called a trypanosome

The trypanosomes live in dogs, cats and other animals as well as people.

These trypanosomes are spread from an infected animal or person to an uninfected person by the bite of an infected reduvid bug (see Figure 18.12). These bugs live in the cracks in ceilings and walls in the poorer houses in rural areas. The bugs bite the faces of people while they sleep at night.

The trypanosomes from the bug enter the body through the mucous membranes of the eye or the mouth or the skin of the face, where they cause a lesion. The organisms then cause a fever and travel in the blood to the lymph nodes, spleen and

Figure 18.12 Diagram to show the means of spread of American trypanosomiasis.

liver. They also enter the heart and nervous system and cause both acute and chronic disease in these places.

The acute disease affects children more often than adults.

A lesion appears where the organisms enter the body. This is usually on the face. There is often swelling of the eyelids of the eye on that side of the face; the lids are firm and red and swollen enough to close the eye. There can be a painful red swelling with much hard oedema around it on the skin. The nearby lymph nodes are enlarged. The swelling and the enlarged lymph nodes stay for some weeks.

One to three weeks after the infection, the patient develops a high fever and the liver, spleen and lymph nodes may be swollen. The pulse is often fast, even when the fever is not present, because by then the heart is also damaged. The organisms can often be found in the blood or the fluid aspirated from the swelling on the face or from an enlarged lymph gland, if it is examined under the microscope.

After some time the patient usually improves slowly; but the organisms stay in the body. They stay especially in the heart and in the nerves of the oesophagus and large intestine.

After many years the patient may get heart failure or the patient may suddenly die because his heart stops. The patient may also develop difficulty swallowing or severe constipation. These things are due to the organisms causing chronic damage to the heart, to the nerves going to the heart and to the gastro-intestinal tract.

Diagnosis and treatment are often difficult. If you suspect the disease, send the patient to a medical officer for diagnosis and treatment unless you have been specially trained in the use of the drugs used for treatment.

Control and prevention is as follows; but mostly by making better houses.
1. Kill the parasite in the body of the original host or reservoir.
   Kill dogs etc. which are known to be infected.
2. Stop the means of spread.
   The bug can be killed by gamma BHC applied to the house. This however is expensive and has to be repeated every few months. It is cheaper to rebuild better houses with smooth walls and non-thatched roofs which have no hiding places for the bugs. Sleeping under a net will also stop bugs biting the face.
3. Raising the resistance of people is not yet possible.
4. Chemoprophylaxis is not yet possible.

Schistosomiasis (Bilharzia)

Definition and cause

Schistosomiasis is the disease caused by worms called schistosomes. These are small worms, like very short threads of cotton, which live in the veins of the pelvic organs. The female worm lays many eggs and these eggs damage the bladder, large intestine and liver.

Epidemiology

Three main types of schistosome affect people. (Figure 18.13 shows the distribution of the different types.)
1. *Schistosoma haematobium* effects mainly the bladder in people in Egypt, the Middle East and Africa only.
2. *S. mansoni* affects mainly the large bowel in people (and baboons) in Egypt, the Middle East, Africa, and South America.
3. *S. japonicum* affects the large and small bowel and other parts of people and many domestic and wild animals in China, Japan, South-east Asia and the Philippines.

S. mansoni and *S. japonicum* live mainly in the pelvis in the veins which come from the bowel. The eggs cause ulceration of the wall of the bowel. This causes diarrhoea and dysentery. It also allows the eggs to enter the bowel and be passed in the faeces. *S. haematobium* lives mainly in the pelvis in the veins which come from the bladder. The eggs cause ulceration of the wall of the bladder. This causes blood in the urine (and it also damages the urethra, bladder, ureters and kidneys). It also allows the eggs to enter the bladder and be passed in the urine.

If the eggs in the urine or the stool go into water, the eggs become worms, now called miracidia. These miracidia swim around until they find certain snails in which they can grow. Then the worms leave the snail and are called cercariae. These cercariae swim in the water until they find a person. They can go through the skin of a person

Figure 18.13 The distribution of schistosomiasis. (Source: WHO Technical Report Series, No. 728, 1985 (Report of a WHO Expert Committee on the Control of Schistosomiasis))

S. haematobium

S. japonicum

S. mekongi

Figure 18.13   The distribution of schistosomiasis (continued).

124

Eggs in stool ◄——— Adult schistosome worms
or urine   in bladder or bowel ◄—┐
  │   veins of man   │
  ▼   │
(if reach water)   │
Miracidia   Cercariae ──┘
                                      in water
  │   ▲
  └──────────► Snail ────────────────────┘

Figure 18.14 Diagram to show the life cycle of schistosomes.

or through the mucous membrane of the person's mouth. The worms then travel around the body of the person until they enter the pelvic veins, where they develop into adult schistosome worms. (See Figure 18.14)

Some of the eggs laid by the female do not enter the bladder or intestine. Some are carried away in the blood in the veins from the bladder and intestine. These veins join to form the portal vein which runs to the liver (See Chapter 24 page 239). The eggs then damage the liver. Some eggs can be carried to other parts of the body as well as to the liver – especially the lungs and the nervous system – and damage these parts too.

Symptoms and signs

1. A mild skin itch and rash may come where the cercariae go through the skin.
2. Several weeks later there may be fever, malasie, cough, abdominal pain and allergic-type symptoms and signs. These are caused by the worms travelling around the body to the pelvic veins. These symptoms last for 1–2 weeks. They are common only in S. *mansoni* and S. *japonicum* infections.
3. Then the patient is quite well until either urinary (see 4 below) or intestinal (see 5 below) schistosomiasis develop. Either urinary or intestinal schistosomiasis may be followed by other complications (see 6 below).
4. Urinary schistosomiasis is caused by S. *haematobium* laying eggs in the veins of the wall of the bladder. Ulcers of the bladder wall cause blood in the urine. Usually the patient notices the blood in the urine when he has nearly finished passing urine. The patient also

notices more blood after excercise. If there is a lot of blood in the urine, clots may form and there may be much pain (especially in boys). If there are not many worms the patient may slowly improve and have blood in the urine only sometimes. He may even get better. However if there are many worms and especially if the patient gets new infections, then other problems develop. The bladder cannot stretch and the patient has to pass urine often (urinary frequency). Bacterial urinary tract infection may develop (see Chapter 26 page 286). After years the ureters may become narrowed and cause chronic kidney failure (see Chapter 26 page 289). The urethra may become blocked and cause urinary retention (see Chapter 26 page 293). Cancer may grow in the damaged bladder. The female pelvic organs and the bowel can also be damaged.

5. Intestinal schistosomiasis is caused by S. *mansoni* or S. *japonicum* laying eggs in the veins of the wall of the intestine. Ulceration of the intestine causes abdominal pain, diarrhoea and dysentery (blood and pus in the faeces). If there are not many worms and no new infections there may be no symptoms or the symptoms caused may go away. If there are many worms or if there are new infections, the symptoms may be severe. Infected lumps on the inside of the bowel may prolapse (come out) through the anus.

6. Complications can develop if the eggs are carried in the blood to the liver, lungs or nervous system.

   (a) The eggs can damage the blood vessels in the liver and cause portal hypertension (see Chapter 24 page 243). The liver becomes large at first; but later small. The spleen becomes very large. The patient can become anaemic. Fluid collects in the abdomen (ascites) and in the legs and back (oedema). The patient can vomit blood and bleed to death.

   (b) The eggs damage the lung. The right side of the heart cannot pump the blood through the lungs and heart failure develops (see Chapter 27 page 301).

   (c) The eggs can damage the brain or spinal cord. The patient can develop paralysis or epilepsy or blindness or coma, etc. (see Chapter 25 page 264). This is more frequent in S. *japonicum* infections.

Tests

1. Eggs may be seen through the microscope when the urine or stool is examined. The last part of the urine passed is the best to examine . A concentration method and repeat examinations may be needed for the stool.
2. If laboratory tests are not available at the health centre, add boiled then cooled water to a sample of urine or a sample of stool in a test-tube or bottle. Allow the urine to stand for 1 hour or the stool to stand for 1 night then examine the tube through a magnifying glass against a dark background. Miracidia will be seen swimming in the tube if eggs are present.

Differential diagnosis

1. Fever.
   See Chapter 36 page 395.
2. Blood in the urine.
   In an area where schistosomiasis is common, almost all cases of blood in the urine are due to schistosomiasis.
   If there are
   • no eggs (or miracidia) in the urine, or
   • other urinary symptoms present, or
   • symptoms present in other systems.
   then transfer the patient to a medical officer for diagnosis and treatment. See also Chapter 26.
3. Diarrhoea/Dysentery
   Bacillary and amoebic infections and cancer of the intestine also cause dysentery or large intestinal symptoms and signs.
   If eggs or miracidia are not present in the stool and if the dysentery continues or keeps on coming back and does not improve after treatment with metronidazole, then refer or transfer the patient to a medical officer. See also Chapter 23 page 225.

Treatment

Do not spend a lot of time and money treating patients with mild infection and few symptoms of schistosomiasis if they are likely to become infected again soon. Give health education to these patients on how not to get more infections.

Also, many of the drugs to treat schistosomiasis have serious side effects, which are more common if the patient has liver disease. Some of the drugs are expensive. Some newer drugs may soon be available which are much easier to use.

Also the best drug for your area depends on which type of schistosome worm is the most common in your area.

You must therefore find out the Health Department policy for
• which patients you should treat,
• which drugs you should use,
• the doses, side-effects and precautions you should take for these drugs.

Refer patients who have urinary problems or rectal problems which are not helped by the drugs to the next visiting medical officer. Surgery may help some of these patients.

Control and prevention

You can use most of the normal methods of control and prevention. However experts need to study each area to find out which method is best. So again you must find out the Health Department policy for your area.

1. Kill the parasite in the bodies of the original host or reservoir. Patients may be treated. The whole population may be treated. This is helpful only if all the population is co-operative and other methods are also used.
2. Stop the means of spread of the parasite.
   (a) All people (including children) must use a toilet at all times.
   (b) Control or eradicate the vector (the snail). This is the main method used. There are many ways of doing this. Find out what way is best for your area.
   (c) Stop contact with water which has cercariae in it. Safe drinking water should be supplied. If water is left to stand in pots for 2–3 days before drinking, cercariae will die. No one should swim or wash in infected water. People should not work in infected water – this is almost impossible for many farmers.
3. Raise the resistance of the people.
   Immunisation is not yet possible.
4. Prophylactic treatment.
   This is used only in special circumstances.

19

Sexually Transmitted Diseases

Figure 19.1 (*top*) Diagram of the male reproductive system.

Figure 19.2 Diagram of the female reproductive system.

Pathology

Sexually transmitted diseases (STD) (also called veneral diseases (VD)) are *usually* spread by sexual intercourse. (But they are sometimes spread by non-sexual means.)

Sexually transmitted diseases *usually* show themselves in two ways:

1. Urethral or vaginal discharge.
2. Sores or lumps in the mucous membrane or skin of the genitalia or in the skin near the genitalia or in lymph glands near the genitalia.

Urethral or vaginal discharge

Urethral or vaginal discharge which is caused by a sexually transmitted disease is usually caused by either:

1. gonorrhoea, or
2. non-gonococcal urethritis usually of the non-specific urethritis type, or
3. trichomonal infection.

Vaginal discharge which is caused by a non-sexually transmitted disease is common. Causes of this include:

1. pelvic inflammatory disease after childbirth or miscarriage,
2. Candida (Monilia or thrush) infection,
3. foreign body in the vagina,
4. vesico-vaginal fistula (after difficult delivery) and
5. cancer.

Genital sores or lumps

Sores or lumps on or near the genitalia which are sexually transmitted have a large number of causes. You must find out which are the common ones in your country. In all countries syphilis is the most important cause. Causes include:

1. syphilis,
2. granuloma inguinale (also called granuloma venereum or donovanosis),
3. lymphogranuloma venereum (also called lymphogranuloma inguinale),
4. chancroid (also called soft sore),
5. herpes genitalis,
6. condylomata accuminata (also called venereal warts),
7. amoebic ulcer (not always sexually transmitted),
8. pubic lice (not always sexually transmitted), and
9. scabies (not always sexually transmitted).

Non-sexually transmitted conditions often affect the genitalia. These include:

1. traumatic sores,
2. balanitis,
3. cancer,
4. amoebic ulcer,
5. pubic lice;
6. scabies, and
7. many of the other skin conditions which can affect any part of the body.

History, examination and tests

When a patient with either a genital sore or lump or an urethral or vaginal discharge or other condition which may be sexually transmitted is seen, you should take a full history, do a full physical examination and do the necessary tests.

History (See Chapter 6 page 16)

This history must include a history of all the people the patient has had sexual intercourse with in the last few months: and how long after intercourse with any particular person the patient's complaint started.

Physical examination (See Chapter 6 page 18)

Special things to note in the examination include:

All patients:

Wear disposable plastic gloves (which you throw away after seeing each patient) or reusable gloves (which you have sterilised before you use them again) to protect yourself.

Male patients:

Look at the pubic hair for lice.

Examine the groin for ulcers or lymph gland enlargement.

Look at the penis for sores or ulcers. Feel if a sore is hard or soft and if it is tender. If the patient is not circumcised, pull back the foreskin so that you can examine the glans too.

Squeeze the urethra gently to see if any discharge comes out of the urethra. Take a smear of any discharge.

Look at the scrotum for sores or ulcers. Gently feel the testes for swelling, lumps or tenderness.

Put the patient onto his side and ask him to lift his knees so that you can look at the perianal region for sores or discharge. Do a pelvic examination through the rectum (PR). (See Chapter 26 page 284.)

Female patients:

Look at the pubic hair for lice.

Examine the groins for ulcers or lymph gland enlargement.

Examine the abdomen (see Chapter 36).

Examine the perineum and genitalia. Ask the patient to lie on her back and bend her knees until the heels touch the buttocks. When the patient parts her knees you have a good view of the external genitalia.

Examine the vulva for any sores, ulcers, swelling or discharge.

Examine the perianal region.

Examine the internal surface of the labia after gently separating them.

Feel if any sores are soft or hard and if they are tender.

Use a speculum to examine the vagina and cervix.

Take a smear from the urethra and from inside the cervix.

Do a pelvic examination through the vagina (PV). (See Chapter 26 page 282.)

Tests

1. Take 10 ml of blood and send the serum to the laboratory with a request for the VDRL test.
2. Make slides from swabs from the urethra and (in the female) inside the cervical canal.
3. Test the urine (see Chapter 26 page 284).

Control and prevention

If after the history and examination and tests you think that the patient has a disease which may have been sexually transmitted, then you should:
1. treat the patient,

2. control and prevent the spread of the disease, as follows:

Kill the organism in the body of the original host or reservoir

All patients and all 'contacts' need to be found and investigated and treated if necessary.

'Contacts' include the person who gave the patient the disease and anyone else the patient may have given the disease to, i.e. all persons the patient has had intercourse with as well as the patient's husband/wife.

Give health education to encourage all people who have the disease to come for treatment. Health education should include:
1. how the diseases are spread;
2. the symptoms and signs of the diseases;
3. the serious results if no treatment is given; and
4. that the treatment is safe, effective and free.

Ask the patient for the names and addresses of *ALL* contacts as soon as STD is diagnosed. Do this before giving treatment. Write the names in the STD Register.

You *must* find, examine and test the contacts and treat any who have the disease. If any contacts have the disease, they are new cases and all *their* contacts must be found. If contacts will not agree to be examined and tested, you should treat them anyway.

It is difficult to get the names and addresses of contacts from patients. It is also difficult to find contacts. There are some things which will help your attempts. Let the patient know that what he or she tells you will be confidential (i.e. you will not tell anyone). Do not be critical of the patient – treat the patient like any other patient. Give the patient *proper* health education about sexually transmitted diseases (see above and below). Ask the patient to bring or send you his or her usual sexual partner, anyone else the patient has had intercourse with, and anyone else the patient 'thinks' may have the disease. If you do this properly it will save you a lot of work as many of the contacts will be brought to you. Patients will often bring persons whose names they would not give. But this does not mean that you need not ask for the names and addresses of contacts and them look for those contacts.

Stop the means of spread

Give health education so that people know that:
1. The means of spread is intercourse (with an infected person).
2. Many people with the disease have no symptoms or signs that could warn of the risk of infection.
3. If they use a condom and wash with soap and water immediately after intercourse it is less likely that they will catch disease from intercourse with an infected person.

Raise the resistance of susceptible people

Immunisation is not yet possible.

Prophylactic treatment

Prophylactic treatment with the proper treatment dose after intercourse with a person who is known to have a sexually transmissable disease is wise.

Common sexually transmitted diseases

Gonorrhoea and other forms of urethritis

Gonorrhoea is a bacterial infection which usually causes an urethritis. It can also spread within the genital organs and to other parts of the body to cause serious disease.

Gonorrhoea is common.

The cause is the gonorrhoea bacterium (*Neisseria gonorrhoae*).

The original host is an infected person. Some infected people have symptoms and signs; but some men and many women are carriers with no symptoms.

The means of spread is direct contact. In adults this is almost always by sexual intercourse. It can infect the eyes of a child if the mother's cervix or urethra is infected at the time of birth. It can infect the throat if infected genitalia are kissed.

Infection does not give any immunity.

Symptoms and signs, course and complications in the male

Symptoms and signs usually develop within a

Figure 19.3 Gonorrhoea in the male. The usual symptom and sign of gonorrhoea – urethral discharge.

week; but they can take longer or never develop.

There is an urethral discharge (Figure 19.3). It is usually white or yellow (pus) and often a large amount. Dysuria and urinary frequency occur. The symptoms slowly improve over weeks or months, although a little white discharge may continue to be present each morning. But the infection does not go.

Complications include:
- abscess around urethra,
- inflammation of the testis,
- septicaemia,
- skin rash, and
- acute infective arthritis.

These complications usually occur soon after infection. Urethral stricture with difficulty in passing urine and distended bladder occurs after many years.

Symptoms and signs, course and complications in the female

Symptoms and signs usually develop within a week; but they can take longer or never develop.

There is usually dysuria and urinary frequency and increase in vaginal discharge (Figure 19.4). This is often mistaken for an urinary tract

Figure 19.4 Gonorrhoea in the female. Urethral discharge may be seen. On speculum examination of the cervix, discharge may be seen (inset A). However, the patient will not complain of these. She may have symptoms of urinary tract infection or of a vaginal discharge.

Figure 19.5 Methods of collecting specimens for examination in the laboratory for gonococci. Use a sterile swab to collect pus from the urethra. If there is not enough pus to be collected on a swab then use a 100L sterile bacteriological wire loop *but only if you have been trained how to use it*. Use a sterile swab to collect secretions from the inside of the cervix. If you have Stuart's transport medium, collect specimens and put them in the transport medium and send them to the laboratory for culture and sensitivity testing. However in a health centre all you can do yourself is to make a smear.

infection. After treatment with sulphadimidine (which does not cure the infection), or after no treatment, the symptoms slowly improve over weeks or months. But the infection does not go.

Complications include:
- acute salpingitis,
- pelvic peritonitis,
- pelvic abscess
- sterility (due to blocked Fallopian tubes),
- abscess in labia,
- septicaemia,
- skin rash, and
- acute infective arthritis.

Tests
Smear some discharge from the urethra *and* (in the female) from inside the cervix, onto a glass slide, fix it by heat and send it to the hospital laboratory for examination for gonorrhoea bacteria.

Send also the serum from 10 ml of blood with a request for a VDRL examination (for syphilis).

Diagnostic features
- Intercourse within previous week.
- Urinary pain and frequency.
- Urethral or vaginal discharge.

Differential diagnosis
Females:
1. Pelvic inflammatory disease after childbirth or miscarriage.
   - Recent childbirth or miscarriage.
   - Discharge 'yellow pus.
   - Pelvic tenderness and or masses.
   - Uterus enlarged and tender.
   - General symptoms and signs of infection.

2. Trichomonal infection.
   - Vulval and vaginal itchiness.
   - Discharge yellow and frothy.
3. Monilia (Candida) infection (thrush).
   - Vulval and vaginal itchiness.
   - Discharge white and thick.
4. Non-gonococcal urethritis of non-specific urethritis type.
   - No diagnostic features in the female.
   - Often mild or no symptoms or signs in the female.
5. Early pregnancy with increase in 'normal' vaginal discharge.
   - Periods late or missed.
   - Uterus enlarged.
   - No pus or trichomal or monilial discharge.
6. Others. See page 128 and a gynaecology book.

Males
1. Non-gonococcal urethritis of non-specific urethritis type.
   - Discharge often less and more watery than gonorrhoea.
   - Discharge often has come after apparently successful treatment of gonorrhoea.
   - Common.
2. Trichomonal urethritis.
   - Rare.
3. Other types.
   - Rare.

Treatment
Treat for gonorrhoea *ALL* clinical cases of gonorrhoea including:
1. All persons with urethral discharges.
2. All persons with 'urinary tract infections' especially young adults if there is a possibility of gonorrhoea.
3. All persons with vaginal infections especially young women if there is a clinical possibility of gonorrhoea.

Find out if there is or was also a sore on the genitalia or anus. If so, treat for syphilis too. Treatment for gonorrhoea is not adequate treatment for syphilis (see page 135).

Treatment for gonorrhoea needs a high concentration of the antibiotic but for only a short time. Treatment for syphilis needs only a low concentration of the antibiotic but for a long time.

Treat the patient immediately.
Give:
1. Ampicillin 3.5 g (7 of the 500 mg capsules or 14 of the 250 mg capsules) *in one dose,* once.
   OR
   Aqueous procaine penicillin 2.88 g 4,800,000 units (16 ml) (2,400,000 units in each buttock) in one dose, once.
   AND
2. Probenecid 1 g (2 tabs) once, together with the ampicillin or the procaine penicillin.

Ask the patient to come back to be checked for cure in 1 week, 3 weeks and 3 months. At the three months visit also check the VDRL again.

If the patient is not cured, or if at first he or she seems to be cured but the condition comes back again, the 3 most likely possibilities are:
1. The 'contact' was not found and treated and the patient is still having intercourse with this infected person.
2. The patient has penicillin (including ampicillin) resistant gonococci.
3. The patient has one of the other causes of urethritis (see Differential Diagnoses above).

Check the patient for all of these possibilities. Take another smear for gonococci.

Treat Monilia (Candida or thrush) vaginitis with nystatin vaginal tablets or pessaries 1 each night for 2 weeks. If these or other antifungal vaginal tablets are not available all that can be done is paint inside the vagina daily with 1% crystal violet solution in water.

Treat trichomonal infection with metronidazole 2000 mg (10 tablets) in one dose or with 200 mg (1 tab) three times a day for a week. Give to both the patient and the patient's sexual partner.

Treat non-gonococcal urethritis of non-specific urethritis type or penicillin resistant gonococci with tetracycline 500 mg (2 caps) four times a day for 10 days. (See below if pregnant or could be pregnant.) Give to the patient and the patient's sexual parther.

Do not give tetracycline or metronidazole to a patient who is pregnant – refer or non-urgently transfer the patient to a medical officer.

Refer/Transfer
Refer or non-urgently transfer to a medical officer:
1. Patients not cured by the proper management;

2. Patients who cannot be managed by the above management, e.g. both allergic to penicillin and pregnant.

Control and prevention
See page 129.

In gonorrhoea all sexual contacts for 2 weeks before the patient developed symptoms should be found, examined if possible, but treated anyway (as not all infected people have symptoms).

Syphilis

Syphilis is a bacterial infection which causes a sore where the organism enters the body. This sore heals without treatment. However, the bacteria spread all through the body and cause serious subacute and chronic disease of many organs.

Epidemiology
Syphilis is common especially among young adults. The cause is the syphilis bacterium (*Treponema pallidum*). The only host is man.

The disease usually spreads from an infectious lesion (chancre, mucous patch or condyloma) during sexual intercourse. The organisms can enter a new person through broken skin or normal unbroken mucous membrane of the genitalia or mouth.

Previous infection with the similar yaws bacterium gives some immunity against syphilis.

Symptoms and signs, course and complications
Primary syphilis causes a chancre and enlarged lymph glands.
1. The chancre is the lesion at the site of infection (usually genitalia but can also be anus or mouth) (see Figures 19.6 and 19.7). First a painless lump develops. It soon ulcerates in the centre and clear fluid oozes from it. It is firm and hard, 'like a button' in the skin. It usually heals after 2–6 weeks, even without treatment. It may look different if secondary bacterial infection occurs.

> Therefore any ulcer of the genitalia is treated as syphilis no matter what it looks like.

A female patient may not know she has a chancre if occurs in the vagina or on the cervix.
2. The nearby lymph glands are usually hard but not tender.

Figure 19.6 Primary syphilis. A chancre on the penis. Note however, that any ulcer on the genetalia is first treated as syphilis no matter what it looks like.

Figure 19.7 Primary syphilis. Chancre on the vulva. Note the fairly typical appearance (see text). However all ulcers in the genetalia are treated first for syphilis. Note also that in females the chancre may be in the vagina or on the cervix and not be noticed by the patient.

Secondary syphilis usually comes about 6 weeks after the primary sore heals. (But it can be earlier or much later.) There may be any or all of these common lesions:

1. A skin rash with bilateral (on both sides) round, red, non-itchy flat patches 5–10 mm in diameter.
2. A skin rash with bilateral red, non-itchy lumps which may become scaly or turn into pustules.
3. A skin rash called condylomata lata in warm moist areas such as the perineum, vulva (see Figure 19.8), scrotum, inner thighs, under breasts, etc. The above lumps here get bigger and the surface skin comes off to produce large painless raised moist grey areas. However, secondary infection may occur and change the appearance.

> Therefore any wet skin lesions in groin, perineum, axilla, etc. must be suspected of being syphilis.

Figure 19.8 Secondary syphilis condylomata lata of vulva and perineum.

4. Mucous patches are painless, shallow grey ulcers with a narrow red margin (or edge). They occur on the lips or mouth, vulva, vagina, scrotum and penis.
5. Painless enlargement of all lymph nodes of the body.
6. General symptoms and signs of infection, e.g. malaise, fever, loss of appetite, loss of weight.

Any of these symptoms of the secondary stage are present for 2–6 weeks and then go away, even without treatment. But they may return again many times.

Tertiary syphilis occurs many years later, in 1 out of every 2 or 3 cases. Disease of the heart or brain or other organs occurs. (In some tropical developing countries there have only been a few cases of tertiary syphilis. This is probably because syphilis has not been common for very long, as infection with yaws used to give some immunity to syphilis.)

Congenital syphilis. A child may be infected through the placenta, if his mother has syphilis. The child may be born dead or develop any of the signs of secondary or tertiary syphilis.

Tests
Send the serum of 10 ml of blood to the laboratory for a VDRL test.

The VDRL is positive in 2 out of 3 cases of primary syphilis.

The VDRL is positive in nearly all cases of secondary syphilis.

Diagnostic features
- Sexual contact about 3 weeks before.
- Hard, painless ulcerated sore on genitalia (or other area) with enlarged non-tender lymph nodes nearby. The sore heals after 2–6 weeks. However, you should suspect syphilis in all ulcers on the genitalia.
- Two to six weeks later, skin rashes, condylomata lata, mucous patches, general symptoms and signs, and possibly disease of other organs can occur.

Treatment
Before giving treatment ask the patient about previous or present symptoms of gonorrhoea. If the patient has symptoms of gonorrhoea do tests and give treatment for gonorrhoea (see page 132) as well as the treatment for syphilis (which will not cure gonorrhoea).

> Treatment for syphilis needs only a low concentration of the antibiotic but for a long time. Treatment for gonorrhoea needs a high concentration of the antibiotic but for only a short time.

The best treatment for syphilis is an immediate injection of a long acting penicillin in case the patient does not come back for the results of tests or for further treatment.

Give IMI benzathine penicillin 2,400,000 units (5 ml) immediately once. The dose can be divided into 2½ ml into each buttock.

If benzathine penicillin not available, *use* instead *either*:

1. Aqueous procaine penicillin 600,000–900,000 units every day for 8 days *or*
2. Procaine penicillin in oil with 2% aluminium monosterate (PAM) 2,400,000 units (8 ml) immediately then 1,200,000 units (4 ml) 3 days later and again 6 days later.

Ask the patient to return for another clinical examination in 2 weeks. If the patient is not cured, investigate and treat for the other likely causes (see page 128).

Even if the patient appears to be cured, ask him or her to return for another clinical examination and another VDRL in 3 months, 9 months and 2 years to make sure he is cured. If the patient is not cured, refer or transfer him non-urgently to a medical officer.

Control and prevention

See 'Control and Prevention' page 129.

1. Before you give treatment, write the patient's name and address in the STD Register. Also write down the names and addresses of the patient's regular sexual partner and all other sexual contacts since the sore appeared and for 3 months before this.
2. Find and treat *all* the patient's contacts (most importantly his regular sexual partner). Also examine them, if possible.
3. If the sore is cured by treatment, you can assume the diagnosis to be syphilis. Confirm the diagnosis in the STD Register.
4. You should examine and test all groups of people who have a high risk of being infected,

and treat them if necessary. These groups include:
   (a) patients who think that they have STD,
   (b) industrial and plantation workers (every year),
   (c) prostitutes (every month), and
   (d) people in prisons and similar institutions.
5. In areas where yaws is uncommon and syphilis occurs, do a VDRL on all pregnant women. Treat the woman if the VDRL is positive to stop congenital syphilis in her baby.

Granuloma inguinale or Donovanosis

Donovanosis is caused by a bacterial infection; but the organism is not very infectious.

The first lesion is usually a lump on one part of the genitalia. The lump soon develops into an ulcer. The ulcer is usually irregular at its edges and bright red, because it is full of granulation tissue and is not covered with a crust. The ulcer is not painful. The ulcer only slowly (many weeks) gets bigger. (See Figure 19.9)

New lesions can appear on the genitalia; especially in places the first lesion touches.

The lymph nodes in the groin become enlarged and then ulcerate through the skin. An ulcer similar to the one on the genitalia develops and

Figure 19.9 Donovanosis. Ulcer on the penis filled with areas of granulation tissue.

Figure 19.10 Donovanosis. Vulval ulcer and granulations with spread of the disease to the lymph glands in the groin, which have ulcerated.

slowly gets bigger. (This is why the disease is called granuloma inguinale.) (See Figure 19.10.)

If not treated, the lesions all slowly get bigger and destroy a lot of tissue. Occasionally the organism can spread to other parts of the body and start ulcers there too. After many years, if not treated, cancer can form in the edges of some lesions.

Diagnosis is often possible by a simple test which can be sent to the laboratory. Clean the sore with saline. Local anaesthetic is not needed. Cut a *small thin* slice from the top of the edge of the sore with a sterile scalpel or razor blade. Smear the cut side on a glass slide. Fix it with alcohol. Send it to the laboratory with a request for examination for 'Donovan bodies'. This is often positive if the disease is Donovanosis. A proper biopsy would be diagnostic; but it is not usually needed.

For differential diagnosis and management see pages 128 and 140.

Treatment is by tetracycline 500 mg (2 caps) four times a day for 2 weeks. Chloramphenicol may be needed in some countries where the organism is resistant to tetracycline. Streptomycin is effective; but do not give streptomycin as you should keep it for only tuberculosis (see Chapter 11 page 43). See page 141.

Control and prevention (see page 129): you need only trace and examine the regular sexual partner, as the disease is not very infectious.

Amoebic ulceration of the genitalia

Amoebic ulcers are caused by a protozoal organism which normally lives in the bowel (see Chapter 23 page 231).

The lesion starts on or near the genitalia because of: direct spread of the organism from the anus; or rectal intercourse; or intercourse with a person who has a genital amoebic ulcer.

The lesion is usually a fast growing (in days to weeks) painful ulcer which destroys much tissue. The ulcer is usually reddish in colour and covered with grey-white pus. If it is very acute, the discharge may be like watery blood. The lymph nodes nearby are usually enlarged and tender. (See Figure 19.11.)

Occasionally the lesion may grow more slowly and look like a cancer of the penis, vulva or cervix.

Diagnosis can be made by immediate microscopic examination of discharge from the edge of the ulcer for *Entamoeba histolytica*; but this is not possible in a health centre. A biopsy would be diagnostic, but is not usually needed.

Treat with metronidazole 800 mg (4 tablets) three times a day for 5 days. If nausea occurs, reduce the dose of metronidazole to 400 mg (2

Figure 19.11 A small amoebic ulcer of the penis. The ulcer did not improve after penicillin or after tetracycline. The patient was therefore treated with metronidazole and was cured. (A smear taken from the edge of the ulcer before metronidazole was given and immediately examined under the microscope showed amoebae.) Often amoebic ulcers are much larger than this ulcer.

tablets) three times a day but continue for 10 days. Warn the patient not to drink alcohol while taking metronidazole. Give tetracycline together with the metronidazole if acute inflamation is present.

Lymphogranuloma venereum

Lymphogranuloma venereum is caused by a bacterial infection.

One to three weeks after infection, a small blister or ulcer appears on the genitalia which is usually not noticed. About 2–6 weeks later the lymph nodes in the groin become enlarged and inflamed. Pus forms in the lymph nodes which then burst. (See Figure 19.12) As more and more nodes are affected, many abscesses discharging whitish fluid develop. Abscesses can join to make large ulcers. The area affected increases. Some times abscesses and ulcers form in the anal region.

During this time the patient may have general symptoms and signs of infection such as malaise, fever, etc.

After some months the ulcers usually get better. But there is often a lot of deformity left. There may be strictures (narrowing) of the rectum or urethra or vulva. There may also be chronic oedema of the genitalia.

Special tests are needed for definite diagnosis. Biopsy would also be diagnostic; but it is not usually needed.

Treatment is with either tetracycline 500 mg (2 caps) four times a day until the infection goes; but you can also give sulphonamides. You should aspirate any pus from lymph nodes. Treatment may be needed for some weeks.

Control and prevention – see page 129.

Chancroid (soft sore)

Chancroid is an infection caused by special bacteria.

A small lump appears on the genitalia. The lump is on the surface of the skin or mucous membrane (different from syphilis, which is in the skin). The lump soon ulcerates. The edge of the ulcer is irregular and red, and it is covered with dirty pus (see Figure 19.13). The sore is very painful. Where the ulcer touches other parts of the body, new ulcers may appear. The ulcers are soft (again different from syphilis).

The lymph nodes in the groin on one or both sides become swollen, painful and tender. These inflamed lymph nodes often form a fluid-filled (fluctuant) mass which bursts to leave a large ulcer.

Figure 19.12 Lymphogranuloma venereum.

Figure 19.13 Chancroid (soft sore).

Diagnosis is possible in a laboratory by examining the discharge from an ulcer under the microscope.

Treatment is with a sulphonamide (e.g. sulphadimidine 1 g (2 tabs) four times a day) or tetracycline 500 mg (2 caps) four times a day until cured (usually about 2 weeks). If lymph nodes look as if they will burst, then aspirate (suck out) the pus through a needle before this happens.

Control and prevention – see page 129.

Venereal warts (condylomata accuminata)

Venereal warts are caused by a virus infection.

The warts are most common under the foreskin and on (and often around) the glans penis of the male. They are found on (and often around) the vulva and in the vagina and on the cervix of the female. They may also occur in the urethra and around the anus in both sexes.

The warts are soft pink fleshy growths like a cauliflower. There may be very many of them. They may grow very big. (See Figures 19.14 and 19.15.)

Figure 19.15 Venerial warts (also called condylomata accuminata) of the vulva and anus.

Figure 19.14 Venerial warts (also called condylomata accuminata) of the penis.

Treatment is difficult. You should treat any genital discharge (see page 132). Regular washing with soap and water will help. Paint the warts with podophyllin 20% in tincture of benzoin or touch them with a silver nitrate stick. Do not use podophyllin during pregnancy. Do not put any podophyllin or silver nitrate on any normal part of the body. Repeat the treatment each week or two until the warts are gone.

Control and prevention – see page 129.

Herpes genitalis

Herpes genitalis is a viral infection.

Infection with herpes genitalis virus causes a number of small vesicles (blisters) to come up on the mucous membranes of the genitalia (glans penis, labia, cervix). The vesicles burst, and shallow ulcers develop (see Figure 19.16). Some ulcers join. The ulcers look like the 'cold sores' which appear on the lips during fever. The surface of the ulcer is green-grey or white. Near the ulcer

Figure 19.16 Herpes genitalis of the penis. Note the small vesicles on the glans. They soon burst to become ulcers and are very painful.

the mucous membrane is red. The ulcers are very painful, especially if urine touches them. The ulcers may look different if they have secondary bacterial infection.

The lymph nodes in the groin are sometimes large, firm and tender.

During a first infection the patient may have the general symptoms and signs of infection – fever, malaise, etc.

The condition usually goes away after some weeks; but it may return many times.

If a pregnant woman has the infection at the time of birth, the child may be infected at birth and get a severe infection and die. Caeserian section may be needed. Discuss such cases with a medical officer.

No treatment available in health centres cures the condition. Keep the affected area clean and dry. You can give the patient crystal violet 1% in water solution to put on the ulcers.

Control and prevention – see page 129. But as there is no treatment possible, it is not usually necessary to find contacts.

Other genital conditions

Balanitis

Balanitis is inflammation of the glans penis and the foreskin. It is more common in those who are uncircumcised, those who have phimosis, those who have diabetes and those who do not regularly wash under the foreskin. The inflammation can be caused by various types of organisms including bacteria, fungi and trichomonas.

The patient complains of a penile discharge; but on inspection the discharge is seen to come from under the foreskin and not the urethra. The glans penis is red, inflamed and some times ulcerated. The foreskin is inflamed and some times gangrenous.

Test the urine for sugar and refer or non-urgently transfer the patient for treatment, if he has diabetes.

Treatment includes benzathine penicillin 2,400,000 units (5 ml) IMI immediately in case it is syphilis.

The patient should wash the area regularly twice every day and apply gentian violet in water solution twice every day.

If the patient does not improve quickly give treatment with tetracycline and metronidazole (see page 141).

Prevention is by good personal hygiene.

Traumatic sores of penis or vulva

There are many causes for these, including small tears during intercourse.

Secondary bacterial infection can occur.

Give local treatment to the sore, e.g. 1% crystal violet in water solution twice daily after washing. As syphilis cannot usually be excluded, give 2,400,000 units (5 ml) of benzathine penicillin. See also page 140. Ask about previous or present symptoms of urethritis. See page 130 if there are symptoms.

Cancer of the penis or vulva

You should suspect cancer in elderly patients who have had an ulcer for some weeks or months. The ulcer is often full of growing tissues with raised, turned out edges (see Figure 19.17). If it has

Figure 19.17 Cancer of the penis. Note that any ulcer which has recently formed and does not get better after treatment with penicillin and then tetracycline and if necessary metronidazole, as well as any chronic ulcer must be referred or transferred to a medical officer for a biopsy to see if it is a cancer.

spread to the lymph nodes, they will be very hard like stones.

Any patient with a very suspicious ulcer should be transferred non-urgently for biopsy or biopsied and the biopsy sent for examination at the laboratory. While waiting for the result, you should treat the patient for amoebic infection as on page 231. If the disease is cancer the only treatment is non-urgent transfer for surgery.

Common diagnostic and treatment problems

All non-specific sores or ulcers on the genitalia or anus

There are three problems in diagnosing and treating patients with genital or anal sores in a health centre.

1. The patients often have secondary infection of the lesions. The lesions therefore do not always look typical of the primary disease.
2. No tests are immediately available. Results of tests sent to the laboratory may take a long time to come back.
3. Patients may not complete a course of treatment. If the patient has syphilis and is not given a curative dose of treatment on his or her first examination, the patient may not recieve long enough treatment with tetracycline or other drugs to cure syphilis. It is best therefore always to treat the patient for syphilis with benzathine penicillin when you first see them.

The following is a regimen which may suit the conditions in which you work.

Send the serum from 10 ml of clotted blood to the laboratory with a request for the VDRL test.

Write the patient's name and address in the STD Register.

Write down the names and addresses of the patient's regular sexual partner and all other sexual contacts since the sore appeared and for 3 months before this.

Educate the patient to bring or to send all his or her contacts (and anyone else the patient thinks may have the disease to) the health worker.

Ask about previous or present symptoms of gonorrhoea (discharge or urinary pain or frequency). If they are present, do tests (page 131) and give treatment (page 132) for gonorrhoea *as well as* the following treatment.

Do all this before giving treatment.

Treatment

1. (a) Treat as an outpatient.

(b) Give benzathine penicillin[1] 2,400,000 units (5 ml) (1,200,000 units (2½ ml) IMI each buttock) stat once. (Treatment for syphilis and traumatic or non-specific sore.)

(c) Give the same treatment to the patient's regular sexual partner. If possible, also examine him or her.

(d) See the patient again in 7 and in 14 days. If the sore is imprived by 7 days and healed by 14 days, see 1 (e) below. If the sore does not get better, see 2 page 141.

---

1 If benzathine penicillin is not available *use:*
either aqueous procaine penicillin 600,000–900,000 units (2–3 ml) daily for 8 days.
or
procaine penicillin in oil with 2% aluminium monosterate (PAM) 2,400,000 units (8 ml) stat then 1,200,000 units (4 ml) 3 days later and again 6 days later.

(e) If the sore gets better, assume the diagnosis is syphilis. Write the patient's diagnosis in the STD register (mark definitely syphilis). Then check that the patient's sexual contacts have been found, examined (if possible) and treated with penicillin (even if they had no symptoms and signs or if they refused examination).

(f) Ask the patient to return for another clinical examination and another VDRL 3 months, 9 months and 2 years after treatment to make sure he is cured. If he is not cured, transfer him non-urgently to a Medical Officer.

2. If sore does not improve in 7 days or heal in 14 days:

(a) Treat as an inpatient.

(b) Make a smear for Donovan bodies (see page 138).

(c) Give tetracycline 500 mg (2 caps) four times a day for two weeks. If the sore is healing, continue the tetracycline until the sore is healed. (This is treatment for Donovanosis, lymphogranuloma venereum, chancroid and traumatic or non-specific sore.)

Aspirate (suck out) through a needle pus from any fluctuant lymph gland.

Give local treatment to the skin lesion

(d) Examine the patient's regular sexual partner again and treat if the disease is present.

3. If the sore is not healing well after 2 weeks of tetracycline, continue the tetracycline.

Also treat with metronidazole 800 mg (4 tabs) three times a day for 5 days. (This is treatment for amoebic ulcer.)

4. If the sore is not healed or is not still improving after 1, 2 and 3, arrange either biopsy or transfer to medical officer care of diagnosis and treatment (non-urgent).

Urethral discharge

See page 128.

Acquired immune deficiency syndrome (AIDS)

Acquired Immune Deficiency Syndrome (AIDS) is not a true sexually transmitted disease. It is included in this chapter because sexual transmission is a significant means of spread. Also, in large hospitals, AIDS is usually the concern of clinics dealing with sexually transmitted diseases.

AIDS can be an acute but is usually a chronic disease. Some monkeys are infected; but in them the infection may cause little disease. The infection probably passed from monkeys to man recently. However, AIDS was not recognised until 1981. AIDS has affected many ordinary adults and children in an epidemic in sub-saharan Africa over the last 10 or so years. It has caused small epidemics in certain other populations especially Haitians, male homosexuals and intravenous drug addicts.

AIDS is caused by infection with a special virus (HTLV-III).

The virus is spread in a way similar to Hepatitis B (serum hepatitis). The AIDS virus is present in the blood of infected people who may be either sick with AIDS or apparently healthy carriers. The virus *may be* in some of the body secretions such as semen. Infected blood or possibly other infected secretions (and only a very small amount of blood is needed) from a person infected with the AIDS virus may get into the body of another person through sexual intercourse (both normal heterosexual intercourse and even more easily by male homosexual intercoures). Transmission can also result from close physical contact, such as occurs in overcrowed schools and houses, if the infected person has an open wound or abrasion or sore. Transmission of course occurs from an infected blood transfusion or from needles or syringes not properly cleaned and sterilised after use.

Some weeks after infection a non-specific influenza-like illness may occur. There may be fever, sweating, malaise, tiredness, loss of appetite, pain in muscles or joints, headache, sore throat, diarrhoea, enlargement of all the lymph nodes in the body or a vague, flat, reddish rash on the trunk. The virus has spread all over the body. There is no way this illness can be diagnosed as AIDS in the health centre.

Infants may not fully recover from the above illness and may 'fail to thrive' or within weeks or months they may develop one or more of the complications below. However, most adults seem to recover and stay apparently well for months or years. Nevertheless the virus is alive and in the infected person's body and is able to infect others. It often also slowly damages special parts of the body including the brain and some of the immune system (including T lymphocytes) in the blood, lymph nodes, spleen and liver.

After some months or years, symptoms or signs may develop due to: (1) damage to some of the body's organs such as the brain or lymph nodes by the virus and/or (2) unusual infections which have developed because of loss of part of the body's immune system; and/or (3) unusual tumours. These symtoms and signs of AIDS include any one or group of the following.

1. Encephalitis (see Chapter 25 page 260) or chronic organic psychosis (see Chapter 35 page 388) or chronic infections of the meninges or brain (see Chapter 25 page 256) or tumour in the brain.
2. Enlarged lymph nodes (other than the inguinal or groin nodes which are often enlarged from chronic bacterial or filarial infections).
3. Kaposi's sarcoma. When this develops there may be an itching or burning feeling in part of the skin or an area of swelling in the skin for several weeks. Later a firm tender nodule about 0.5 cm in diameter comes up under the skin. It is often dark and can look like a bruise. It often seems to empty if it is pressed, but fills again when the pressure is taken away. The nodule is often surrounded with swelling due to oedema. Some lesions can be larger and flatter. Nodules can ulcerate through the skin. The nodules usually come first on the hands or feet. The main complaint is pain. New nodules then come up in surrounding areas. All parts of the body can have nodules in or on them.
4. Weight loss.
5. Fever ('PUO') (often due to a virus infection if not due to one of the following infections).
6. Lung infection with unusual organisms when symptoms and signs can vary from those of only a cough and fever with no abnormal chest signs, to an illness which looks like tuberculosis, to a pneumonia.
7. Gastro-enteritis because of infection with unusual organisms, which can cause chronic diarrhoea, weight loss, abdominal pain and other symptoms; as well as thrush (*Candida* or *Monilia*) infection in the mouth.
8. Miliary tuberculosis.
9. Malaria in persons previously 'immune'.
10. Septicaemia.

The diagnosis of AIDS could be suspected if the following things occur. The more of the following things that are present, the more likely it is for AIDS to be the diagnosis.

1. If the influenza-type illness or any of the above conditions occurred in your patient.
2. If the patient would not be expected to get a serious illness (was an otherwise healthy adult).
3. If AIDS is common in your area.
4. If the patient is from one of the groups of people who are likely to get the disease (male homosexuals, prostitutes, etc.).
5. If the illness does not get better with the usual treatment or comes back after treatment.

There is no test possible for the disease in the health centre. In some countries a special and expensive blood test for HTLV-III antibodies can be done in large hospitals. As the antibodies do not kill the virus which is present in the body cells, most of the patients with a positive antibody test do have the infection and are infectious.

No treatment is possible to cure the HTLV-III virus infection. Not all patients who have the infection have yet developed one of the conditions (see above) caused by the infection. The drugs needed for treatment of some of the chest and bowel and other infections and cancers caused by

Figure 19.18 Kaposi's sarcoma. Note the typical features – a nodule which is dark, surrounded with oedema, is painful, is on the hands or feet and is in a young man. Think of AIDS in such a patient.

AIDS are not available in a health centre and are expensive and have serious side effects, and may not be given even in a hospital. As well as this, the infection often returns after treatment. In most health centres the usual treatment outlined in other sections of this book is all the treatment possible.

Patients are usually treated in a normal health centre ward. However, if AIDS is suspected or proven then all the measures as for Hepatitis B (see Chapter 24 page 243) and as set out below are taken.

1. Kill the organisms in the body of the original host or reservoir. This is not yet possible.
2. Stop the means of spread. General measures that always apply:
   • Do not transfuse anyone with blood unless it is really needed (in case the donor blood is infected)
   • Always clean and sterilise needles and syringes properly after every patient before using on another patient (in case the first patient is infected).
   • Make sure health workers do not accidently get injuries from needles before they are sterilised.
   • Encourage people not to become drug addicts and especially not to use syringes and needles shared with other people.
   • Do not allow health workers to get blood on them from patients in case the patient's blood is infected. If this does happen, gently wash off the blood.
   • Encourage people to cover wounds and sores so that if the blood is infected it cannot get onto other people.
   • Clean all blood from contaminated instruments etc. (whilst wearing gloves and gown and mask) and sterilise by boiling for 10–30 minutes; or sodium hypochlorite solution, 10,000 ppm chlorine for 30 minutes; or alcohol 70% with either cetrimide 5% or chlorhexidine 0.5% or both for 1 hour; or gluteraldehyde 2% solution (prepared no more than 24 hours before) for 1 hour.
   • Encourage people not to have sexual intercourse with prostitutes or other people likely to have AIDS; or if they do, to at least use a condom.
   • Discourage male homosexuals from having sexual intercourse with other males and especially many partners; or if they do, to at least use a condom.

If a patient is known to have AIDS:
   • Advise this patient not to have sexual intercourse with other than his/her spouse or present partner and that the use of a condom may give some protection to the partner.
   • Advise this patient against pregnancy.
   • Advise this patient he or she must not donate blood.
   • Advise this patient to cover sores and wounds and not get his or her blood on other people.
   • Take measures, such as the use of masks, to avoid inhaling secretions coughed out by patients with AIDS who have a chest infection, especially if they have haemoptysis.
3. Increase the resistance of possible new hosts. This is not possible.

At the time of writing it seems that the action a health worker should take about AIDS will depend on how common the disease is in his or her area, how it is spread in that area and what facilities for diagnosis and treatment exist. You should discuss these with your medical officer. Write down what you should do under this heading and also under the appropriate other headings of 1–10 above.

20

Disorders of the Respiratory System

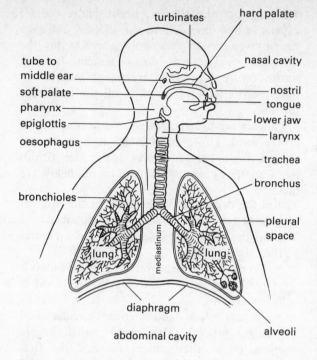

Figure 20.1 Anatomy of the upper and lower respiratory tracts.

Anatomy and physiology

All the cells of the body need oxygen. The cells make carbon dioxide while they work, which must be taken away. If the carbon dioxide is not taken away, it will poison the cells.

Air is about 20% oxygen, 80% nitrogen and much less than 1% carbon dioxide. The body cells take oxygen from the air and excrete carbon dioxide into the air (where it is used by plants which make it into oxygen again).

The oxygen and carbon dioxide are taken to and from the body cells in the blood. The respiratory system is where the body takes the oxygen from the air and puts it into the blood and the carbon dioxide from the blood and puts it into the air. Taking air in and out of the respiratory system is called ventilation. Exchanging the oxygen and carbon dioxide is called respiration.

The respiratory system is in two parts – the

Figure 20.2 Diagrams to show the position of the paranasal sinuses.

Figure 20.3 Diagrams showing the nasal cavity as if the head were cut in half from the front to back in the centre. The top diagram shows structures of the lateral (side) wall. In the bottom diagram parts of the conchae are removed to show the way the paranasal sinuses and naso-lacrimal duct (see Figure 31.1) drain into the nasal cavity.

upper respiratory tract and the lower respiratory tract (see Figure 20.1).

The upper respiratory tract is above the lowest part of the larynx or voice box. The work of the upper respiratory tract includes taking air to and from the lower respiratory tract, and warming, moistening, filtering and purifying the air; also and speech, hearing and other things. The upper respiratory tract is often called the 'URT' or the ear, nose and throat 'ENT'. Figures 20.2, 20.3, 20.4 and 20.5 show the parts of the upper respiratory tract.

The lower respiratory tract consists of the trachea, bronchi and lungs (see Figure 20.1).

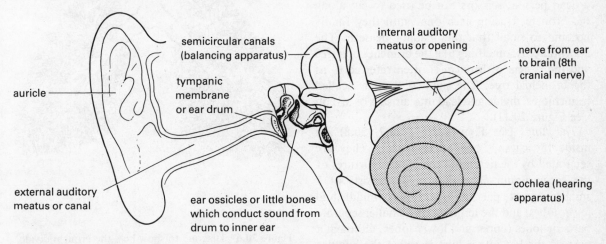

Figure 20.4 Diagram to show the ear especially its subdivisions into outer middle and inner ear and its anatomy. The middle ear is connected to the nasopharynx (back of the nose and throat) by means of the Eustachian or pharyngo-tympanic tube or canal.

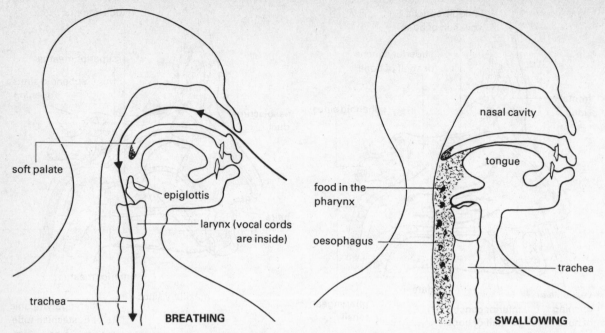

soft palate

epiglottis

larynx (vocal cords are inside)

trachea

BREATHING

nasal cavity

tongue

food in the pharynx

oesophagus

trachea

SWALLOWING

Figure 20.5 This diagram shows the changes in the upper respiratory tract during breathing and swallowing. Note the positions during swallowing of the soft palate (to stop food going into the nose) and of the epiglottis (to stop food going into the larynx and trachea, bronchi and lungs). This does not occur when the patient is deeply unconscious.

Air is taken to the lungs by air passages. Air enters the mouth or nose, goes through the larynx then down the trachea, which divides into two main bronchi. Each main bronchus divides into smaller and smaller bronchi (see Figures 20.1 and 20.6). The smallest bronchi end in little air bags or sacs known as alveoli. If the lungs are taken from a dead person, scissors can be used to cut along the bronchi, tracing each one, until they finally become so small that they cannot be seen. The appearance is something like the branches of a tree and the system of bronchi is often referred to as the bronchial tree. The smallest bronchi, called bronchioles, divide and lead into air sacs or alveoli (see Figure 20.11).

The lungs (see Figures 20.1, 20.7, 20.8) are inside the chest – one on each side. They are separated by the heart and the other structures of the mediastinum. The right lung consists of 3 smaller separate parts or lobes (upper, middle and lower lobes) and the left lung of 2 smaller separate parts or lobes (upper and lower lobes, although a part of the left upper lobe is called the lingular lobe). Each lobe has one bronchus bringing air to and from it.

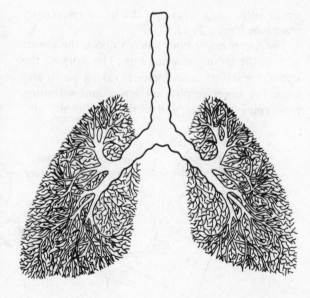

Figure 20.6 Diagram to show how the bronchi divide to form smaller and smaller bronchi (like branches of a tree). The smallest air passages lead into air sacs or alveoli (see Figure 20.11).

146

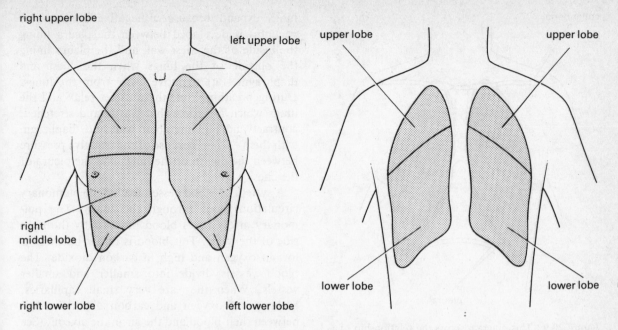

Figure 20.7 Diagrams to show the position of the lungs in the chest and to show which lobes of the lungs are affected when abnormal signs are found during examinaton of the front and back of the chest.

Each lung is surrounded by a thin but strong airtight membrane called the pleural membrane or the pleura. The pleura surrounding and fastened to each lung is in turn surrounded by another layer of pleura which is on the inside of and fastened to the chest wall and the mediastinum. The 2 layers of pleura are not fastened to each other and so can easily move over each other. There is normally nothing between the two layers of pleura, except a thin layer of slippery fluid. (See Figure 20.9.)

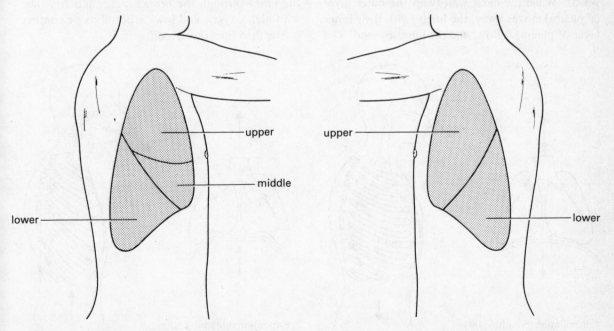

Figure 20.8 Diagram to show the position of the lungs in the chest and to show which lobes of the lung are affected when abnormal signs are found during examination of the lateral (side of the) chest.

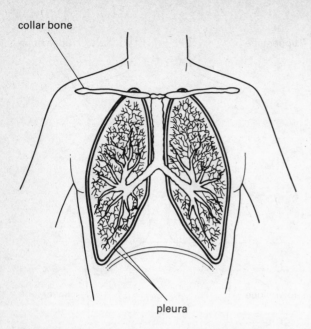

collar bone

pleura

Figure 20.9 This diagram shows the relationship of the two layers of pleura to each other. (See also Figure 20.1.) There is normally no air and only a little fluid in each pleural space or cavity.

Breathing is done by the muscles of the chest wall and the diaphragm (see Figure 20.10). During breathing in, the muscles pull the rib cage outwards and upwards and the diaphragm downwards. When the chest wall (with the outer layer of pleura) moves away, the lungs (with their inner layer of pleura) follow, and the lungs expand. The lungs expand because a negative pressure (or vacuum) is developed between the pleura lining the inside of the chest wall and the pleura lining the outside of the lungs when the chest and diaphragm start to move away from the lungs. During breathing out, the muscles relax and the lungs which are somewhat elastic and stretched, contract and pull the chest wall and diaphragm with them – again because of the negative pressure between the pleura of the lungs and the pleura of the chest wall.

A system of blood vessels (called the pulmonary circulation) goes through the lungs. The pulmonary artery takes blood pumped by the right side of the heart. This blood is rather blue and is low in oxygen and high in carbon dioxide. The blood vessels divide into smaller and smaller vessels. When they are very small capillaries, exchange of oxygen and carbon dioxide occurs between their blood and the air in the alveoli. (See Figure 20.11.) The capillaries then join up to form veins. The blood in them is taken back to the left side of the heart by the pulmonary veins.

The blood in the pulmonary vein is more red, as it has a high content of oxygen and a low content of carbon dioxide.

The left-over air with high carbon dioxide content and low oxygen content is breathed out of the lungs through the bronchi, etc. and fresh air with high oxygen and low carbon dioxide content is breathed into the alveoli.

1. INspiration (breathing in)   2. EXpiration (breathing out)

Figure 20.10 Diagram showing how the ribs and diaphragm are used to ventilate the lungs.

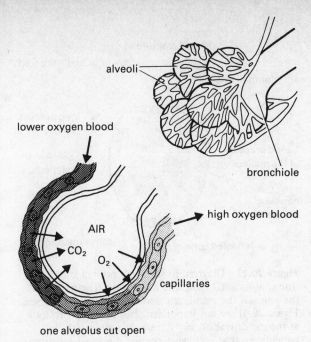

alveoli

lower oxygen blood

bronchiole

high oxygen blood

AIR

CO_2

O_2

capillaries

one alveolus cut open

Figure 20.11 Diagrams showing anatomy and physiology of the small air sacs and blood vessels.

Pathology of the respirtory tract

Most diseases of the respiratory tract are caused by infection. These infections are usually caused by viral, bacterial or tuberculosis organisms; but there are others. Some diseases are caused by allergy, some by smoking and some by dust and fumes in mines or factories. A few are caused by other things known and unknown.

Symptoms and signs of diseases of the respiratory tract

Symptoms of diseases of the upper respiratory tract

Ear
- pain in ear
- discharge from ear
- deafness

Nose
- nasal discharge
  - clear fluid
  - pus
  - blood
- pain in face or forehand (over paranasal sinuses)

Throat
- sore throat
- hoarse voice or loss of voice

All
- cough

For causes and management of these symptoms, see page 158 onwards.

Signs of diseases of the upper respiratory tract

Ear
- external canal
  - discharge (clear fluid, pus, blood)
  - foreign body
  - injury
  - dermatitis
  - inflammation of the whole canal
  - furuncle (pimple or boil)
- drum
  - retraction (pulled in)
  - bulging (pushed out)
  - inflammation (dilated vessels, dull or red or yellow, loss of light reflex, red or yellow)
  - perforation (hole)
- hearing – all degrees of deafness

Nose
- discharge
  - watery fluid
  - pus
  - blood
- mucous membrane
  - inflammation
  - thickened blue-pink 'allergic' appearance

Mouth and throat
- inflammation of all or a part (especially tonsils)
- pus over a part (especially tonsils)
- post-nasal discharge

All
- cough

Use the auriscope to insepct the external ear canal and the ear drum like this:

Hold the auriscope in your right hand. Pull the pinna (outside ear) upwards and backwards with the finger and thumb of the left hand to straighten the external ear canal. Rest your right hand on the side of the patient's face. Then, if the patient suddenly moves, your hand will also move, and the auriscope cannot push into his ear and damage it. Use the largest speculum possible to push into the ear without hurting the patient much.

It may hurt the patient a little to push the speculum of the auriscope into the canal. There may be wax in the canal. Both of these things are normal.

Pain on moving the ear, swelling and redness of the skin lining the canal (either in one area or involving the whole canal), or pus in the canal itself, all suggest inflammation of the external canal (external ear inflammation)

The ear drum is normally white. It also reflects the light, in its lower part, as a bright white triangle called the 'light reflex'.

The ear drum may be retracted (pulled back) if the Eustachian tube is blocked.

The ear drum may be pink or red, small dilated blood vessels may be seen running in from the edge, the light reflex may not be present and fluid levels may be seen behind the drum in early acute inflammation of the middle ear.

A little later in acute middle ear inflammation the drum usually bulges (is pushed out). As it cannot bulge where it is held in the centre by a little bone, the drum then looks like the buttocks of a baby at a breech birth!
The drum may be perforated (broken) and pus may come out of the hole and even fill the ear canal in late acute middle ear inflammation.

If you cannot see the eardrum clearly because of wax or pus in the canal, gently clean the canal with a swab (or by syringing) until you can see the drum clearly.

To test the hearing of an ear
Block the other ear of the patient with one of your fingers which you keep moving in his ear (to make a noise so that he can hear nothing else with that ear); do not let him see your mouth; ask in a quiet voice questions which need answers that are more than just 'yes' or 'no'.

Examination of the nose using a torch
Put the patient's head back and press gently on the end of his nose. This will open the nostrils and allow you to look in.

Red, swollen mucous membrane will be seen in acute rhinitis. If the infection is viral, you may see watery discharge on the mucous membrane. If the infection is bacterial, you may see pus on the

Figure 20.12 Diagram to show the normal left ear drum, also called tympanic membrane. The names of the parts of the membrane and of the small bones (see Figure 20,4) are not important. It is important to look at the ear drums of may normal as well as sick patients, so that you can recognise a normal ear drum.

mucous membrane.

A blue or pale, swollen, watery-looking mucous membrance suggests an allergic rhinitis or hay fever.

Tenderness of sinuses
Tenderness can be tested for by pressing firmly or tapping the bones containing the sinuses (above and below the eyes).

Examination of the mouth and throat, using a torch and tongue depressor.
Examine the inside of the mouth, the tongue, the soft palate, the tonsils and the back of the throat for redness and swelling and pus from acute inflammation. You may need to press the tongue down and ask the patient to say 'Ah' to see the back of the throat wall. You may see pus from the nose running down the back of the throat (called post-nasal discharge or drip).

Symptoms of disease of the lower respiratory tract (lung)

Cough
Sputum
– white (mucus)
– yellow or green or brown (pus)
– jellylike (mucus)
Haemoptysis (blood in sputum)

Table 20.1. Summary of the symptoms and signs of the common lung diseases

	Pneumo-thorax	Fluid in pleural cavity	Lobar pneumonia	Broncho-pneumonia	Acute bronchitis	Asthma	Chronic bronchitis (COLD)**	Bronchiec-tasis	Laryngeal or tracheal obstruction
Temperature	varies	varies	*raised	often raised	*often raised	*normal NOT raised	*normal	sometimes raised	varies
Sputum	varies	varies	*pus	pus	*pus sometimes	*thick mucus NOT pus	*mucus	*pus or mucus	varies
Respiration rate	sometimes fast	sometimes fast	*fast	often fast	sometimes fast	slow	usually normal	normal	slow
Respiration type	sometimes shallow	sometimes shallow	*shallow	often shallow	normal	deep	usually normal	normal	*deep stridor
Movement	*decreased	*decreased	*decreased	normal	normal	decreased	decreased	normal	normal or decreased
Percussion	very resonant	*very dull 'stony' dull	*dull	normal	normal	normal or more resonant	normal or more resonant	normal	normal
Breath sounds	*reduced or absent	*reduced or absent	*reduced	normal	normal	normal or reduced	normal or reduced	normal	normal or reduced
Type of breath sounds	varies or absent	varies or absent	*bronchial	normal	normal	normal	normal	normal	normal
Wheezes or rhonchi	none	none	none	none	usually present	*present	present	none	*stridor
Crackles or crepitations	none	none	*present	*present	usually absent	usually absent	usually absent	*present	none

* These are the important signs for this condition
**Chronic obstructive lung disease (COLD)

151

Pain in chest
- tracheal (in the front of the neck or centre of the chest present only on coughing)
- pleural (at the side of the chest more on breathing or coughing)
Shortness of breath
Wheezing
For causes and management of these symptoms, see page 158 onwards.

Table 20.1 summarises the symptoms and signs of the common lung diseases.

Signs of disease of the lower respiratory tract (LRT)

Examine for
- Rate of respiration (normal 16–20/minute)
- Type of respiration (deep or shallow; use of extra muscles; insuction; grunting; prolonged expiration, etc.)
- Deformity of chest or spine.

Palpate for
- Decreased movement of (1) all of chest, (2) part or parts of chest.

Percuss for
- Dullness or abnormal resonance of all of chest or part or parts of chest.

Auscultate for
- Amount of breath sounds normal or decreased
- Breath sounds (bronchial instead of normal) in
- Crackles (or crepitations)
- Wheezes (or rhonchi)

all of chest

part or parts of chest

Ask the patient to cough. Listen to type of cough.
Examine any sputum (pus? mucus? blood?)

Examination of the rate and type of respiration (or breathing)

The normal rate is 16–20 breaths/minute. The type of respiration is, however, often more important than the rate.

Is the patient distressed or not? Is the patient taking rapid shallow respirations which suggest pneumonia, or deep wheezing respirations which suggest asthma? Is there any indrawing of the soft tissues above and below the clavicle and between

and below the ribs ('insuction') and dilation of the nostrils on breathing in? Is there grunting during breathing out? Insuction, dilation of the nose and grunting mean that the patient is having to do much extra work in order to breathe. This is common in pneumonia (especially in children), and in asthma and chronic respiratory disease (especially in the old).

Wheezing is when you hear the whistling noises of the air moving through the air passages without the stethoscope. The causes are the same as for rhonchi or wheezes heard with a stethoscope (see page 155).

Stridor is when you hear a loud whistling or crowing noise during breathing *in*. (Noisy breathing *out* is not as important.) It is caused by obstruction of the larynx or trachea. Stridor is always dangerous. Stridor is very dangerous if there is also insuction, rib recession (lower ribs moving *in* not *out* during breathing in), and the neck and abdominal muscles are being used for breathing.

Ask the patient to take a deep breath and look at the chest movement once again. Stand back from the patient when looking for these signs. See how well the chest moves. If he has great difficulty in moving the chest wall, it is said the chest wall is 'fixed'. This is a sign of chronic respiratory disease. Is one side moving and the other not moving? The side which does not move is the side with the disease in it.

Palpation of the chest

Palpate the chest to find out if there is decreased movement of (1) all of the chest, or (2) part or parts of the chest.

You must find out from examining many normal people how much chest movement is normal – it is usually more than 1 cm on each side.

Disease affecting all of the lungs will cause decreased movement of all of the chest and the same amount of decrease on both sides. This decreased movement of all the chest is caused by chronic obstructive lung disease and acute asthma.

Disease of one part of the lung causes decreased movement of the chest on the same side. This decreased movement of one part of the chest is caused by lobar pneumonia, tuberculous pneumonia, pleural fluid, lung cancer and pneumothorax.

Figure 20.13 Photographs to show method of palpation of the chest for movement. Press your finger-tips firmly into the lateral chest wall so that they stay in the same place between the ribs. Put your finger-tips in such a position that when the patient breathes right out, then the ends of your thumbs just meet in the midline of the spine. (See left photograph.) Then get the patient to take slow deep breath in (and out). Let the palms of your hand and your thumbs slide over the skin; but do not let your finger-tips move. The movement of each side of the chest is shown by how far the ends of your thumbs move away from the spine in the midline. (See right photograph.)

> The side of the chest which moves less is the abnormal side.

Percussion of the chest

Press the middle finger of the left hand firmly over the area you are percussing. Place the finger in the same line or direction as the ribs in that area and between the ribs (over the muscles between the ribs). Percuss or hit the middle of this finger in a light and loose fashion with the bent middle finger of the right hand.

Percuss the chest wall in a systematic fashion. Percuss the sides front and back of the chest wall (see Figure 20.14).

Percuss the *same* part of *each* side of the chest and decide if the percussion note is normal or not and equal or not on both sides before percussing another part.

Feel *and* listen for the type of percussion note. The percussion note may be either dull or resonant (hollow sounding).

Normally the chest over the lungs is resonant, but it may be a little dull if the person is very muscular or fat. The area of resonance moves down 2 to 5 cm during breathing in as the diaphragm moves down and the lungs expand.

Percussion over the heart, liver and large muscle masses in the shoulders will give a dull note.

Percussion over the air in the stomach will give a very resonant note. (see Figure 20.15.)

The percussion note will be dull if anything more solid than lung filled with air is underneath.

The percussion note will be dull over an area of pneumonia because there is a lot of fluid in the alveoli. The percussion note will be very dull when there is pleural fluid as no air is under the chest wall there.

In patients who are acutely ill with breathlessness and fever, see if the precussion causes pain. Pain on percussion is a sign of pleurisy usually due to pneumonia.

The percussion note will be very hollow if only air and not air and lung are underneath the chest wall, e.g. pneumothorax.

Auscultation of the chest

Listen in all areas including the axillae using a

Figure 20.14 The left photograph shows sites for percussion and auscultation of the posterior and lateral chest wall. The right photograph shows sites for percussion and auscultation of the posterior and lateral chest wall.

Figure 20.15 Quality of percussion note over the normal chest. 1. Flat or 'stony' dull. 2. Dull. 3. Resonant (hollow). 4. Very resonant (very hollow).

stethoscope (see Figure 20.14).

Listen in one place and then in the same place on the opposite side of the chest next. Decide if the breath sounds are present or not (air entry is normal or not), if they are normal or not, and if crackles or wheezes are present or not in the *same* places on *both* sides, before you listen to another place on the chest.

It is better to use the bell of the stethoscope when you listen to the breath sounds. Do not press hard when you use the bell.

Listen for three things when you auscultate:

1. *The quantity of the breath sounds* (amount of air entry).

   Compare both sides of the chest and see if breath sounds are the same. The breath sounds may be loud, or soft, or absent. Breath sounds are softer or absent, if less air is entering that part of the lung under the stethoscope. Breath sounds may be softer (or less) over an area of pneumonia and may be softer or even absent over a pleural effusion or empyema. Breath sounds may be soft in all areas if not much air is entering any part of the lung e.g. severe chronic obstructive lung disease or very severe asthma.

2. *Quality of the breath sounds* (type of breath sounds).

   The breath sounds normally have a quality which is a bit like the sound of rubbing the hands together (or the rustling of leaves in a tree). These types of breath sounds are called 'vesicular'.

   Over the trachea the normal breath sounds you hear are louder, and sound something like blowing air over the top of a bottle. These types of breath sounds are called 'bronchial'.

   You hear bronchial breath sounds or bronchial breathing at the chest wall only if something solid *in the lung* (not in the pleura) conducts these breathe sounds from the trachea to the chest wall.

   You hear bronchial breathing only over large areas of pneumonia or tumours (and very occasionally over very large tuberculous cavities, or at the upper level of plural fluid). You do not often hear bronchial breathing in diseases other than pneumonia. Bronchial breath sounds are not always easy to hear; but are very helpful if they are heard.

3. *Added sounds*.

   Added sounds are sounds which are not normally present. There are three kinds of added sounds which you may hear – 'crackles' which used to be called 'crepitations' (crackling or bubbling sounds), 'wheezes' which used to be called 'ronchi' (whistling sounds) and a 'pleural rub' (a rubbing or scraping sound).

   Crackles or *crepitations* are the crackling noises made by alveoli or bronchi which are closed but snap open and vibrate by air bubbling through fluid in alveoli and bronchi. Causes include:

   (a) acute infections of the alveoli (lobar pneumonia, broncho-pneumonia);

   (b) chronic infections of the alveoli (tuberculosis);

   (c) chronic damage to the bronchi with fluid in the bronchi (bronchiectasis);

   (d) oedema of the lungs (left heart failure); and

   (e) Some cases of obstructive lung disease, and after some attacks of asthma.

   Wheezes, which used to be called *ronchi,* are whistling sounds made by air going through narrowed bronchi. (These sounds are also called wheezing, when you do not need a stethoscope to hear them.) They are often louder during breathing out. Causes include:

   (a) asthma,

   (b) acute bronchitis, and

   (c) chronic obstructive lung disease.

   A *pleural rub* is a creaking, grating or rubbing noise usually heard in breathing in and out over one area. It is not changed by coughing (wheezes often are), but may be changed by pressing hard on the chest and thereby changing the position of the pleura. It is caused by pleural inflammation.

The important conditions which produce abnormal chest signs

1. Obstruction of the trachea or larynx e.g.
   • foreign body inhaled,
   • infections e.g. croup, acute bacterial epiglott-itis or laryngo-tracheo-bronchitis,
   • allergy (angio-oedema).
2. Obstruction of the bronchi e.g.
   • pus e.g. acute bronchitis,

- mucus e.g. chronic obstructive lung disease,
- spasm of the muscles e.g. asthma.
3. Fluid in the alveoli e.g.
   - heart failure (left heart),
   - pneumonia (all types).
4. Solid lung (consolidation) e.g.
   - lobar pneumonia.
5. Fluid in the pleural cavity e.g.
   - water – effusion,
   - pus – empyema,
   - blood – haemothorax.
6. Air in the pleural cavity e.g.
   - pneumothorax.

Positions of lung lesions (See Figure 20.7)

Upper lobes or parts	– Suspect tuberculosis
Lower lobes or parts	– Suspect bacterial pneumonia
Right middle lobe or lower front right side of chest	– Suspect tuberculosis and inhaled foreign body as well as ordinary bacterial pneumonia

General symptoms which may be caused by respiratory disease

1. Fever
2. Weight loss
3. Malaise

General signs which may be caused by respiratory disease

1. The temperature may rise in any infective disease.
2. The pulse rate may increase in any infective disease, or any disease of the lungs which does not allow the body to receive enough oxygen.
3. The respiration rate and type of respiration may be abnormal (see page 152).
4. Cyanosis is the blue colour of the blood caused by low oxygen concentration in the haemoglobin of the blood.

   It is easiest to see cyanosis where blood is close to the surface of the body, and there is little or no pigment (e.g. the mucous membranes of the conjunctivae, the tongue and inside the mouth and under the finger nails and toe nails). Cyanosis is caused by haemoglobin which does not have oxygen. (Haemoglobin with oxygen is red. Haemoglobin without oxygen is blue.)

There must be 1.5–5 g of haemoglobin without oxygen in each dl (100 ml) of blood to make the blood look blue. In a very severely anaemic person (with a haemoglobin of less than 5 g/dl) you may not see cyanosis, even if their hoemoglobin does not have much oxygen. They may not have the necessary amount of haemoglobin without oxygen to show the blueness of cyanosis.

If the blood in all parts of the body is blue, i.e. there is cyanosis of the tongue *and* the finger nails and toe nails, this may be caused by:

(a) the patient not breathing enough (for any reason);

(b) some diseases of the lungs, especially pneumonia;

(c) some diseases of the heart;

(d) some poisons in the blood which stop the haemoglobin combining with oxygen (e.g. sodium nitrite in 'anti-rust' tablets).

If only part of the body is cyanosed and blue but the tongue is a normal pink, then the blood must be circulating slowly through the cyanosed area, and most of the oxygen is being taken out before the blood leaves that area.

Be careful not to mistake the blue colour in the pigment or normal colouring of some person's mouths for cyanosis of the lips.

5. Clubbing of the nails. When clubbing occurs, the normal angle between the nail and the finger goes. Later on, the end of the finger may become swollen, and look like the head of a drumstick, (see Figure 20.16.)

Clubbing is usually caused by chronic respiratory diseases, but usually only those caused by chronic infection or cancer. It sometimes occurs in heart disease (especially infective or congenital), chronic liver and bowel disease and other conditions. Very occasionally it is inherited.

Do not confuse clubbing with curved finger nails (which are not important). With curved nails there is still a normal angle between the base (or back or top) of the nail and the back of the finger.

Clubbing does not occur with usual chest infections or even tuberculosis or with chronic obstructive lung disease or with asthma. If clubbing is present look for a serious chronic disease, especially chronic infection of the chest.

Figure 20.16 A patient's hands with severe clubbing of the nails. Note that there is no angle between the proximal (body) end of the thumb nails and the back of the thumb. In this severe clubbing the whole of the end of the finger is swollen. The finger nail does not seen to be firmly attached and seems to be floating (or be fluctuant) on top of the tissues at the end of the finger.

Tests in respiratory disorders

Chest X-ray

A chest X-ray is not possible in a health centre. It also takes a lot of training to be able to understand and use an X-ray properly. Fortunately most conditions can be accurately diagnosed and treated without the use of an X-ray.

Sputum examination for AFB

See Chapter 14 page 69.

Summary of methods of treatment of respiratory diseases

1. Treat infections with antibiotics or, if tuberculosis, anti-tuberculosis drugs.
   Use penicillin first. It is usually effective.
   Give chloramphenicol instead of penicillin if the infection is severe and may cause death.
   Use tetracycline if penicillin does not work and

the patient is not likely to die soon from the infection and especially if he may need repeated courses of antibiotics.
Give chloramphenicol if penicillin and then tetracycline do not work; but look first for reasons why the antibiotics are not working.
Give streptomycin *only* for tuberculosis. Do not use it for any other respiratory infection.
Give at least two antituberculosis drugs to all cases of tuberculosis for at least 12–18 months.

2. Treat bronchial narrowing (causing wheezing and/or rhonchi) like this:
   (a) Treat the cause if possible (antibiotics if infection; stopping smoking if COLD etc.).
   (b) Give adrenaline or salbutomol or terbutaline or orciprenaline or ephedrine (never more than one of these at a time). If these drugs are not effective *add*:
   (c) Aminophylline or theophylline by tablet *or* suppository or IVI or IV drip

3. Remove sputum or pus (if present) like this:
   (a) encourage a patient to breathe deeply and cough sputum up,
   (b) suck out the pharynx if the patient cannot cough,

(c) physiotherapy,

(d) postural drainage,

(e) postural sleeping (with head of bed down). *But* do not continue with any of these methods if less than 15 ml of sputum is produced.

4. Treat a cough like this:

(a) Treat the cause.

(b) Remove the sputum from the chest (See 3 above)

(c) Do *not* give an effective anti-cough drug (e.g. codeine) if the patient has sputum.

(d) Cough medicine ('Mist. tussi') does not help. Give it only if the patient wants medicine very much, and does not need effective drugs.

5. The patient should stop smoking.

It is very important that he does not start smoking again if he has chronic obstructive lung disease (COLD).

6. Treat low oxygen in the blood, which has caused cyanosis of the whole body including the tongue, with intra-nasal oxygen 1–4 litres/minute. Do not give more than 1–2 litres/minute if patient has COLD.

7. Treat swelling of the nasal mucous membrane with:

(a) ephedrine or other vasoconstrictor nasal drops, which narrow the blood vessels and make the swelling of the mucous membrane less

(b) oral antihistamines (e.g. promethazine).

8. Analgesics may be needed for pain. If the pain stops the patient coughing up sputum, give analgesics, but you *must* then make the patient cough up the sputum.

9. Rest and nursing are important for acute severe diseases.

Diseases of the respiratory system

The common cold

The common cold is an acute viral infection of the upper respiratory tract. It can be caused by one of many viruses.

Symptoms may include sneezing, watery nasal discharge, sore throat, cough, watery eyes, mild fever and malaise.

On examination there may be mild fever and red swollen watery mucous membranes of the upper respiratory tract.

There are no abnormal signs in the chest and there is no purulent sputum. There are no signs of severe general disease.

Complications can occur including acute otitis media, acute sinusitis, tonsillitis, acute bronchitis and pneumonia caused by bacteria. (These complications need treatment with antibiotics.)

Treatment

Examine all the respiratory tract to see if there is a complication which needs treatment (especially otitis media).

Treat as an outpatient.

Tell the patient to come back if a complication develops (especially pain in the ear or deafness; or shortness of breath or pus in sputum).

You can only treat the symptoms:

1. Rest may be needed.

2. Give aspirin 300–600 mg (1–2 tablets) each 6 hours if needed for headache or aches and pains.

3. Give ephedrine or other nasal drops, which narrow the blood vessels, if the nose is blocked.

4. Cough mixture does not help. Give it only if the patient wants medicine.

5. Give antimalarials (usually chloroquine) if there is any fever. (See Chapter 13 page 55.)

Influenza

Influenza is an acute viral infection of *all the respiratory tract*. It is caused by one of only a few viruses.

Usually it is an epidemic disease.

Severe general symptoms and signs of infection occur:

- sudden start of the symptoms,
- fever,
- pains all over the body,
- loss of appetite, and
- feeling too sick to walk around.

But only mild respiratory tract infection symptoms and signs occur:

- cough (but no sputum),
- sore throat,
- tracheal pain, and
- slight redness of the upper respiratory mucous membranes.

There is improvement after a few days; but the patient may not get better for two weeks.

The patient may get suddenly worse if he

develops a complication, especially pneumonia or other bacterial infection of the respiratory tract. Pneumonia is more common in old people, or patients with chronic obstructive lung disease. Bacterial pneumonia is the usual cause of death in influenza epidemics.

Treatment

Examine all the respiratory tract, and look at any sputum. Find out if there is a complication (especially pneumonia) which needs treatment.

Treat as an outpatient.

Tell the patient to come back if any complication develops (especially bad cough, shortness of breath or pus in sputum).

Treat the symptoms as for a common cold (see page 158); but rest, aspirin and antimalarial drugs will probably all be needed for some days.

Admit for inpatient treatment if any complications develop (especially pneumonia) and treat these complications in the usual way.

Notify the Health or Medical Officer if an epidemic occurs (e.g. more than 20 cases in 1 month).

Control and prevention are not possible in most places. During an epidemic you may be told to give procaine penicillin (900,000 units (3 ml) daily) to everyone who has a cough. This will help to reduce the number of deaths from secondary bacterial pneumonia.

Immunisation against influenza is possible, but it is expensive and difficult to organise and is usually not possible in most developing countries.

Acute middle ear inflammation (acute otitis media)

Acute middle ear inflammation is a common acute inflammation of the middle ear. It is often caused by bacteria and pus often forms in the middle ear.

Acute middle ear infection often develops with or after a viral or bacterial upper respiratory tract infection, especially if these block the Eustachian tube.

Symptoms include:
* pain and a feeling of fullness in the ear,
* deafness,
* discharge from the ear, if the drum bursts, and
* general symptoms of infection sometimes e.g. fever, malaise, gastro-enteritis.

Signs (see Figure 20.17) can include:
* inflammation of the ear drum (the drum may be pink or red, there may be small blood vessels seen running in from the edge and the normal white colour and light reflex are not seen),
* fluid or pus seen behind the ear drum,
* bulging of the ear drum,
* rupture of the ear drum, with a hole in the drum and pus in the external canal,
* deafness, and
* general signs of infection including raised temperature and pulse rate.

Many cases get better without treatment. Some cases develop complications. These include:
* 'Glue ear' with partial deafness (the acute

Finger 20.17   Left: normal ear drum. Middle: acute otitis media. Right: Otitis media with perforated drum.

infection settles but thick fluid is left filling the middle ear).
• Chronic otitis media (continuing infection in the ear that usually causes the ear drum to burst)
• Acute mastoiditis (a tender swelling of the bone (not just the lymph node) behind the ear develops).
• Meningitis.
• Acute tonsillitis

Treatment
Treat as an outpatient. Admit for inpatient treatment if there is discharge from the ear.
1. Give procaine penicillin 900,000 units (3 ml) IMI daily until cured (6–10 days). Use tetracycline if penicillin is not successful.
2. Give ephedrine or other vasoconstrictor nasal drops four times a day.
3. Tell the patient to blow his nose often (to try to open up the Eustachian tube).
4. Give aspirin 300–600 mg (1–2 tablets) *or* codeine compound tablets (2 tablets) every 6 hours if needed for pain.
5. Give an antimalarial drug (such as chloroquine) if fever (see Chapter 13 page 55).
6. Do ear toilet and put in ear drops (see below) *if* the ear is discharging. Do this daily or more often if there is a lot of discharge. Continue the ear toilet and ear drops until the discharge stops.

Method for ear toilet
Cut the end off a clean size 8 feeding tube (or cut the needle off a used scalp vein set) so that it is about 5 cm (2 inches) long. Put this on to a clean 5 ml or 10 ml syringe.

Draw up 2 ml of clean water (or better still normal saline made with 2½ ml (½ teaspoonful) of salt in 200 ml (1 cup) of clean water).

Put the cut end of the feeding tube *gently* into the ear.

Do not put the tube deep into the ear or you will damage the ear.

Inject the water *slowly* into the ear. Then suck out the water and pus from the ear into the syringe. Throw away this dirty water. Refill the syringe with clean water again. Repeat the treatment until no more pus comes out.

Dry the ear like this – roll up a small piece of soft toilet paper, put it into the ear, leave it there for 1 minute, then take it out.

Look with an auriscope at the canal and drum. If there is still pus, etc., repeat the cleaning with the syringe and the drying with toilet paper. Continue until the drum is seen and the drum and canal are clean and dry.

After use, clean the syringe and feeding tube very well. Then soak them in antiseptic soloution.

This method is very effective and not dangerous.

Another method of doing ear toilet
Clean inside the canal with a *small* piece of cotton wool wrapped around the end of a *very thin* swab stick. Do not push it into the drum. Use a new piece of cotton wool when the cotton wool on the stick becomes dirty or wet. Continue until you can see the canal and drum are clean and dry (through the auriscope). This method is harder for most health workers in health centres to do, and is also less effective.

After the ear toilet put 5 drops of boric acid 3% in alcohol ear drops into the ear.

Transfer
Transfer to Medical Officer care if:
1. the ear drum does not return to normal after 3 weeks of treatment (non-urgent), or
2. acute mastoiditis develops (urgent).

Chronic middle ear infection (chronic otitis media)

Chronic middle ear infection is a chronic infection of the middle ear by bacteria.

It is usually a complication of untreated or badly treated acute middle ear inflammation.

There are symptoms and signs of discharge of pus from the ear from time to time. The ear drum is perforated (has a hole in it) and does not heal. The patient is partly deaf.

Treatment
Treat as an outpatient. Admit for inpatient treatment, if necessary for ear toilet.

Ear toilet and drops daily as for acute middle ear inflammation (see above), until the discharge stops.

Treat as for acute middle ear inflammation (see above) if it suddenly gets worse. Tetracycline

250–500 mg (1–2 caps) four times a day may help if penicillin does not improve the acute infection.

Tell the patient that he must try to keep inside his ear dry (no swimming, care with washing, dry carefully if water does get inside, etc.).

Refer (do not normally transfer) the patient to the next visiting Medical Officer, as some cases need an operation.

External ear inflammation (otitis externa)

External ear inflammation is an acute or a chronic inflammation of the skin of the external canal of the ear. The inflammation is usually caused by an infection with bacteria and occasionally with fungi. This infection often complicates an injury or a chronic non-infective dermatitis (see Chapter 32 page 369) of the skin inside the ear.

There may be inflammation of all of the skin of the canal, often with pus formation. At other times there is a furuncle (pimple or boil) in one area.

Treatment
Treat as an out-patient.
1. Ear toilet and ear drops daily (see page 160).
2. Insert glycerine and ichthammol 10% on a gauze wick deep into the ear canal daily, until the condition is cured or improved enough to use ear drops:
3. Boric acid 3% in alcohol ear drops (3–5 drops after ear toilet). If this does not work, give: crystal violet 1% in alcohol solution (3–5 drops twice daily after ear toilet).
4. Tell the patient to keep the ear dry (no swimming, care with washing) and to dry the inside of the ear carefully if water does get in.
5. Give aspirin 300–600 mg (1–2 tablets) or codeine compound tablets (1–2 tablets) if required every 6 hours for pain.
6. Antibiotics are not usually needed.

If the external ear inflammation returns many times, tell the patient to always keep the inside of the ear dry (no swimming, care during washing, dry carefully if water does get inside, etc.) and to use boric acid 3% in alcohol ear drops or even just alcohol ear drops once or twice weekly even when the ear seems to be well.

Foreign body in the ear

A foreign body in the ear may cause pain or discharge or no symptoms.

If the foreign body is an insect, put an oil into the ear; when the insect is dead, syringe the ear. You can syringe many other foreign bodies out of the ear. However do not put water into the ear if the foreign body is vegetable (e.g. dry bean) and may swell. Instead try sucking on it with the end of a small tube attached to a strong sucker. If you use forceps you can easily push the foreign body further into the ear and damage the ear drum. If the patient is unco-operative or has a lot of pain and you have to use forceps, give a general anaesthetic first.

Acute sinusitis

Acute sinusitis is an acute bacterial infection of one or more of the paranasal sinuses. (See Figures 20.2 and 20.3.)

There are often general symptoms and signs of infection – fever etc.

Local symptoms and signs of inflammation are almost always present as follows.

Pain over the affected sinus. Sometimes there is also a general headache or pain in the nearby teeth or eye.

Tenderness over the affected sinus.

There is often nasal mucous membrane swelling, and pus in the nose and throat.

Treatment
1. Procaine penicillin 900,000 units (3 ml) IMI daily until cured.
2. Ephedrine or other vasoconstrictor nasal drops, 2–3 drops into each nostril four times a day.
3. Aspirin, 300–600 mg (1–2 tablets) or codeine compound tablets (1–2 tablets) every 6 hours if required for pain.
4. Antimalarial drug (usually chloroquine), (see Chapter 13 page 55) if there is fever.
5. If these are not successful, wash out the nose with saline (see page 175).

Foreign body in the nose

The most common symptom caused by a foreign body in the nose is a discharge of pus from one side of the nose.

> If a patient has discharge of pus from one side of the nose always look for a foreign body in the nose.

If you can see the foreign body remove it with forceps. Sometimes you will need general anaesthetic to see and remove the foreign body. If you cannot see the foreign body or if the foreign body is hard or round and you cannot easily hold it with forceps, then try to remove it with a probe. Gently push a thin round-ended metal probe along the floor of the nose (i.e. almost straight in; but pointed a little downwards as well as backwards) until it touches the back of the throat. Then press the end you are holding downwards until the end in the patient's throat hits the top of the back of the nose. The foreign body will then be on top of and in front of the probe. Slide the probe out, keeping your end gently pressed down as far as possible. The foreign body often comes out in front of the probe.

Bleeding nose (epistaxis)

Causes of a bleeding nose include:
1. a cause not found (common),
2. a small crusted area on septum (just inside the nose) which has cracked (common),
3. trauma,
4. strong nose blowing or sneezing,
5. others – snake bite, rare blood diseases, diptheria etc.

Treatment
1. Treat any underlying cause found.
2. Sit the patient up.
   Pinch his nose tightly together between finger and thumb.
   Let the blood run out of his mouth into a dish. Do this for 10 minutes by the clock. Do not stop before 10 minutes are over.
   If this does not stop the bleeding, then:-
3. Put in anterior nasal pack. Soak a long strip of narrow gauze bandage in 1 in 10,000 solution of adrenalin (mix 9 ml of saline with 1 ml of the 1 in 1000 adrenalin solution used for injection). Use long narrow forceps to pack the gauze in layers into the nose. Start off by putting the first layer as far back as possible. (See a

reference book for details.) If this does not stop the bleeding, remove this anterior nasal pack, put in a posterior nasal pack (see below) and then another anterior nasal pack, starting off as far back as possible and pressing it onto the posterior nasal pack.
4. A posterior nasal pack can be made with a Foley's urethral self-retaining balloon catheter. Push the catheter through the bleeding side of the nose until the tip can be seen at the back of the throat when the patient opens his mouth. Inflate the balloon of the catheter with 4–10 ml of air or saline. Make sure the balloon is not behind or below the tongue. Then pull the catheter forward as far as it will go until the balloon is stuck in the back of the nose. Fasten the catheter to the face with sticking plaster to keep the catheter pulled firmly forward so that it will press on any bleeding site at the back of the nose. Then put in an anterior nasal pack.
5. Treat for shock or anaemia if necessary. (See Chapter 27 page 305 and Chapter 21 page 182)
6. When the bleeding has stopped, gently put ointment (e.g. antibiotic compound ointment) into the nose, three times a day for a few days, to soften and heal any hard cracked area.

Allergic rhinitis (hay fever)

An allergic reaction of the mucous membrane of the nose is called allergic rhinitis or 'hay-fever'. The allergic reaction often affects the eyes too (allergic conjunctivitis) and the throat.

The allergy is usually to something breathed in – often house dust or a pollen.

The nose (and eyes and throat) become itchy, watery and sore.

The patient often sneezes a lot and rubs his nose and eyes.

On examination the mucous membrane is thickened, bluish-pink and has watery material covering it. There is no pus in the nose and no fever.

The condition may continue for hours or days or weeks or months.

Try to discover what is causing the reaction. The patient must try to avoid this. But, this is not often possible.

Treat with an antihistamine e.g. promethezine 25 mg (1 tablet) at night.

Acute tonsillitis and diphtheria

Acute tonsillitis is an acute bacterial or viral infection of the tonsils and surrounding area of the throat. This causes acute inflammation and usually pus formation in the throat and the general symptoms and signs of infection.

The patient complains of a sore throat worse on swallowing or turning the head, and headache and fever.

The patient may be quite sick with a high temperature and fast pulse. The tonsils and inside the throat are red and swollen and usually there are spots of white or yellow pus on the tonsils. The lymph glands in the neck are often swollen and tender.

Complications can occur including an abscess behind the tonsil or at the back of the throat or under the chin. Any of these can block the airway. After 1–3 weeks rheumatic fever (See Chapter 27 page 303) or acute glomerulonephritis (See Chapter 26 page 289) can occur.

Diptheria is a special kind of upper respiratory tract infection, although it can infect other areas including the skin. It usually causes tonsillitis but can cause infection of the larynx (voice box) or nose. It is caused by a special bacterium spread by droplet infection. It is much more common in children than adults. The diagnostic feature is a greyish covering or membrane over the affected area, usually the tonsils, which is firmly stuck on and cannot be pushed off with a tongue depressor as pus can be. Around the edge of the grey covering is an area of inflamation which sometimes bleeds. The illness can vary from mild to severe. In severe cases death can occur within the first couple of weeks from shock or from complete blockage of the larynx. Heart failure can occur in the next couple of weeks. Damage to nerves, which control muscles, can result in things swallowed coming back up the nose, difficulty seeing and even weakness of the arms and legs some weeks later.

Treatment
1. Procaine penicillin 900,000 units (3 ml) IMI daily for ten days.
2. Aspirin 600 mg (2 tablets) four times a day, if needed for pain.
3. Antimalarials usually chloroquine (see Chapter 13 page 55).

If the patient has a very acute severe infection, give benzyl (crystalline) penicillin.

If an abscess starts to block the airway see below.

If you think the patient has diptheria, treat with penicillin but immediately contact the medical officer about the use of diptheria antitoxin, examination or treatment of contacts and immunisation with toxoid. If there is difficulty in breathing or if stridor occurs arrange urgent transfer as tracheostomy may be urgently needed. Diptheria can be prevented by immunisation, especially triple antigen given during childhood.

Acute bacterial throat or laryngeal or tracheal infections

Acute bacterial infections in these structures can cause death by blocking the airway. This block may be caused by an abscess or infective swelling or membrane or secretion which can be seen; but sometimes one of these things is so far inside the throat or in the larynx or trachaea that it cannot be seen.

Suspect possible block of the airway if:
1. You can see a swelling which could block the airway.
2. The patient has difficulty in breathing. Stridor means death may be close.
3. The patient looks very 'sick'.

If a block of the airway is possible, treat like this:
1. Immediately give antibiotics as for septicaemia (IVI chloramphenicol, see Chapter 12 page 46).
2. Nurse carefully (suck out when needed; give oxygen when needed; etc.) Observe carefully every 15 minutes.
3. Give adrenaline and antihistamines if allergy is possible (see Chapter 27 page 308).
4. Transfer patient if he does not quickly improve.
5. Incise and let the pus out of any swelling which will cause death before transfer is possible; or do an emergency laryngostomy if incision is not possible.

Acute tracheitis and bronchitis

Acute bronchitis is a common acute inflammation of the mucous membrane lining the inside of the bronchi (see Figure 20.18). If the trachea is inflamed, acute tracheitis is also present.

Acute bronchitis is usually caused by an infection with bacteria; but viruses and chemicals can also cause the inflammation.

General symptoms and signs of infection may be present, including
- malaise and
- fever.

Symptoms of a chest infection may be present, including
- cough,
- tracheal pain (pain in the front and middle of the neck and upper chest during coughing),
- sputum, and
- shortness of breath and wheezing.

Signs of bronchial obstruction (wheezes) are usually present but there are no signs of pneumonia:
- chest movement unchanged,
- percussion note unchanged,
- air entry unchanged to all areas, but
- wheezes (and occasionally coarse creps) in all areas.

Treatment

Treat as an outpatient.
Tell the patient to return if shortness of breath gets worse (pneumonia or asthma).
1. Procaine penicillin 900,000 units (3 ml) IMI daily until cured (usually 5–7 days).
2. Aspirin 600 mg (2 tablets), every 6 hours if required for pain.
3. A 'bronchodilator' e.g. salbutamol 4 mg or orciprenaline 20 mg (1 tablet) each 6 hours *if* wheezing present.
4. Inhalation (the breathing in) of steam (from a cup or tin of boiling water), for five minutes three or four times a day.
5. An antimalarial drug usually chloroquine (see Chapter 13 page 55) if there is fever.

Bronchopneumonia

Bronchopneumonia is an acute infection of groups of alveoli in the lungs (see Figure 20.19).

Figure 20.18 Diagram showing the changes in acute tracheitis and bronchitis. The mucous membrane lining all the air passages is inflamed and swollen and sometimes coverer with pus. These things cause narrowing of all the airways to all parts of the lung. The alveoli themselves are normal.

Figure 20.19 Diagram showing the changes in bronchopneumonia (in this case of both lower lobes – the most common places affected). Scattered groups of alveoli are involved. Bronchi are usually normal. However disease of the bronchi can also be present.

Bronchopneumonia is usually caused by bacteria.

Bronchopneumonia usually develops as a complication of another condition which has either:
1. stopped the patient moving around and breathing deeply and/or
2. has allowed bacteria to come into the lungs from the upper respiratory tract e.g.
   - after anaesthetics, operations, accidents,
   - old or sick people lying in bed, or
   - measles or whooping cough.

There are the general symptoms and signs of infection:
- the patient has another condition but is not as well as he or she should be or is getting worse,
- fever (but not always),
- fast pulse etc.

Symptoms of a chest infection are usually present (but not always):
- cough,
- sputum (made of pus), and
- shortness of breath.

Signs of the chest infection include:
- sputum made of pus,
- respiratory rate usually fast and shallow,
- normal movement, normal percussion note and normal air entry, but scattered crackles or crepitations throughout the lungs, often mostly low down at the back.

Treatment

1. Antibiotics – procaine penicillin 900,000 units (3 ml) IMI daily until cured. (See page 166.)
2. Physiotherapy – tell the patient to breathe deeply and cough, while you hit his chest.
3. Tell the patient to move around in bed and if possible make him get out of bed.
4. Antimalarials usually chloroquine if any fever. (See Chapter 13 page 55.)
5. Treat any underlying conditon.

Prevention of bronchopneumonia is by encouraging activity in old, ill or post-operative patients.

Lobar pneumonia

Lobar pneumonia is a very common cause of sickness and death in the tropical and developing world.

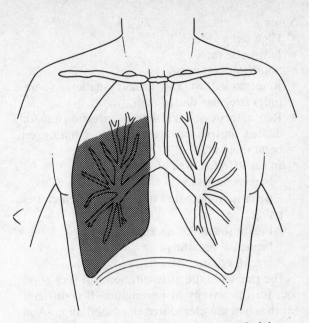

Figure 20.20 Diagram showing the changes in lobar pneumonia (in this case the right lower lobe). One whole lobe (or section) of lung is solid (bronchi and alveoli filled with organisms, fluid and blood cells). The solid lung extends from large central airways to the edge of the chest wall.

Lobar pneumonia is caused by an acute infection of all the alveoli in one lobe or one part of the lung by bacteria (usually pneumococci). (See Figure 20.20.)

The affected part of the lung becomes filled with bacteria, plasma and blood cells and becomes 'solid' (often called 'consolidation').

Symptoms

- The start of the infection is usually sudden; but sometimes there has been an upper respiratory tract infection.
- A rigor at first is common.
- Cough is almost always present.
- Sputum – rusty looking (from blood) or made of pus.
- Pleuritic chest pain (pain at the sides of the chest but occasionally in the shoulder or in the upper abdomen, worse when the chest moves, for example on deep breathing or coughing and relieved by keeping the chest still, for example by holding or lying on the painful side).
- Shortness of breath.

Signs

- High temperature.
- Fast pulse rate.
- Sometimes cyanosis.
- Respiration fast and usually shallow, sometimes irregular due to pain.
- Respiratory distress if severe – insuction and/or dilated nostrils on breathing in; grunting on breathing out.
- In the affected area of the chest
  - movement less,
  - percussion note dull (percussion often causes pain)
  - breath sounds or air entry less,
  - bronchial breathing,
  - crackles or crepitations.

The rate and type of respiration is a very good sign for the severity of pneumonia. It is difficult for the chest muscles to stretch a 'solid' lung. And chest movement often causes pleuritic pain. So the patient often takes shallow breaths which do not exchange as much oxygen and carbon dioxide as normal respiration with normal lungs. So breathing is usually also fast when it is shallow.

If the pneumonia is more severe (and the patient has to do much extra work to breathe and his lungs do not exchange oxygen and carbon dioxide well and the body needs more oxygen than when it is not fighting an infection) there are signs of respiratory distress:

1. indrawing of the soft tissues between the ribs and below and above the clavicles when the patient breathes in, (called 'insuction');
2. use of neck and shoulder muscles when he breathes in;
3. dilation of the nostrils when he breathes in; and
4. grunting when he breathes out.

The earliest signs in the chest are usually decreased movement of the affected side and decreased breath sounds. Percussion at this stage often causes pain. At first there may be no, or only a few, crackles or crepitations. It is often a day or two before many crackles are heard. Not all the signs do develop in every case. If you give antibiotic treatment early fewer signs develop. Sometimes you can hear a pleural rub if inflamation of the pleura (pleurisy) has developed.

Complications

- Heart failure (see Chapter 27 page 301).

- Septicaemia sometimes with shock (see Chapter 12 page 46).
- Jaundice (see Chapter 24 page 241).
- Pleural effusion (see page 168).
- Empyema (see page 168).
- Pneumothorax (see page 169).
- Lung abscess.
- Infections in other organs especially meningitis (see Chapter 25 page 256) and arthritis (see Chapter 29 page 315).
- Others.

Tests

Tests are not usually necessary. But, always do sputum examinations for AFB in any case which is unusual (see Chapter 14 page 69). This is especially important if the pneumonia does not get better when it should.

Without treatment, 20–40% of severe cases result in death.

Treatment

Management includes:
1. Antibiotics until cured.
   Procaine penicillin, if it is a mild case.
   Benzyl (crystalline) penicillin, if it is a moderate case.
   Tetracycline if benzyl penicillin does not cure but it is not a severe case.
   Chloramphenicol, if it is a severe case, or if penicillin and tetracycline do not cure a moderate case.
2. Antimalarial drugs as indicated.
3. Treatment of symptoms, especially pain.
4. Oxygen, if necessary.
5. Physiotherapy, if very much sputum.
6. Look for and treat complications, especially
   - heart failure,
   - septicaemia/shock,
   - infections in other parts, especially meningitis and arthritis,
   - pleural fluid, and
   - pneumothorax.
7. Look for and treat other important conditions (e.g. severe anaemia).
8. Look for tuberculosis in unusual cases.
9. Transfer the patient if necessary.

Treat according to severity.

Mild
- no respiratory distress[1] and RR < 30 and < PR 100 and
- no cyanosis and
- no complications[2]
  See below

Moderate
- respiratory distress[1] but not severe and RR < 40 and PR < 120 and/or
- cyanosis if present but not marked and
- no complications[2] except, if there is COLD, the patient may have heart failure. See below

Severe
- respiratory distress[1] and RR > 40 and PR > 120 and/or
- cyanosis and/or
- complications[2]
  See below

Mild case

Treat as an outpatient.
1. Procaine penicillin 900,000 units (3 ml) IMI daily until four days after fever and symptoms have gone (usually 5–7 days).
2. Antimalarial drug as indicated (see Chapter 13 page 55) usually chloroquine 450–600 mg (3–4 tabs) daily for 3 days.
3. Aspirin 300–600 mg (1–2 tabs) every 6 hours if necessary for pain.

If the patient is not much improved after 5 days, or if he gets worse, look for a complication especially a pleural effusion. If no complication that needs special treatment is found, then treat as a moderately severe case.

Moderate case

Admit for inpatient treatment.
1. Benzyl (crystalline) penicillin 1,000,000 units (2 ml) IMI every 6 hours until improved, then

---

1. Respiratory distress
   is (1) indrawing of soft tissues between the ribs and below and above the clavicles when the patient breathes in (insuction); (2) use of neck and shoulder muscles when he breaths in; (3) dilation of the nose muscles when he breathes in; (4) grunting when he breathes out. It is not distress from pain during breathing.
2. Complications include:
   (1) heart failure, (2) shock/septicaemia, (3) infections in other organs, (4) pleural fluid, and (5) pneumothorax.

procaine penicillin 900,000 units (3 ml) IMI daily until four days after all fever has gone.
2. Antimalarial drugs as indicated (Chapter 13 page 55) usually chloroquine 450–600 mg (3–4 tablets) daily for 3 days.
3. Aspirin 600–900 mg (2–3 tablets) or codeine compound tablets 2 tablets every 6 hours if necessary for pain.

If the patient is not much improved after 2–5 days, but is not worse and is not severly sick, then:
1. change pencillin to tetracycline 500 mg (2 caps) every 6 hours, and
2. send sputum for examination for AFB.

If the patient gets worse at any time treat as a severe case with chloramphenicol (see below).

Severe case
Use this treatment for severe cases (the patient will die soon if the treatment is not successful) and moderate cases not cured by treatment.
1. Chlorampheniclo 2 g immediately, then 1 g every 6 hours until much improved, then 750 mg every 6 hours. Give chloramphenicol for 10 days or until cured – which ever is longer.
   If the patient has shock or is *very* sick or cannot swallow or is vomiting, give IV or IM chloramphenicol 2 g immediately and 1 g every 6 hours until he can take oral chloramphenicol (if shock, IV needed).
   In other cases give oral chloramphenicol 1 g (4 caps) immediately and 1 g (4 caps) every 6 hours until much improved; then 750 mg (3 caps) every 6 hours until cured.
2. Antimalarial drugs as indicated (see Chapter 13 page 55) usually chloroquine 450–600 mg (3–4 tablets) daily for 3 days. You should give quinine first to *very* sick patients (see Chapter 13 page 56).
3. Oxygen at 2 litres per minute by intranasal prongs or catheter, if the patient is cyanosed or very short of breath.
4. Codeine compound tablets, 2 tables every 6 hours for pain.
5. Look for complications (see page 166). Treat in the usual ways.
6. Look for other conditions which need treatment, especially severe anaemia. Treat in the usual ways (see index).

Look for tuberculosis in all cases of pneumonia

Send sputum for AFB if:

1. Previous chronic cough (ask *all* patients if they had a chronic cough before the present illness).
2. Pneumonia is in an upper lobe or in the (right) middle lobe.
3. Patient not as acutely sick as you would expect when he has marked chest signs.
4. Past or family history of tuberculosis, or other history that suggests tuberculosis.
5. Wasting or lymphadenopathy or other sign that suggests tuberculosis.
6. Patient does not get better as quickly as expected, or patient not cured after 2 weeks of proper treatment.

Send sputum for AFB (3 smears) from these patients. If the smear is negative and you still suspect tuberculosis, send 3 more smears for AFB after 1–2 weeks of treatment with antibiotics.

Transfer

Transfer these cases to Medical Officer care:

1. severe cases which do not improve, or get worse after 2 days' chloramphenicol (urgent);
2. cases not cured or much improved after 2 weeks chloramphenicol (non-urgent);
3. those with complications that you cannot treat at the health centre (urgent).

Prevention

Prevention is not usually attempted. But, there are vaccines which give protection against the common pneumococci which cause pneumonia and their use may be valuable in some populations.

Pleural fluid

There are often no symptoms of fluid in the pleural cavity, but there may be shortness of breath and/or pleuritic pain. (See Figure 20.21)

Signs of fluid in the pleural cavity include (on the affected side):

- movement less,
- percussion note very dull ('stony dull')
- breath sounds or air entry less (usually none), and
- no crackles or wheezes but occasionally a pleural rub.

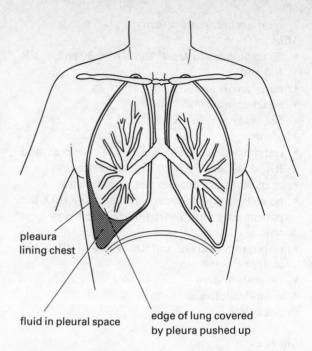

pleaura lining chest

fluid in pleural space

edge of lung covered by pleura pushed up

Figure 20.21 Diagram showing the changes with pleural fluid to the right in the standing position. The fluid in the pleural space pushes the lung up. The fluid can fill almost all the chest and squash (collapse) almost all of the lung so that no ventilation is possible.

There may *also* be symptoms and signs of the cause of the pleural fluid.

When you diagnose fluid in the pleural cavity,

1. *Always do a diagnostic pleural aspiration* to find out what kind of fluid it is i.e.
   (a) clear (usually yellow) fluid ('effusion'),
   (b) pus ('empyema')
   (c) blood ('haemothorax')

You must transefer all patients with pus or blood to a medical officer immediately.

2. *Always find out the cause*
   (a) Pneumonia can cause an effusion (clear yellow fluid).
   (b) Tuberculosis can cause an effusion (clear yellow fluid).
   (c) Many other conditions can cause fluid, pus or blood in the pleural cavity, all of which need transfer to a medical officer for diagnosis and/or treatment.

> If the patient does *not* have clear fluid *and* pneumonia or sputum positive for AFB, then you *must* transfer the patient to a Medical Officer (even if the effusion goes away – early tuberculosis often causes an effusion which goes away without treatment).

Pneumothorax

A pneumothorax is when there is air in the pleural cavity (see Figure 20.22).

Symptoms may include pleuritic pain and/or shortness of breath.

Signs may include (on the affected side):

* movement less,
* percussion note very resonant or hollow (difficult to be sure of this), and
* breath sounds or air entry less.

There may also be symptoms and signs of the cause of the pneumothorax.

Contact your Medical Officer urgently for management of any case you diagnose.

Transfer all cases urgently.

If there is severe shortness of breath, put a plastic cannula (or a needle) into the pleural cavity immediately. The best place is in the mid-clavicular line in the 2nd intercostal space (i.e. 2–3 cm below the middle of the clavicle.) Make a valve for the cannula or needle before you put it into the chest with part of a surgical rubber glove, like this:

1. Take a rubber surgical glove and cut a small 1 cm slit at the top of one of the glove fingers.
2. Then cut that glove finger from the glove, where it joins the palm of the glove.
3. Put the glove finger, where it joined the glove palm, around the hub of the needle which is to go in the chest (i.e. where the needle can join onto a syringe).
4. Tie the glove finger onto the cannula or needle with suture material or cotton around the hub of the needle.

Asthma

Asthma is a condition which causes episodes (or times) when all of the bronchi are narrowed (see Figure 20.23). This causes episodes of shortness

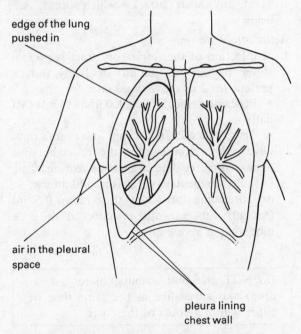

Figure 20.22 Diagram showing the changes in a pneumothorax. The air in the pleural space pushes the lung towards the trachea. The air can fill almost all the chest and completely collapse (squash) the lung so that no ventilation of that lung is possible.

Figure 20.23 Diagram showing changes during on attack of asthma. All the bronchi going to all parts of the lung are narrowed by a thick layer of thick mucus, swelling of the mucous membrane, and contraction of the bronchial muscles. Between attacks the bronchi return to normal.

of breath and wheezing called attacks of asthma. Between attacks the bronchi are not narrowed and there are then no symptoms.

You often cannot find the cause of a patient's asthma in a health centre. There may be a family history of asthma or allergies. There may be a past history of attacks of shortness of breath or of allergies (see Chapter 10 page 37) to things breathed in, or swallowed (including drugs), or touched. Often asthma is caused by allergy to dust (especially house dust). Sometimes it is caused by allergy to organisms which cause respiratory infection.

The bronchi are narrowed by bronchial muscle spasm, swelling of the bronchial mucous membrane, and thick layer of jelly-like mucus on the bronchial walls.

Symptoms include:
- sudden shortness of breath,
- a feeling of tightness in the chest,
- wheezing,
- sometimes repeated coughing, and
- usually a history of having previous attacks and of being well in between attacks.

Signs include:
- temperature normal (no fever),
- respiration slow and deep with wheezing and sometimes coughing,
- pulse rate fast if a severe attack,
- jelly-like sputum (not pus),
- chest – rhonchi or wheezes in all areas especially when the patient breathes out.

There are two very important exceptions to the above:
1. In some patients the asthma does not ever go away completely (especially people who do not have the allergic type of asthma and whose asthma started when they were in middle or láte adult life). These patients do have acute attacks of asthma. But between acute attacks they may have chronic shortness of breath and wheezes may be heard on examination of the chest. This is called 'chronic asthma'.
2. Some patients have very severe attacks when almost no breath sounds or breathing in can be heard. In this case the patient is very anxious, has respiratory distress (see page 167) has very

fast pulse rate is cyanosed, has decreased breath sounds or air entry and few wheezes or rhonchi can therefore be heard. This patient is near death.

Treatment
Chronic asthma
1. Give a bronchodilator e.g. salbutamol 4 mg or terbutaline 5 mg or orciprenaline 20 mg or ephedrine 30 mg (1 tablet) four times a day.
   Reduce the dose if side effects occur (shaking, nervousness, sweating, giddiness or palpitations).
   Increase the dose slowly if no side effects but still asthma. Do not give more than 2 tablets four times a day.
2. Add aminophylline or theophylline if necessary. Give 100 mg (1 tablet) four times a day. Increase the dose until:
   - the asthma is controlled or
   - there is nausea, or other side effects (reduce dose a little) or
   - you are giving 400 mg (4 tablets) four times a day (do not give more).
3. Find and avoid or treat the cause if possible.
4. Treat any acute attacks which occur (see below).

Acute attack asthma
1. If infection of the respiratory tract is present (fever or pus in sputum) or likely (attack present for 2 or move days) give:
   - Procaine penicillin 900,000 units (3 ml) IMI daily or
   - Tetracycline 250 mg (1 cap) four times a day.
2. Give *either* salbutamol 4 mg or terbutaline 5 mg or orciprenaline 20 mg or ephedrine 30 mg (1 tablet) immediately if it is a mild attack,
   or adrenaline tart. 1–1000 solution 0.5 ml (½ ml) subcutaneous injection if it is a moderate or severe attack.

> Do NOT give both salbutamol (or similar drug) and adrenaline at the same time or either within 4 hours of the other.

3. Give intra-nasal oxygen 2–4 litres/minute for a moderate or a severe attack.
4. Give aminophylline or theophylline orally or aminophylline IV for a moderate attack or IV

for a severe attack. *Give IV slowly* – take 10 minutes by the clock.

Small adult (<50 kg) 300 mg (3 tabs) orally *or* 250 mg (10 ml) IV

Large adult (<50kg) 400 mg (4 tabs) orally *or* 375 mg (15 ml) IV.

> Do not give this large dose of aminophylline or theophylline if the patient has taken regular oral aminophylline or theophylline or had a large oral dose in the last 12 hours. In these cases start an aminophylline drip (see below).

5. Do *not* give morphine, pethidine or phenobarbitone. Instead, if mentally abnormal, treat as a severe attack; also look for other causes of mental abnormality (see Chapter 35 page 384).
6. If the attack is moderate or severe and the patient has been taking prednisone, prednisolone or other cortisone-like drug, urgently consult the Medical Officer. If the patient does not quickly improve, give 60 mg (12 tabs) of his prednisolone (or 6–12 times his usual total daily dose of other cortisone-like drug) immediately and daily until you get further advice from the Medical Officer.
7. Find and avoid or treat the cause, if possible.

> IF the symptoms and signs go within 2 hours THEN discharge on orciprenaline 20 mg or salbutamol 4 mg (1 tab) four times a day for 5 days; then four times a day it necessary.
> IF symptoms and signs do not all go in 2 hours or
> IF it is a severe attack from the start,
> THEN immediately treat as follows (as well as 1–7).

8. Start an aminophylline drip
   Add aminophylline solution
   • 150 mg (6 ml) for a small adult (<50 kg) *or*
   • 225 mg (9 ml) for a large adult (>50 kg)
   to 1 litre of 4.3% dextrose in 0.18% sodium chloride. Use only half of these doses of aminophylline if the patient has heart failure or liver disease.
   Give 1 litre every 8 hours. Continue until the attack has completely gone.

If the patient is a smoker *and* if the asthma does not improve *and* if there are no toxic effects, you can double the dose of aminophylline.

If, however, there is continuous nausea or headache or any vomiting, then slow the drip to half (½) the rate, or (better) reduce the dose of aminophylline in each flask to half the previous dose and continue to run the drip at the same rate.

9. Give adrenaline every 4–6 hours (see page 170)
10. Give antibitoics (see page 170)

When the patient improves:
1. Stop oxygen.
2. Change adrenaline injections to salbutamol 4 mg or similar tablets (1 tablets) four times a day.
3. Change aminophylline drip to aminophylline or theophylline tablets four times a day. Start 100 mg (1 tablet) four times a day. Increase the dose if necessary.
4. Continue salbutamol and aminophylline until the attack is clinically cured and then for 5 days more.

When the patient is better he can go home, with a supply of:
1. salbutamol 4 mg or similar tablets, 1 tablet four times a day (or more) if necessary, *and*
2. aminophylline tablets or theophylline if necessary (see chronic attack page 170).

Transfer to medical officer care if there is:
1. very severe asthma which does not improve, or is worse, after 8 hours of proper treatment for a severe case, i.e. if
   • PR 120 or more,
   • severe shortness of breath and respiration distress, or
   • cyanosis
   (urgent – emergency);
2. severe asthma after two days of full treatment (urgent);
3. repeated acute attacks needing repeated inpatient care during several months, (non-urgent).

Chronic obstructive lung disease

Chronic Obstructive Lung Disease (COLD) (also

Figure 20.24 Diagram showing the changes in COLD. The bronchi going to all parts of the lung are narrowed by (1) a thick layer of mucus on the surface of the mucous membrane, (2) the mucous membrane itself is thickened and (3) the irregular size of many damaged bronchi, many of which collapse when the patient breathes out thus trapping air in the lungs.

called Chronic Obstructive Airways Disease (COAD) or Chronic Bronchitis and Emphysema) is a common chronic non-infective disease of the bronchi and lungs.

The mucous membrane lining the bronchi is thickened and covered by a thick layer of mucus. These narrow the bronchi and cause shortness of breath, a cough and sputum. The walls of the bronchi are of irregular size and are also weak. When the patient breathes out, many of the bronchi collapse before the air from the alveoli can go through them. This traps air inside the lung. This also causes shortness of breath (See Figure 20.24.)

COLD is caused by repeated attacks of lung infections, smoking, air pollution (and other things that are not known yet).

Symptoms
- Chronic cough (on most days for at least 3 months for at least 2 years).
- Sputum which is white (except if there is also acute chest infection).
- Shortness of breath – at first during exercise, but later all the time.
- Wheezing at times.

Signs
- Middle aged or old person who has been a smoker or had repeated chest infections.
- Normal temperature.
- Normal pulse.
- Increased respiratory rate (if severe).
- Wasting (if severe).
- Chest – abnormal use of neck and shoulder and abdominal muscles for breathing and drawing in of the skin and soft tissues above and below the clavicles and over the upper and lower chest during breathing in ('insuction') (if severe).
- Only a little but equal movement on both sides (the chest is almost fully expanded *all* the time).
- The percussion note often more resonant (hollow) than normal but on both sides.
- Breath sounds air entry often decreased equally on both sides.
- Wheezes or rhonchi and sometimes crackles or crepitations – heard equally on both sides and more often low down in the chest.

Complications
- acute bronchitis (see page 164) and pneumonia (see page 164)
- asthma (see page 169) is very common
- heart failure (see Chapter 27 page 301)

The patient usually gets worse slowly over years, and dies of one of these complications.

Tests
Always send 3 sputum smears to the laboratory for examination for AFB.

Do not diagnose COLD until smears have been negative for AFB.

Treatment
Treat as an outpatient.

Admit for inpatient treatment only if a complication (pneumonia, moderate or severe asthma or heart failure) develops.

1. Tell the patient to stop smoking (or to smoke less).
2. If there is wheezing or rhonchi then supply:
   (a) salbutamol 4 mg or similar tablet, one tablet three or four times a day and if necessary –
   (b) aminophylline or theophylline tablets

regularly (see page 170) if there is shortness of breath all the time, or as required (see page 170) if there are only attacks or shortness of breath.

See Asthma, page 169.

3. *Show* the patient how to look for pus in his sputum (yellow or green colour).

   Tell the patient to look every day and to come for antibiotics immediately if he sees pus.

   Treat any chest infection immediately, until there is no pus in the sputum (it is white again).

   Treat as follows:

   procaine penicillin 900,000 units (3 ml) IMI daily for 5–10 days. If this fails give:

   tetracycline 250–500 mg (1–2 caps) four times a day.

   Use chloramphenicol only for infections which threaten life.

4. Look for heart failure. If it is found start hydrochlorothiazide 50–100 mg (1–2 tables) daily, and see Heart Failure (Chapter 27 page 301).

5. Do not give oxygen unless there is a complication (e.g. pneumonia). Do not give oxygen faster than 2 litres/minute intra-nasally. (Too much oxygen may make the patient unconcious and cause death.)

6. Never give morphine, pethidine or phenobarbitone (as these may stop the patient breathing and cause death).

Transfer to Medical Officer care is not necessary as no more treatment is possible at a hospital.

Control and prevention

1. Treat chest infections quickly and properly.
2. Tell everyone never to smoke tobacco.

Lung diseases caused by worms

A number of lung diseases can be caused by worms.

Bronchitis and pneumonia can be caused by the larvae of worms (e.g. hookworm or roundworm) as they travel through the lung.

Asthma and other chest pains and other symptoms can be caused by worm larvae (e.g. roundworm or hookworm) as they travel through the body, or by some of the filarial worms.

Chronic lung disease with heart failure can be caused by schistosomiasis.

Haemoptysis, pneumonia or chronic lung disease can be caused by lung flukes

None of these conditions can be diagnosed outside a laboratory. Do not worry. If one of these conditions is very common in your area, you will be taught about it. Otherwise the condition will be diagnosed when you refer or transfer the patient to a Medical Officer (usually when the patient does not get better with your treatment).

Bronchiecatasis

Bronchiectasis is a condition when there is permanent damage to the bronchi of part of the lung. The bronchi are permanently dilated (widened) and do not work properly. They often become infected and finally become just like tubes or bags of pus, (see Figure 20.25).

Bronchiectasis is caused by obstruction and infection of bronchi which are not treated and cured quickly. This infection and obstruction may be caused by tuberculosis or pneumonia or

Figure 20.25 Diagram to show the changes in bronchiectasis affecting some of the bronchi of the left lower lobe. The bronchial walls have been weakened or destroyed. The bronchi therefore became irregular in size and shape. The bronchial mucous membrane has been destroyed. The bronchi therefore cannot move secretions out through the bronchial tree. The bronchi therefore become filled with secretions. The bronchial secretions often become infected and form pus.

bronchitis (especially attacks complicating measles or whooping cough which are not treated quickly or properly).

Symptoms include:
- Chronic cough which is present every day and worse after waking in the morning or after exercise.
- Sputum in large amount (e.g. 20–200 ml or more daily) which is often made of pus (e.g. green or yellow or brown and often smells bad).
- Sometimes blood in the sputum.
- Shortness of breath; but only late in the disease.

Signs of bronchiectasis are few early in the disease. Often there is only one sign – crackles or crepitations in the affected part of the lung which stay there after deep breating and coughing and are always in the sample place every time the patient is examined.

Signs which come later include: wasting, anaemia, and clubbing of the fingers and toes.

The symptoms and signs of attacks of acute bronchitis and pneumonia are common.

Send sputum for AFB to check the patient does not have tuberculosis.

Treatment includes:
1. Postural drainage and physiotherapy for 15–30 minutes once or twice *every* day of the patient's life. Most patients will not do this; but without this, any other treatment is of no real help. Show the patient how to raise the foot of a straight bed by using blocks of something about 0.2–0.5 m high; lie on this with the affected side of his lung uppermost (as well as his head end downwards); and take deep breaths and cough up the sputum as he (or someone else) hits the affected part of the lung with the palm of the hand. Tell the patient to do this for 15–30 minutes each morning and also if possible each evening. Also tell the patient to sleep on a straight bed if possible.
2. Antibiotics if there is an acute bacterial infection (but do not continue the antibiotic if it does not cure the infection).
3. Surgery can help only very occasionally.

Discuss treatment of the patient with the next visiting medical officer.

Some problems of diagnosis and management

Deafness

Causes include:
1. any condition blocking the external ear canal, including wax, foreign body or external ear inflammation;
2. any condition damaging the middle ear, including blocked Eustachian tube and acute and chronic middle ear infection;
3. any condition damaging the inner ear, the nerve to the ear or the brain, including side effects of streptomycin and trauma of the head;
4. others. If the cause is not one of these see a specialist book.

Always look in the ear with an auriscope.

Do ear toilet or syringing until you can see the ear drum. Treat any condition in the usual way (see index).

Ear pain

Causes include:
1. external ear infection (otitis externa);
2. foreign body in the external ear canal;
3. middle ear inflammation (otitis media), acute or chronic;
4. mastoiditis;
5. acute parotitis – mumps or acute bacterial;
6. infection of teeth;
7. others. If the cause is not one of these see a specialist book.

Always look in the ear with an auriscope. Do ear toilet and syringing until you can see the ear drum. Examine behind the ear (mastoid) in front of the ear (parotid) and below the ear (in the mouth).

Treat any condition in the usual way (see index).

Ear discharge

Causes include:
1. external ear inflammation (otitis externa);
2. foreign body in external ear canal;

3. middle ear infection (otitis media), acute (with perforated ear drum) or chronic;
4. others. If the cause is not one of these see a specialist book.

Always look in the ear with an auriscope.

Do ear toilet or syringing until you can see the ear drum. Treat any condition in the usual way.

Nasal discharge – both sides

Causes include:
1. virus infections of the upper respiratory tract and measles (watery discharge);
2. bacterial infections of the upper respiratory tract e.g. sinusitis (pus);
3. foreign body in the nose (pus or blood);
4. allergy ('hay fever') (watery discharge);
5. irritation by dust, smoke etc. (watery discharge);
6. others. If the cause is not one of these see a specialist book.

Treat any condition in the usual way (see index). You can sometimes improve chronic infections by irrigation (washing out the nose twice daily with normal saline solution) (2½ ml or ½ teaspoon of salt in 200 ml or 1 cup of clear water). Tell the patient to pour the saline through the nose; let it run into the mouth, then spit it out.

Nasal discharge – from one side only

Always look for a foreign body in the nose.
See also nasal discharge both sides (above).

Acute loss of voice or hoarse voice (present for less than 4 weeks)

Causes include:
1. shouting, singing or talking too much;
2. smoking too much;
3. acute viral throat/larynx/tracheal/bronchial infections (the patient is usually not 'sick');
4. acute bacterial throat/larynx/tracheal/-bronchial infections (the patient is usually 'sick');
5. others. If the cause is not one of these see a specialist book.

Treat any condition found in the usual way.

Chronic loss of voice or hoarse voice (present for more than 4 weeks)

Causes include:
1. tuberculosis of lung;
2. cancer of neck;
3. others.

You must transfer all patients with this so that the Medical Officer can examine the patient's larynx, except patients with sputum positive tuberculosis (who you will treat at the health centre).

Sore throat

Causes include:
1. common cold, and other viral upper respiratory tract infections;
2. acute tonsillitis, and other bacterial upper respiratory tract infections;
3. one of the causes of a painful ear (see page 174).

Always look in the mouth and throat with a tongue depressor and light, and in the ear with an auriscope.

If these conditions are not present see a specialist book. Treat any condition found in the usual way (see index).

Cough

The cause is usually obvious from the history and examination.

Do full history and examination (see Chapter 6).

Look at sputum (?pus ?blood).

Always ask how long the cough has been present see below. If it has been present for more than four weeks send sputum for examination for AFB.

Cough present for less than four weeks

Upper respiratory tract infection
• No other chest symptoms.
• Respiratory rate normal and no respiratory distress (see page 152).
• No chest signs.

Asthma
- Shortness of breath. Previous similar attacks.
- Sputum not made of pus i.e. not yellow or rusty.
- Wheezes or rhonchi in chest.
- No fever.

Acute bronchitis or pneumonia
- Fever.
- Sputum is pus or of rusty colour.
- Respiratory rate fast.
- Respiratory distress may be present.
- Other chest signs.

Cough present for more than four weeks
Where tuberculosis is common
Make 3 sputum smears for examination for AFB – specimen 'A' collected immediately; specimen 'B' collected by the patient the next morning as soon as he wakes; specimen 'C' collected when the patient returns with 'B',

Where tuberculosis is not common
- Treat for 1 week with procaine penicillin, 900,000 units (3 ml) daily IMI.
- If the cough is not cured treat for 1 week with tetracycline 250 mg (1 cap) four times a day.
- If the cough is still present continue the tetracycline and send sputum specimens 'A', 'B' and 'C' for examination for AFB.

If one or more sputum examinations positive for AFB
Tuberculosis. See Chapter 13.

If all sputum examinations negative for AFB
1. Repeat sputum for AFB × 3 again if:
   (a) past or family history of tuberculosis or other history suggests tuberculosis;
   (b) there is wasting or lymphadenopathy or other signs of tuberculosis.
2. Otherwise, and if repeat sputum examinations negative for AFB, check for:
   (a) Chronic Obstructive Lung Disease;
   (b) smoker's cough;
   (c) repeated asthma attacks, upper respiratory tract infections, acute bronchitis or pneumonia;
   (b) chronic sinusitis with pus running down back of the throat;
   (e) whooping cough (the whoop is very rare in an adult with whooping cough);
   (f) bronchiectasis;
   (g) tuberculosis with sputum negative for AFB. If you still suspect tuberculosis transfer non-urgently to Medical Officer.

Treatment of cough
1. Treat the cause (see index).
2. Stop the patient smoking.
3. Physiotherapy often helps; but only if it causes the patient to cough up more than 30 ml sputum every time. See page 174
4. Cough medicines do not help.

Sputum
See causes of cough for causes of sputum.

Always find the answers to these three things:
1. Is the sputum from the lower respiratory tract (which is often serious) or from the upper respiratory tract (which is not as serious)?
2. What is the colour of the sputum?
   - Coloured sputum (yellow, green or brown) usually means bacterial infection, e.g. acute bronchitis, bronchopneumonia, lobar pneumonia, bronchiectasis, sinusitis, etc.
   - White sputum occurs in viral infections (if there is no bacterial infection as well).
   - White sputum is also common from smoking, chronic bronchitis (COLD), asthma and some cases of chronic sinusitis.
   - Bacterial infection needs treatment with antibiotics. Antibiotics will not help other conditions.
3. Is there blood in the sputum (haemoptysis)? If there is blood in the sputum see below.

Blood coughed up – haemoptysis

1. Always check that it is *blood* that is coughed up. Always examine what is coughed up.
2. Always check that the blood was *coughed* up.
   - Check that the blood was not vomited up.
   - Check that the blood was not just from the upper respiratory tract (especially the nose).
3. Always find out *how much* blood was coughed up – if more than one cup, it is an emergency and you must start an IV drip.
4. Always find out the *cause*. Causes include:
   - Tuberculosis. Send sputum for AFB in all cases.

- COLD.
- Any acute lower respiratory tract infection.
- Bronchiectasis or lung abscess.
- Chest injury.
- Others. If the cause is not one of these see a specialist book. Causes such as pulmonary embolus and cancer of the lung are not common in the rural areas of tropical and developing countries but may be common in the cities.

> Tuberculosis is the most common cause of haemoptysis.

If you cannot diagnose the cause at the health centre, transfer the patient for investigation.
5. Treatment of haemoptysis.
(a) Treat the cause.
(b) If there is shock or anaemia, give routine treatment for these (see Chapter 27 page 305 and Chapter 21 page 182).
(c) If the patient has difficulty in breathing (because blood is filling the bronchi)
– put the patient on his side, with the diseased part of the chest down or on his under side,
– tip the head of the bed down,
– suck out the pharynx and larynx if necessary
– give IVI diazepam 5–10 mg (1–2 ml) or (*but only if does not have COLD*) morphine 10 mg (1 ml) by slow IVI or IMI
– give intranasal oxygen,
– transfer as soon as possible to Medical Officer care.

Shortness of breath

Do a full history and examination (see Chapter 6).
Look at any sputum (?pus ?blood).
Test the urine for protein and sugar.
See page 178 for classification
Look at the following 7 headings (page 177 to 178) to see which paragraph will apply to your patient.

1. With stridor (loud noise breathing in)
Block of throat, larynx or trachea by foreign body, acute allergic reaction or acute bacterial or viral infection.
- Emergency. Act immediately.
- If inhaled foreign body or vomit is possible, pull any foreign body out of throat. If not

successful, lay the patient face down, lift up his hips and abdomen and hit his back *very hard* between the shoulder blades.
- If acute allergic reaction is possible, give IM adrenaline 0.5 ml (½ ml) and IV promethazine 50 mg (2 ml) immediately.
- If infection is possible, give IV (or IM) chloramphenicol 2 g immediately, then 1 g each 6 hours.
- Give intranasal oxygen 4 litres/minute.
- Transfer urgently (emergency) unless the patient is cured immediately.

2. With pallor and/or shock (fast PR, low BP, cold hands and feet).
Anaemia +/– blood loss.
- If shock or severe blood loss see Chapter 27 page 305.
- Give routine anaemia treatment to other cases (see Chapter 21 page 182).

3. With fever
Chest infections (cough, sputum made of pus or a rusty colour, crackles or other signs in chest).
- Give penicillin or chloramphenicol (see page 157).
- Send sputum for AFB if cough present for more than 4 weeks.
Malaria if there is no evidence of chest infection.
- Give antimalarials (see Chapter 13 page 55)

4. With wheezing and rhonchi
Asthma; COLD; acute bronchitis.
- Give adrenaline or salbutamol *and*, if needed, aminophylline orally or by IVI. (See page 157.)
- Send sputum for AFB of cough present for more than 4 weeks.

5. With oedema, large liver, raised neck veins
Heart failure.
- Give diuretics – IV frusemide 40 mg (4 ml) immediately if severe or oral hydrochlorothiazide 50–100 mg (1–2 tabs) if not severe and see Chapter 27 page 301.
- Treat the cause (see Chapter 27 page 305).

6. And 'sick' but not distressed by shortness of breath
Dehydration usually from gastro-enteritis.
- Give IV fluids (see Chapter 23 page 224).

Meningitis or septicaemia.
- Give chloramphenicol by IVI or IMI. (see Chapter 12 page 46).

Diabetes mellitus.
- Give IV fluids for dehydration.
- Transfer to Medical Officer urgently.

Chronic kidney failure.
- See Chapter 26 page 289.

7. And very worried by shortness of breath but no abnormalities found on examination

The patient feels as if he cannot get enough air into the lungs – anxiety.

Obvious 'over-breathing' often with dizziness and strange feeling around mouth and in hands and feet – 'acting out'.

See Chapter 36.

Classification

Here is one classification of the causes of shortness of breath.

Shortness of breath is normal after strong exercise or in high areas (on mountains).

Diseases causing shortness of breath include:
1. Respiratory diseases
   (a) of alveoli
   pneumonia including severe or advanced tuberculous pneumonia – shallow quick breathing
   (b) of bronchi
   acute bronchitis
   asthma (deep slow breathing) } sometimes
   COLD } wheezing
   (c) of throat/larynx/trachea/bronchi,
   acute bacterial infections
   acute viral infections
   (e.g. 'croup') } often stridor
   allergy
   foreign body
   (d) of pleura
   effusion or empyema { shallow quick breathing
   pneumothorax
2. Cardiovascular
   (a) heart failure – shallow quick breathing
   (b) shock – gasping breathing.
3. Anaemia – deep fast breathing.
4. Kidney failure } deep slow breathing; but
   Diabetes mellitus } no distress.

5. Anxiety – the patient feels as if he can't get enough air into his lungs; but on examination no abnormalities are found.
   'Acting out' – obvious overbreathing,
6. Others.

Stridor

Stridor is noisy breathing *in*. (Noisy breathing *out* is not as important.) Stridor is usually a crowing noise; but sometimes it is more like snoring.

> Noisy breathing is obstructed breathing. Immediately relieve the obstruction.

Stridor is always serious. Stridor is very dangerous if there is rib recession (insuction) during breathing in, and/or if the patient uses his neck and abdominal muscles to keep breathing.

Always think of these things and treat any present like this:
1. If the patient is weak or not fully conscious (often like 'snoring'):
   (a) lay the patient on his side,
   (b) tip his head back,
   (c) pull his jaw forward,
   (d) suck out his throat.
2. Infection of throat and/or epiglottis and/or larynx and/or trachea and/or bronchi
   (a) IVI (or IMI) chloramphenicol urgently *or* IVI (or IMI) crystalline penicillin urgently as for septicaemia (See Chapter 12)
   (b) Make the patient breathe moist air by boiling water near him if the air is cool and/or dry.
   (c) Nurse him carefully (suck out if necessary; give intranasal oxygen).
   (d) Observe him carefully.
   (e) Transfer urgently (emergency) if he does not quickly improve.
3. Foreign body
   (a) Tip the patient with head and neck down. Hit his back very hard between shoulder blades. See Chapter 37 page 415
   (b) Transfer urgently if he does not cough up the foreign body.
4. Allergy
   (a) IVI antihistamine e.g. promethazine 50 mg (2 ml).

(b) IMI adrenaline (1–1000 solution) 0.5 ml (½ ml).
5. Others.

Chest pain

Do a full histroy (See Chapter 6).

Find out all about the pain:
1. Is it 'pleuritic'? i.e.
   - in the chest wall at the side of the chest
   - worse on coughing or deep breathing
   - helped by holding that side of the chest or lying on the side of pain.
   See this page.
2. Is it tracheal? i.e.
   - in the neck and front of centre of chest
   - present only when coughs.
   See this page.
3. Is it spinal? i.e.
   - also in the back
   - worse on bending or lifting.
   - tenderness of spine
   See Chapter 29 page 325.
4. Is it constant and in the lower chest, and are abdominal symptoms also present?
   See Chapter 36 page 407.
5. Is it in the lower chest and comes or goes with eating food?
   See Chapter 23 page 215.
6. Has it been present for more than four weeks, and has cough also been present for four weeks?
   See this page.

Do a full examination (see Chapter 6).

Ask the patient to cough.

Listen to the cough.

Observe if coughing causes pain (pleuritic or tracheal pain).

Examine any sputum (?pus).

Diagnose and manage according to the 6 types of pain (see above) that the patient has, like this:

Pain is pleuritic
1. *If* ± cough ± sputum (pus or rusty colour) ± shortness of breath ± fever ± fast pulse ± crepitations in chest, *then* pneumonia. See page 164.
2. *If* history of injury to chest, tender place on chest, *then* fracture of rib.
3. *If* no abnormality found, *then* chest wall pain. Observe the patient daily for a few days.

Pain is tracheal
1. *If* cough ± sputum ± shortness of breath ± fever ± rhonchi in chest, *then* tracheitis/bronchitis. See page 164.
2. *If* no abnormality found, *then* viral upper respiratory tract infection or too much smoking or shouting etc. See page 158.

Pain is spinal
1. *If* pain gets worse over weeks, *then* ?tuberculosis, transfer urgently to Medical Officer.
2. *If* pain is sometimes present and sometimes not present, *then* ?osteoarthrosis. See Chapter 29.
3. *If* spinal tenderness on percussion or stiffness (will not bend properly) especially if lump, *then* ?tuberculosis. Transfer non-urgently to Medical Officer.
4. *If* weakness of legs, not able to pass urine properly, *then* ?tuberculosis, ?fracture. Transfer urgently to Medical Officer.

Pain is constant in lower chest and there is tenderness or mass in upper abdomen
Then abdominal condition with referred pain. See Chapter 36 page 407.

Pain in lower chest that comes or goes with eating
Then peptic ulcer. See Chapter 23 page 215.

Pain and cough present for more than 4 weeks
Then ?tuberculosis. See Chapter 14 page 64.

21

Disorders of the Blood and the Blood Forming Organs

Anatomy

Blood is made of many cells, called blood cells, and a liquid, called plasma. There are 2 kinds of blood cell – red blood cells (RBCs) and white blood cells (WBCs). Platelets are detached broken off) parts of cells. These cells stay in the bone marrow. (See Figure 21.1) The blood cells are suspended (or 'float') in the plasma. The plasma is

Figure 21.1 A blood slide as seen through a microscope. The blood was smeared on the slide, dried, fixed and stained. The plasma cannot be seen. You can see many RBCs, two WBCs and some platelets.

made of water which carries many things ('dissolved') in it. Proteins, sugars, fats and salts are all carried in the plasma.

Blood is made in these parts of the body.
1. Bone marrow – the red marrow in the ends of the long bones and in the flat bones (e.g. sternum and pelvis) is most important for making blood. RBCs and most WBCs are made in the marrow.
2. Spleen.
3. Liver.
4. Lymph nodes.

The bone marrow needs iron, folic acid, protein and other things to make blood. These things are all in a good diet which includes protein foods (meat, fish, eggs, milk, peanuts etc.) and protective foods (dark green leafy vegetables, fruit etc.). Without enough iron and folic acid and protein in the diet, even a normal bone marrow cannot make enough blood.

Physiology

The body circulates blood to all its organs. The blood keeps the cells of these organs alive and functioning properly. Blood takes food and oxygen and hormones to the cells. Blood takes used and waste material and carbon dioxide away from the cells. Blood contains many parts of the body's defence system against infection. Different parts of the blood have difference functions:

Red blood cells (RBCs) containing haemoglobin (Hb)
– carry oxygen.
White blood cells (WBCs)
– fight infection.
Platelets
– make the blood clot to stop bleeding.
Serum proteins
antibodies
– fight infection,
albumin
– keeps water inside the blood vessels,
clotting proteins
– make the blood clot to stop bleeding,
body building and repair proteins
– build and repair the body.
Sugar (glucose)
– for body nutrition and energy.

Fats
– for body nutrition and energy.
Hormones
– carry messages from one part of the body to another part.
Salts ⎱
Water ⎰
– contain the other parts of the blood and also make up the main volume of the blood.

Pathology

Disease may make the blood have too much or too little of one of its parts. Too much or too little of parts of the blood may cause these conditions:

- too few RBCs or low Hb – Anaemia
- too few WBCs – Infection
- too few platelets – Bleeding
- too little antibody protein –Infection
- too little albumin protein – Oedema
- too little clotting protein – Bleeding
- too little body building and repair protein – Wasting (body becomes thin)
- too much sugar – Diabetes (see Chapter 30 page 333)
- too little fat – Wasting
- too much water and salt – Oedema, Heart failure
- too little water and salt – Dehydration, Shock

Most of the conditions affecting the blood are caused by pathology in the organs which make the blood (i.e. marrow, spleen and liver).

1. *The marrow*
   The marrow may not make enough blood cells or may make abnormal blood cells because:
   (a) The marrow was abnormal from birth (i.e. the patient inherited an abnormal marrow).
   (b) The marrow does not get enough 'food' to function.
   (c) The marrow has been affected by disease or drugs.

2. *The spleen*
   If the spleen gets larger than normal for any reason, it may destroy normal blood cells. Sometimes the spleen makes abnormal antibodies.

3. *The liver*
   If disease affects the liver, the liver may not be able to use and store the food absorbed from the intestine properly. This can affect the protein, sugar, fat, salt and water in the blood.

Some of the conditions affecting the blood are however caused by pathology in organs other than the marrow, liver and spleen. These include:
1. bleeding or loss of fluid from the body,
2. heart disease, or
3. kidney disease.

History and examination

The most important disease of the blood is anaemia (see page 182). Look for anaemia in *all* patients who you see.
   Symptoms of anaemia include:
1. Shortness of breath.
2. Weakness and tiredness.
3. Dizziness.

The sign of anaemia is 'pallor' (i.e. paleness or whiteness). Look for pallor in those parts of the body which are normally pink or red because you can see the red colour of the blood there. Always look at all of these four places for pallor.
1. The conjunctiva under the lower eye lid.
2. The mucous membrane behind the lower lip.
3. The beds of the finger nails.
4. The palms of the hands (especially the skin creases).

If you suspect anaemia or any other disease of the blood examine very carefully the parts of the body where the blood is made:
1. The bones which, of course, are around the bone marrow. Look for lumps.
   Feel gently for tenderness. Examine the sternum carefully.
2. The spleen
   See Figure 22.10
3. The liver
   See Figure 24.6

Tests

1. *Examination of haemoglobin using a comparator (or haemoglobimometer)*
   If you do not have a laboratory worker to do it,

you must do this test yourself. For methods see Appendix 1 and Appendix 2 at the end of this chapter.

2. *Examination of a thin blood film*

This test must be done in a laboratory by a trained laboratory worker. If you do not have a laboratory worker to do it, you must make the blood film yourself and then send the blood film to a laboratory with a letter. The letter must state patient's problem and your diagnosis, and ask for both a report and an explanation of the results.

See Chapter 6 page 22 for the method of making a thin blood film.

Anaemia

Anaemia is said to be present when there is not enough RBC Hb (red blood cell haemoglobin) in the blood.[1] Normally there is more than 10g haemoglobin in each decilitre (or 100 ml) of blood (written as 10 g/dl or 10 g/100 ml or 10 g%).

Anaemia is very severe if the Hb is less than 2.5g/dl.

Anemia is severe if the Hb is less than 5 g/dl but more than 2.5 g/dl.

Anaemia is moderate if the Hb is less than 7.5 g/dl but more than 5 g/dl.

Anaemia is mild if the Hb is less than 10 g/dl[1] but more than 7.5 g/dl.

Anaemia is very common especially in hot wet tropical places where malaria and hookworm are common, where malnutrition is common, in women of childbearing age, and in children.

The common causes of anaemia include:

1. Not enough red blood cells and haemoglobin are made in the bone marrow because:

(a) Not enough iron is absorbed from the food.

(b) Not enough folic acid is absorbed from the food.

(c) Not enough protein is absorbed from the food.

(d) Diseases or drugs or chemicals have stopped the bone marrow functioning properly. The most common cause of this is chronic kidney failure (see Chapter 26 page 289); but there are others.

(e) The patient was born with abnormal bone marrow which cannot make *enough* normal haemoglobin i.e. thalassaemia (see page 190).

2. Red blood cells are destroyed before they are worn out. This is called 'haemolysis'. When red blood cells are destroyed more quickly than new ones are made, this causes anaemia.

Reasons for this include:

(a) Malaria – acute attack.

(b) Malaria – chronic

(c) Malaria – Tropical Splenomegaly Syndrome.

(d) Any cause of a very big spleen as well as malaria e.g. schistosomiasis, kala azar.

(e) Certain drugs or chemicals especially in patients who were born without enough G6PD (a special part of the red blood cells).

(f) Sickle cell anaemia – the patient was born with an abnormal bone marrow, which makes an abnormal haemoglobin which causes the red blood cells to become an abnormal sickle shape (called 'sickling'.)

3. Red blood cells are lost from the body during bleeding. Reasons for this include:

(a) Gastro-intestinal tract bleeding. This is usually caused by hookworm in the small bowel sucking the patient's blood (see Chapter 23 page 217). This is sometimes due to bleeding from a peptic ulcer (see Chapter 23 page 215).

(b) Genital tract bleeding in the female. This is usually caused by an ante-partum or post-partum haemorhage. But it can be caused by having pregnancies close together.

The common causes of anaemia are:
1. not enough iron, folic acid and protein in the diet,
2. hookworm,
3. malaria,
4. repeated pregnancy,
5. sickle cell anaemia – in Africa only.
You must find out the epidemiology of anaemia in your area. If other causes are common in your area, then change this list.

---

1 In countries which have good public health services, anaemia is diagnosed if the Hb is less than the following.
men 13 g/dl
non-pregnant women 12 g/dl
pregnant women 11 g/dl

When you take the history of a patient with anaemia, find out if this patient has any of these common causes of anaemia. Ask about a family history of blood diseases. Ask about a past history of the common causes.

When anaemia is present there is not enough haemoglobin in the blood to carry enough oxygen to any part of the body. No part of the body, therefore, functions properly. The heart pumps the blood through the lungs and through the body more quickly than normal to use the small amount of haemoglobin in the blood to carry oxygen more often – palpitations (feeling the heart beat more quickly or strongly than normal) occur. The patient breathes more deeply or quickly than normal. Shortness of breath occurs. Muscles do not get enough oxygen – tiredness and weakness occur. The brain does not get enough oxgyen – dizziness or headaches occur. The heart, which is also doing more work than normal, does not get enough oxygen – heart failure can happen.

Symptoms of anaemia include:
1. weakness or tiredness,
2. dizziness,
3. shortness of breath.

Signs of anaemia include pallor (or paleness or whiteness) of:
1. the mucous membrane of the mouth inside the lips,
2. conjunctivae under the lower eye lids,

3. finger nail beds, and
4. palms of hands.

Symptoms and signs of (1) the cause of the anaemia, or (2) heart failure (see Chapter 27 page 301) can also be present.

Haemoglobin estimation (see page 191) should always be made. This
1. confirms the diagnosis of anaemia
2. confirms how severe the anaemia is, and
3. gives a starting point to measure the success of treatment.

Management and treatment

Treatment of anaemia will usually cure the anaemia. However, treatment cannot increase the haemoglobin by more than 1 g/dl each week. Often the Hb rises by only 0.5 g/dl each week. As the haemoglobin estimation is often as much as 2 g/dl above or below the real level of the haemoglobin, you cannot tell for at least 4 weeks if the treatment is working. (i.e. 0.5 g/dl × 4 weeks = rise of 2 g/dl). After 4 weeks the haemoglobin should have risen by at least 2 g/dl.

However, if the cause of the anaemia is not stopped the anaemia will usually return when the treatment is stopped. Therefore you must always try to *find out the cause of the anaemia and stop this cause.*

Blood transfusion is not the treatment of anaemia. Blood transfusion does not help the

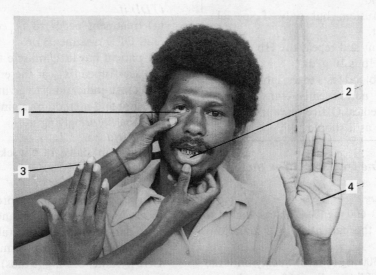

Figure 21.2 Photograph showing the *four* places of the body where pallor *must* be looked for in *all* patients. (1) The conjunctivae under the lower eyelid. (2) The mucous membrane inside the lower lip. (3) The fingernail beds. (4) The palms of the hands.

body make more blood, or stop blood being destroyed, or stop bleeding. Blood transfusion does not stop the cause of anaemia. Blood transfusion is used only if it is needed to keep the patient alive while the cause of the anaemia is found and stopped and the treatment of the anaemia is given time to work.

Admission for treatment is not needed for many patients. Admit for inpatient treatment *if*:

1. very pale or Hb less than 5 g/dl (until Hb 5 g/dl); *or*
2. a lot of dizziness, shortness of breath, weakness, etc.; *or*
3. heart failure (oedema, etc.); *or*
4. patient may get quickly worse (e.g. acute malaria, recent gastro-intestinal bleeding, late pregnancy, etc.); *or*
5. time of stress for patient (e.g. infection, post-partum state etc.).

---

1. Give these six routine treatments for the common causes to all anaemic patients:
   (1) antimalarials.
   (2) iron,
   (3) folic acid,
   (4) nutrition education if needed,
   (5) anti-hookworm drug,
   (6) advice about family planning and antenatal care if needed.
2. Look for other causes. Treat any other cause you find.
3. Blood transfusion; but only if special reasons for it.
4. See the patient and repeat the Hb each 4 weeks until Hb is 10 g/dl.
5. Send special blood tests to the laboratory, or refer (or non-urgently transfer) the patient to Medical Officer care if the Hb does not rise as it should.

Give the six routine treatments for the common causes

1. *Antimalarial drug*
   Chloroquine 450–600 mg (3–4 tablets) daily for 3 days; *then* if the patient is in a malarious area –
   Chloroquine 300 mg (2 tabs) weekly until the Hb is above 10 g/dl (usually 6–12 weeks but up to 2 or more years if Tropical Splenomegaly Syndrome) (supply 8 tabs each 4 weeks); *then* –

Chloroquine to be taken 450–600 mg (3–4 tabs) daily for 3 days if the patient gets any attack of fever. (Supply 9–12 tabs to the patient to keep at home.)

If in chloroquine resistant malaria area use special anti-malarial drugs (see Chapter 13 page 56).

2. *Iron*
   Give ferrous sulphate (200 mg tablets) or ferrous gluconate (300 mg tablets)
   if
   (a) anaemia not severe (Hb > 7.5 g/dl if pregnant *or* Hb > 5g/dl in other persons), *and*
   (b) you think the patient will swallow 3 tablets a day for 3 months.
   Give 1 tab three times a day for whole of pregnancy or for 3 months to other patients.
   Give IMI iron dextran (any brand) to
   (a) all other cases *and*
   (b) if Hb does not rise by 2 g/dl after iron tablets given for 4 weeks.
   But see Appendix 3 at the end of this chapter, *before* giving IMI iron dextran, for contra-indications to giving IMI iron dextan and for method of giving IMI iron dextran. *Give* 5 ml daily for
   • 6 days if weight < 40 kg
   • 10 days if weight > 40 kg, and
   • 2 days extra if pregnant.
   Give IV iron dextran (only 'Imferon') infusion (TDI) if
   (a) treatment needs to be completed quickly (e.g. OPD treatment) *or*
   (b) patient has little muscle for IM injections.
   But see Appendix 4 at the end of this chapter for contra-indications to giving IV iron dextran infusion and method of giving IV iron dextran infusion *before* giving it.

3. *Folic acid*
   5 mg (1 tab) daily for 1 week *then* 5 mg (1 tab) weekly for 12 weeks.

4. *Diet*
   Educate to eat enough protein foods (e.g. meat, fish, eggs, peanuts) and protective foods (e.g. dark green leafy vegetables, fruit) daily.

5. *Pyrantel* or other hookworm treatment
   Give pyrantel 625 mg (5 tabs) in one dose orally once.

6. *Offer family planning and/or antenatal care advice if required.*

Give only half (½) of these doses of iron if the Hb is 7.5 g/dl or above.

Do NOT give oral iron for more than 3 months unless pregnant or told to do so by the Medical Officer.

Do NOT give a course of iron by injections more than once in any twelve-month period

Do NOT give iron injection (IM or IV) while a patient is very sick or has a fever (above 37.5°C).

Wait until malaria, infections and fever have been successfully treated and then give iron injections.

Treat also any other underlying cause found

Arrange transfer for blood transfusion but only for the following patients

1. *If* the haemoglobin is 7.5 g/dl or less
   and
   if the patient is more than 36 weeks pregnant (post-partum haemorrhage possible) *or if* the anaemia is due to haemorrhage which may occur again (e.g. recent haematemesis, melena, or haemoptysis).
2. *If* the haemoglobin is less than 5 g/dl
   and
   if there is also
   acute malaria (fever), *or*
   heart failure (oedema, etc.), *or*
   severe symptoms of anaemia (dizziness, shortness of breath, severe weakness, etc.), *or*
   pregnancy at any stage, *or*
   a severe infection or other illness, *or*
   other time of stress such as the post-partum state.

Repeat Hb estimation each 4 weeks until Hb is 10 g/dl.

The haemoglobin should rise by 2–4 g/dl in 4 weeks.

If the haemoglobin does not rise by at least 2 g/dl, give fully supervised treatment for another 4 weeks including iron by injection and you yourself watching the antimalarial tablets being swallowed and checking for chloroquine resistant malaria.

If the haemoglobin does rise by at least 2 g/dl continue treatment and arrange special blood tests

or referral or non-urgent transfer to a medical officer.

Transfer to Medical Officer Care if Needed

1. If blood transfusion is needed (see page 195) (urgent – sometimes emergency).
2. If the haemoglobin does not rise by 2 g/dl after 4 weeks of correct, fully supervised treatment of the common causes (except Tropical Splenomegaly Syndrome) (non-urgent).
3. If anaemia has returned after full treatment (see page 184) and if necessary adequate treatment of malaria, before 1 year has gone (non-urgent).
4. If the haemoglobin does not rise by 2 g/dl and the spleen decrease in size by 2 cm in 6 months when the patient has Tropical Splenomegaly Syndrome and has had correct prophylactic antimalarial drugs regularly (see page 187) (non-urgent).
5. If the patient has Tropical Splenomegaly Syndrome and becomes pregnant (discuss with Medical Officer first) (non-urgent).

Prevention

Prevention of anaemia is the prevention and treatment of the common causes of anaemia. This includes:

1. Control and treatment of malaria (see Chapter 13 page 54)
2. Control and treatment of hookworm (see Chapter 23 page 217)
3. Good diet with enough iron folic and protein etc. in it. The diet should be a mixed one which has in it protein foods (meat, fish, eggs, peanuts etc.) and protective foods (dark green leafy vegetables, fruit etc.).
4. Good obstetrical advice and care. Advice and help with family planning. Antenatal care including iron, folic acid and anti-malarials for all women during pregnancy. Prevention of post-partum haemorrhage.

Tropical splenomegaly syndrome

Tropical Splenomegaly Syndrome (TSS) is an abnormal reaction by the immune system of the body to chronic malarial infection. It is present when a person who has had chronic malaria for years has a very big spleen, anaemia, wasting and repeated attacks of haemolysis (see below), and these things are not improving but are worsening.

Pathology

When a non-immune person starts to live in an area where there is malaria, first he gets acute malaria and then he gets chronic malaria. (See Chapter 13 page 54.) A person with chronic malaria has a big spleen, anaemia, wasting (or poor growth if a child) and repeated attacks of acute malaria and other infections. If the person does not die from acute or chronic malaria, he develops antibodies against malaria. After about 4–10 years he develops semi-immunity to malaria. Then his spleen becomes smaller, his haemoglobin rises, his wasting gets less (and he grows better if he is a child) and there are fewer attacks of acute malaria and other infections. However, a few people with chronic malaria do not develop normal antibodies and normal immunity to malaria. These people develop abnormal antibodies and abnormal immunity to malaria. This causes Tropical Splenomegaly Syndrome. In these people who develop an abnormal immune reaction to malaria, the big spleen stays big and may get bigger. The big spleen (for no other reason than that it is big) destroys red and white blood cells more quickly than the bone-marrow can make enough new ones.

This causes severe chronic anaemia, low resistance to infections, wasting and chronic ill health. At times the big spleen may suddenly destroy many more red blood cells than it usually does. This causes acute very severe anaemia (acute haemolysis) and fever and splenic pain.

Clinical features

The patient is usually a young adult from a malarious area. The condition happens more commonly in certain places and certain families.

Symptoms include those of:

1. anaemia (malaise, inability to work, weakness, dizziness, shortness of breath);
2. enlarged spleen (swelling of abdomen, abdominal discomfort); and
3. episodes of acute haemolysis (severe weakness etc. often with fever and sometimes with pain in the abdomen over the spleen).

wasting (thin arms) and chronic ill health

large liver

very large spleen (gr. 4) tender when acute haemolylic attacks occur

anaemia (pale nails, palms, inside lips and conjunctivae)

Figure 21.3 Tropical splenomegaly syndrome. Note the features in an adult who has lived all her life in an area where malaria is always present.

Signs include (see Figure 21.3):

- anaemia,
- wasting (thin muscles, little fat),
- spleen very enlarged, firm and usually non-tender,
- liver usually enlarged,
- episodes of fever, jaundice and tender spleen during which the patient is more anaemic than before (acute haemolytic episodes).

The patient has chronic ill health. He becomes worse from time to time because of haemolytic episodes. The condition does not improve by itself while the patient stays in a malarious area. Death usually occurs from acute malaria or acute severe bacterial infection or an haemolytic episode.

Management

You are not able to change the patient's abnormal reaction to malaria parasites to normal. You can, however, stop this abnormal reaction, by curing the patient of malaria and then giving him malaria prophylaxis so that no more malarial parasites are in his body. The patient must take the malarial prophylaxis until all the symptoms and signs of Tropical Splenomegaly Syndrome are gone – this usually takes at least 2 years. After this, he will have to take malarial prophylaxis for life if the condition starts to return when he stops the prophylaxis. Details of the management of a patient with Tropical Splenomegaly Syndrome are set out below.

Do a haemoglobin estimation (see page 191). Write down the result. Do this each time you see the patient.

Send a thin blood smear (and if possible 4 ml of blood in an EDTA bottle and enough blood on blotting or filter paper to cover a thumb nail) to the hospital laboratory and ask them to look for sickle cell anaemia, chronic leukaemia, thalassaemia and other rare blood diseases. (Result is not urgent.)

Measure the size of the spleen before starting treatment. Write down the size. Do this again each time you see the patient.

Admit for inpatient treatment if

- the haemoglobin is less than 5 g/dl, or
- the patient has had recent acute haemolytic episode, or
- the patient is sick, or
- the patient is pregnant.

Give routine treatment for anaemia with chloroquine, iron, folic acid, pyrantel, education about diet, and family planning (see anaemia page 182). However, do not give total dose infusion of iron during pregnancy if the patient has Tropical Splenomegaly Syndrome.

Give explanations and health education about the need for regular treatment for many years. Give chloroquine 300 mg (2 tabs) weekly or 125 mg (½ tab) daily for at least 2 years and probably for life.

Give quick, effective treatment for any acute attacks of bacterial infections or malaria as they occur.

Transfer to Medical Officer care the following patients:

1. If the patient has haemolytic episode at any time, but especially during pregnancy (i.e. sudden increase in anaemia often with fever, increased weakness, and possibly jaundice and spleen pain). Transfer for blood transfusion and prednisolone (urgent – at times emergency).
2. If a patient with Tropical Splenomegaly Syndrome becomes pregnant. (Discuss with Medical Officer the need for this first.) (Non-urgent.)
3. If after 6–8 months of treatment the Hb has not risen by 2 g/dl and the spleen has not decreased in size by 1 grade or 5 cm (transfer for investigation for other diseases) (non-urgent).

Sickle cell anaemia

Sickle cell anaemia is a severe inherited disease which causes chronic anaemia, episodes of severe pain and tenderness of bones and other parts of the body, and often death.

Sickle cell anaemia is common only in people from parts of Africa and people of African descent.

Pathology

Sickle cell anaemia is due to a large amount of an abnormal haemoglobin called, Hb S, in the red blood cells (instead of normal adult haemoglobin). This abnormality must be partly

Figure 21.4 Photograph of normal red blood cells and sickle cells.

present in both parents for a child to get the severe abnormality. A small amount of Hb S helps protect a person against malaria. A large amount of Hb S does not protect against malaria and also causes sickle cell anaemia. As the abnormality that makes Hb S (instead of normal haemoglobin) is inherited, there is no cure for the disease.

When a red blood cell which has a lot of Hb S in it gives up its oxygen, it changes to an abnormal long thin 'sickle' shape (see Figure 21.4). If the sickled cell is quickly given oxygen again, it goes back to the normal shape. If the sickled cell is not given oxygen for more than a couple of minutes, it cannot ever go back to the normal shape.

Sickling of red blood cells causes two groups of problems.

1. The abnormal red blood cells are destroyed in the body (mostly in the spleen) more quickly than normal red blood cells (called chronic haemolysis). This causes chronic anaemia and a big spleen.

   From time to time, sometimes because of an infection, but often for no obvious reason, the spleen may destroy many more red cells than normal, the anaemia becomes much worse with jaundice and more enlargement of the spleen. This is called a haemolytic crisis. The bone marrow makes as many red cells as it can to replace the ones being destroyed by the spleen. The marrow in the bones gets bigger. This may make the bones get bigger and give an unusual appearance to the bones of the skull and face. The bone marrow often needs more folic acid

than it can get to make all the extra blood. All the body then becomes short of folic acid. This shortage of folic acid may stop the patient growing and stop puberty (a child developing into a man or woman).

2. The red blood cells become sickled as they give up their oxygen in the capillaries of the body tissues. The sickled cells can then get stuck in the capillaries and cannot then return to the lungs to get more oxygen. The blocked capillaries stop other red cells passing through them and these other red cells give up there oxygen and then sickle. The blood then often clots in the blocked blood vessels. The part of the body, which the blocked blood vessels usually supply, gets no oxygen and so becomes inflamed and dies. Death of part of the body like this is called an 'infarction'. The process just described is often called an 'infarction crisis'.

The things which make an infarction crisis more likely are:

(a) infections, (bacterial and malarial);

(b) dehydration;

(c) if less oxygen is breathed in than usual e.g.

• during an operation,

• going high in an aeroplane which is not properly pressurised;

(d) if part or all of the body becomes cold and the blood circulation slows down;

(e) if the blood flow to part of the body is stopped e.g. putting on a torniquet or tight bandage.

However, many infarction crises happen for no reason that can be found.

Some patients have many attacks of infarction – 1 or 2 each week. Some patients have few attacks – 1 or 2 each year.

The parts of the body most often affected by infarction crises are the bones. In infants, the fingers and toes are the most often affected. In older people, any bone or any other part of the body can be affected If the spleen has many infarctions, it may become small.

The parts of the body which have been affected by infarction may be infected by bacteria which cause osteomyelitis, etc.

In pregnancy the above other severe complications can result in death.

Symptoms and signs

Anaemia and related conditions
The usual symptoms and signs of anaemia are present (see page 182).

The haemoglobin is usually about 8 g/dl. (If the haemoglobin is normal (and the patient is not dehydrated) the patient probably does not have sickle cell anaemia.)

The patient may be mildly jaundiced.

The spleen and liver are usually large; though the spleen may become small.

Sometimes the anaemia may become much worse (haemolytic crisis).

The skull and face bones may have an unusual shape.

Growth and puberty may be slow.

Sometimes there are leg ulcers.

Infarction crises
Sudden severe pain and tenderness (and often fever) start in a bone or the spleen or another part of the body. With proper treatment, the pain usually greatly improves within 2 days and goes within 7–9 days.

The bones are affected more often than other parts of the body. Any bone can be affected, but often the fingers and toes are most affected. The infected bone becomes painful and tender.

Old bone infarctions may have made the fingers short and thick with narrow ends. Also the patient may not be very tall, because the trunk of the body is short.

If a joint is affected, acute arthritis occurs.

If the kidney is affected, there is often blood in the urine.

If the spleen is affected, there is a tender swelling in the left upper abdomen.

If the intestine is affected there may be acute abdominal pain and tenderness and vomiting.

If the brain is affected, there may be paralysis.

Infections
If pain and tenderness and fever in an area of infarction does not become much better after 2 days of proper treatment, and is not nearly gone after 7–9 days of treatment, then that part of the body probably has developed a secondary bacterial infection.

Tests

Haemoglobin
The Hb is usually about 8 g/dl.

Sickling test
If you have a laboratory with a microscope, then you can do a simple test for sickling of the blood with sodium metabisulphate.

On one slide a drop of patient's blood is mixed with a drop of freshly prepared 2% sodium metabisulphate solution and placed under a cover slip. The same test is done with normal blood on another slide. Both are examined 20 minutes later. If the patient's blood but not the normal blood shows sickle-shaped or long curved red blood cells, then the patient *has* HbS in his blood.

People who have only a *little* HbS in their blood and do not have sickle cell anaemia *can* still have a positive sickling test.

If the sickling test is *negative*, it is almost certain that the patient does *not* have sickle cell anaemia.

The only *certain* way to diagnose that *the disease* is present is to send the blood to a laboratory where they do a special test for HbS.

Thin blood smear
You can diagnose sickle cell anaemia fairly certainly in most cases if there is (1) anaemia and (2) a typical thin blood smear for sickle cell anaemia.

White cell count
The white cell count is often high (often twice the normal levels) even when there is no infection.

Treatment
There is no cure.

Treat the anaemia
1. Give regular prophylactic antimalarial drugs for life (if in a malarial area) (see Chapter 13 page 35).
2. Give folic acid 5 mg (1 tab) daily for life.
3. Do not give blood transfusions unless the Hb suddenly falls to very low levels or before operations etc.
4. Do not give iron after the first course as it is not usually needed. However ask the laboratory or Medical Officer to do tests to see if iron is needed if you suspect iron deficiency.

Tell the patient how to avoid infarction crises

1. Take prophylactic antimalarials for life (see Chapter 13 page 59).
2. Avoid infections.
3. Avoid dehydration – always drink enough to pass a lot of urine (especially if he or she has vomiting or diarrhoea or it is very hot). He should never take (and health workers should never order) diuretics (e.g. hydrochlorothiazide, frusemide etc.) even for heart failure or high blood pressure etc.)
4. Avoid becoming cold.
5. Avoid tight clothes on the limbs.

Treat infarction crises

1. Give aspirin or paracetamol or codeine as needed (see Chapter 7 page 28). Do not give pethidine or morphine as the patient may become addicted to it.
2. The patient must be fully hydrated. Use and IV drip in severe cases (see Chapter 23 page 224).
3. Make the patient rest.

Treat any infection quickly

If pain from an infarction crisis has not improved in 2 days and and not nearly gone in 7–9 days, there is an infection which you must treat with antibiotics (see Chapter 11 page 40).

Transfer patients who need an operation

The condition may be because of infarction crisis.

The operation may cause an infarction crisis.

The anaesthetic needs high concentrations of oxygen and may need a pre-operative blood transfusion. No tourniquets can be used.

Do not operate on patients who have sickle cell anaemia yourself. Transfer all patients with sickle cell anaemia who seem to need an operation to a Medical Officer.

Transfer pregnant patients

Transfer all patients with sickle cell anaemia who become pregnant to a Medical Officer.

Prognosis

Without treatment most patients would die before they were adults. If proper treatment is given patients may have a reasonable life although they may have many attacks of the problems described.

Thalassaemia

Thalassaemia is an inherited disease in which the bone marrow cannot make enough haemoglobin and the patient becomes anaemic.

Thalassaemia is common around the Mediterranean; but it can occur in all parts of the world.

Thalassaemia must be present, even if only mildly so, in both parents for a child to get severe thalassaemia.

Mild thalassaemia (called 'Thalassaemia minor') causes only a few symptoms and signs. There is a mild anaemia which is like iron deficiency anaemia but which does not improve on routine anaemia treatment (see page 183). If blood tests are sent to the hospital laboratory (a thin blood smear, 4 ml blood in EDTA bottle and blood about 1 cm across on filter or blotting paper) or if the patient is referred or transferred non-urgently to the Medical Officer, the condition can be diagnosed by tests. Treat mild thalassaemia patients with regular prophylactic antimalarials if in a malarious area (see Chapter 13 page 59) for life and with folic acid 5 g (1 tab) daily for life. DO NOT GIVE IRON after the first course unless the medical officer tells you that the patient also has iron deficiency, as may occur in girls on vegetarian diets, women with many pregnancies etc.

Severe thalassaemia (called 'Thalassaemia major') affects children. They have very severe anaemia which does not improve on any treatment. The spleen becomes larger and exentually very large, also the skull and face bones are large and unusual to look at. You can only keep the patient alive by repeated blood transfusions and treatment for mild thallasaemia. The iron from the blood transfusions and the food damages the heart and other organs and can cause death if death is not caused by a complication of the anaemia (usually before adult life is reached).

Appendix 1   Haemoglobin estimation using a comparator

Principle

This is a method for estimating haemoglobin using the eyes.

The test solution is compared with a series of coloured glass standards that show the amount of haemoglobin.

Materials

- Haemoglobin comparator with standards to cover the range 3-13 g of haemoglobin per decilitre (g/dl)
- Two comparator tubes
- 0.05 ml (50 mm³ or 50μl) pipettes
- Haemoglobin diluting fluid. This is made by adding 0.4 ml of strong ammonia solution to 1 litre of distilled water.

Method

1. Fill a test tube with 10 ml of the diluting fluid.

2. Draw venous or capillary blood to the 0.05 ml (or 50 mm³ or 50 μl) mark of the blood

pipette. Do not allow air bubbles to enter. If blood from a bottle is being tested, make sure that it is well mixed by tipping the bottle containing it and the anticoagulant repeatedly for about 1 minute immediately before pipetting it.

3. Wipe the outside of the pipette so that no blood is on the outside, check that the blood is still on the mark, and blow the blood into the 10 ml of diluting fluid. Wash the inside of the pipette 2–3 times with the solution containing the blood.

4. Mix the contents of the tube.
   The fluid will become a clear red as the red cells are haemolysed. The colour of the solution will not fade for a few hours.

5. Fill one of the comparator tubes to the mark with the fluid. Lift the lid of the comparator and place the tube in the right-hand side of the comparator.

6. Fill the other comparator tube to the mark with the diluting fluid and place this in the left-hand side of the comparator. Close the lid.

7. Holding the equipment with the front of the comparator directed towards the daylight, look down through the viewing aperture, (as in the picture).

8. Daylight must be used, but do not hold the comparator in direct sunlight.

9. Starting with the pale-coloured standards, compare each with the colour of the test solution, as seen in the left-hand side of the viewing aperture.

   When the colours are matched as closedly as possible, make a final check by comparing with the standard on each side of the one thought to match best.

10. Read the haemoglobin value in grams per decilitre (g/dl) as shown on the disc used to rotate the standards.

11. When the colour of the test lies between two standards, make an estimate between the two values.

Appendix 2 Haemoglobin estimation by Sahli method

Principle

The blood is diluted in an acid solution, converting the haemoglobin to acid haematin. The test solution is matched against a coloured glass reference. The Sahli method is not an accurate way of estimating haemoglobulin.

Materials

– Sahli haemoglobinometer
– Sahli pipette (graduated to 20 mm³, i.e. 0.02 ml, or 20 μl)
– Small glass rod
– Dropping pipette
– Absorbent paper
– 0.1 mol/l(0.1 N) hydrochloric acid (HCl)

Method

1. Fill the graduated tube to the 20 mark (or the mark 3 g/100 ml) with 0.1 mol/l HCl.

2. Draw venous or capillary blood to the 0.02 ml mark of the Sahli pipette. Do not allow air bubbles to enter. If blood from a bottle is being tested, make sure that it is well mixed by tipping the bottle containing it and the anticoagulant repeatedly for about 1 minute immediately before pipetting it.

3. Wipe the outside of the pipette with absorbent paper to remove all blood. Check that the blood is still on the mark.

4. Blow the blood from the pipette into the graduated tube of the acid solution.
Rinse the pipette by drawing in and blowing out the acid solution 3 times.
The mixture of blood and acid gives a brownish colour.
Allow to stand for 5 minutes.

5. Place the graduated tube in the haemoglobinometer. Stand facing a window. Compare the colour of the tube containing diluted blood with the colour of the reference tube.
If the colour is the same as or lighter than that of the reference tube the haemoglobin value is 4 g/dl or less.

6. If the colour is darker than that of the reference tube continue to dilute by adding 0.1 mol/l HCl drop by drop.
Stir with the glass rod after adding each drop. Remove the rod and compare the colours of the 2 tubes.
Stop when the colours match.

7. Note the mark reached. Depending on the type of haemoglobinometer, this gives the haemoglobin concentration either in g/100 ml (i.e. g/dl) or as a percentage of 'normal'. To convert percentages to g/dl, multiply by 0.146.

193

Appendix 3 Method of giving iron dextran by IMI

Inject only into upper, outer buttock (see Figure 21.5 (A)).

Use a 19 or 20 s.w.g. needle;

First, with the fingers of one hand, slide the skin and underlying tissue over the upper, outer buttock away from this area (See Figure 21.5 (B)).

Insert the needle through the stretched skin (from another area) into the upper, outer buttock (See Figure 21.5 (C)).

If blood comes back along or through the needle withdraw it and try again.

Inject slowly.

Wait 10 seconds after the injection is finished and then withdraw the needle.

Allow the skin to slide back to its proper place (See Figure 21.5 (D)).

Make the patient walk around or move the leg. Do not rub the site of the injection.

Do not give iron by injection until malaria, infections and fever have been successfully treated.

Do not give more than one course of iron by injection in any one 12-month period.

Figure 21.5 Diagrams to show method of giving iron dextran by IMI. See text for details.

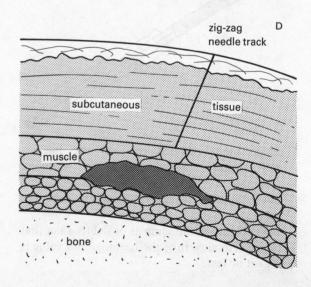

Appendix 4 Method of total dose iron dextran by IV drip (TDI)

Use only 'Imferon'. *Do not* use iron dextran compound unless 'Imferon' is also on the ampoule.

Give only if the patient (1) is past childhood, (2) has no history of allergy or asthma, (3) has no fever or infection and is not sick.

Record pulse rate and blood pressure.

Give promethazine 50 mg (2 ml) IMI first.

Insert the drip – 1 litre of dextrose 4.3% in sodium chloride 0.18% (or ½ – 1 litre of 0.9% sodium chloride; but only if no heart failure). Add only one ampoule of the 'Imferon' to the 1 litre of IV fluid.

Start the drip at 5 drops per minute. Check pulse and blood pressure after 5 minutes and again after 10 minutes.

If
- blood pressure falls more than 15 mm systolic, *or*
- pulse rises more than 15 beats per minute, *or*
- patient becomes restless or breathless or coughs, or has chest pains, sweating, nausea or vomiting;

then immediately stop the drip, change both flask and drip set and treat for shock (Capter 27 page 305).

Give adrenaline 1–1000 solution 0.5 ml (½ ml) IMI.

Give promethazine 50 mg (2 ml) IVI if needed. *Also change to* IM *iron dextran (after patient has fully recovered).*

If none of the above signs come, then add the rest of the total dose of 'Imferon' to the flask. Then observe the patient for another 10 minutes as above. Treat as above if signs of shock or allergy occur.

If none of the signs of shock or allergy (above) come increase the drip rate to 40–60 drop/minute. Check PR and BP each 15 minutes. The drip should finish in 4–6 hours.

Appendix 5 Notes on blood transfusion

Refer to these notes and any other instructions you have been given on blood transfusion before giving blood.

1. One unit of blood usually raises the Hb in an adult by 1–1.5 g%.
2. Transfuse till Hb over 5 g/dl – all patients described on page 185. Transfuse till Hb over 7.5 g/dl – (a) patients who may bleed and bleeding could be difficult to control (after 36 weeks of pregnancy, recent gastro-intestinal bleeding etc.) and (b) patients who have severe infections.
3. Only use blood which has been properly grouped and cross-matched.
4. Make certain the *correct* bag of blood is given to the patient. The labels, etc. must be checked by two senior health workers.
5. Remove a bag of blood from Blood Bank refrigerator only when you can start transfusing it immediately.
6. Never transfuse blood that has been out of the refrigerator for more than 6 hours.
7. Take the temperature, pulse rate, blood pressure and respiration rate:
   - before the transfusion is started,
   - 15 minutes after the transfusion is started, and
   - each hour after the transfusion is started.
   - A responsible health worker must stay with the patient all the time for the first 15 minutes.
   - Observe the patient carefully for any kind of reaction (including low BP, fast PR, back pain, breathlessness, fever, restlessness, skin rash, etc.).
8. If the patient develops any kind of reaction (as above):
   - stop blood transfusion,
   - give promethazine 25 mg (1 ml) IV and 25 mg (1 ml) IM,
   - consult medical officer immediately,
   - see Chapter 27 page 305 if shock.

22

Disorders of the Lymphatic System and Spleen

Anatomy, physiology and pathology

The lymphatic system goes through most of the body. The important parts of it are:

- the lymph vessels,
- the lymph nodes (sometimes called 'lymph-glands' or just 'glands'),
- the spleen,
- the tonsils, and
- the appendix.

A body fluid called lymph flows through the lymph vessels and lymph glands. The lymph system is connected to the blood circulation system (see Figure 22.1).

Lymph vessels are tubes like the blood capillaries and veins. There is a network of very small lymph capillaries over almost all of the body (see Figure 22.2). These capillaries join to make larger lymph vessels as the vessels go towards the centre of the body.

The lymphatic system

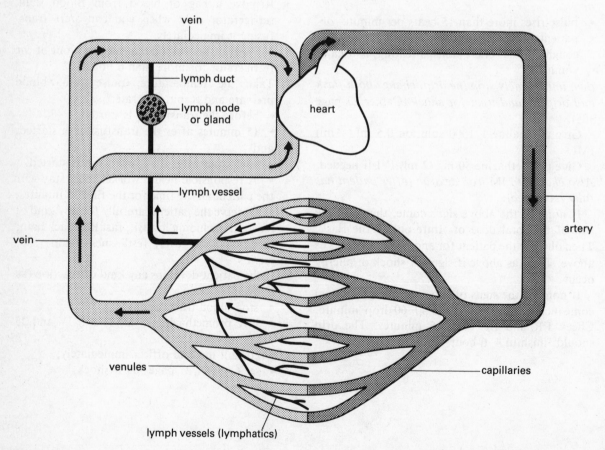

Figure 22.1   Diagram to show the relationship of the lymphatic system to the circulation of the blood.

Figure 22.2 This diagram shows the position of the main groups of lymph glands. It also shows the lymph vessels which carry lymph into the glands. It also shows the lymph glands draining into lymphatic ducts. The largest lymphatic ducts then drain into the large veins.

Lymph nodes are collections of lymphatic tissue along the course of the lymph vessels.

Lymph vessels collect fluid from the capillaries and tissues in the same way as veins. But lymph vessels also collect larger things (such as large proteins and organisms) which veins cannot collect. These proteins and organisms are taken to the lymph nodes, where, if necessary, the lymphatic system cells make antibodies etc. against the protein or organism. (See Chapter 10 page 35.)

The protein or organisms travelling in the lymphatic system can sometimes cause inflammation of parts of the lymphatic system. Inflammation of the lymph vessels is called *lymphangitis*. Inflammation of the lymph nodes is called *lymphadenitis*. If the infection is severe, pus may form in the lymph nodes.

If the lymph nodes are inflamed or destroyed and cannot take fluid and protein from the tissues in the normal way, then the extra fluid and protein in the tissues causes swelling. This is called *lymphoedema*. Lymphoedema is like ordinary oedema except that the fluid has much protein in it, so the oedema does not get a hollow in it, or 'pit', when you press on the area, as easily as ordinary oedema.

History and examination

If you suspect disease of the lymphatic system you must:

1. Examine the lymph nodes in the neck (see Figure 22.3), and axilla (see Figure 22.4), and groin.

    Examine the lymph nodes in the neck and axilla when you examine the head and neck, ENT and thyroid.

    Examine the lymph nodes in the groin when you examine the abdomen for herniae and lymph nodes.

    You cannot examine the lymph nodes in the chest or abdomen in a routine physical examination.

2. Examine the related organs:
    - liver (see Chapter 24 page 241),
    - spleen (see this chapter page 208),
    - bone (see Chapter 28 page 311), and
    - blood for anaemia, bleeding or infection (see Chapter 21 page 181).

3. Examine the areas drained by any abnormal lymph nodes for lymphoedema, infections and cancer.

Figure 22.3 Method of examination of the lymph glands in the neck. The left photograph shows examination of the lymph glands at the back of the neck – from in front of the patient. The right photograph shows examination of the lymph glands at the front of the neck – from behind the patient with the patient's head tipped to the side you are examining to make the muscles relax.

Figure 22.4 Method of examination of the lymph glands in the axilla. Note that the patient must not hold his arms out so that you can feel under them. That makes the muscles tight and you cannot feel the lymph glands under the muscles. The patient's arm must be at his side as in this photograph.

Common clinical conditions of the lymphatic system

Acute infective lymphangitis and lymphadenitis

Acute infection anywhere in the body may enlarge lymph nodes which drain the area. This may be because the nodes are making antibodies etc. (see Chapter 10 page 35).

But in some infections, the organisms defeat the body defences, and then these organisms may grow and multiply in the lymph vessels and/or lymph nodes, and cause inflammation.

In inflammation of the lymph vessels there is a red, hot, tender, swelling in a thin line between the place where the infection started and the lymph nodes. This is called *acute lymphangitis*.

In inflammation of the lymph nodes the nodes are enlarged and tender (and if they are close to the skin, they may be hot and red). This is called *acute lymphadenitis*.

In severe acute lymphadenitis, pus may form and the nodes become fluctuant.

In acute infections of the lymph vessels or lymph nodes, the patient will develop malaise, fever, fast pulse, and the other signs of toxaemia.

Most cases of acute lymphangitis and acute lymphadenitis are caused by bacterial infections. Sometimes they are caused by filarial infection (see page 200) and other causes.

Treatment includes:

1. Antibiotics – usually penicillin. (See Chapter 10 page 34.)
2. If there is pus and fluctuation, aspirate (suck out) the pus through a needle, or incise and drain (if aspiration is not successful).

Bubonic plague

See Chapter 17 page 104.

Chronic infective lymphadenitis

Chronic lymphadenitis can be caused by repeated attacks of acute bacterial infection or by chronic infection.

These can cause (1) enlargement of the lymph nodes and/or (2) block of the lymph vessels and the lymph passages in the lymph nodes.

This block of the flow of the lymph can cause lymphoedema. Lymphoedema is swelling of the area drained by the affected vessels and nodes caused by oedema. (See Figure 22.7.)

Elephantiasis – chronic severe swelling of the affected body parts with thickening and folding of the skin (see Figure 22.7) – can develop if lymphoedema is present for many years. Lymphoedema and elephantiasis are particularly common in the leg and the scrotum.

Other causes of similar clinical lymphoedema and elephantiasis are:

1. filariasis,
2. tuberculosis,
3. cancer,
4. chemicals absorbed from some soil in some countries through repeated cuts in the feet,

{ affecting the lymph nodes.

For treatment see page 202.

Tuberculous lymphadenitis

Tuberculous lymphadenitis is a chronic infection of lymph nodes caused by the tuberculosis bacteria. Always think of tuberculous lymphadenitis if patient is like this:

1. He is a child or young adult (but can be any age).
2. His neck glands are affected (but can be glands in any other area).
3. He has only one symptom – a lump which does not go away but gets bigger.
4. His only signs are enlarged lymph nodes joined or matted together which are not tender or red or hot. Sometimes there is also a sinus discharging pus over the top of the nodes.
5. There is no obvious cause of the enlarged nodes (unless other signs of tuberculosis are present) (see Chapter 14 page 64).
6. He has a positive tuberculin test (see Chapter 14 page 69).
7. Antibiotic treatment does not cure the infection even if continued for 3 weeks.

> Any chronic cervical gland enlargement with no obvious cause (e.g. infection in the ENT or head) which does not improve after 3 weeks treatment with antibiotics must be biopsied to find out if it is caused by tuberculosis, especially if the tuberculin test is positive.

If a biopsy is not possible, and after 6 weeks the condition is still getting worse, a trial of anti-tuberculosis treatment could be started. A full eighteen month's treatment must be completed even if the patient quickly improves.

See Chapter 14 page 71 for management.

Filariasis

Filariasis is a disease caused by infestation with small filarial worms (*Wuchereria bancrofti* and *Brugia malayi*). These worms live in the lymphatic vessels and lymph nodes and cause inflammation, and later block the flow of lymph through them.

Filariasis is only common in some areas in the tropical and coastal and island areas of Africa, Asia, the Pacific and the Americas (see Figure 22.6.)

The adult filaria worms produce larvae called microfilaria. Microfilaria are carried around in the blood near the skin only at the time when certain mosquitoes in that area usually bite people. This is often at night between 10 p.m. and 2 a.m. If these mosquitoes take up the microfilaria in their blood meal, the microfilaria then develop in the mosquitoes. These mosquitoes later pass on the filaria larvae, which are infective to people they bite. (See Figure 22.5).

The adult filarial worms irritate the lymph vessels and lymph nodes in which they live. This causes repeated acute inflammation, acute lymphangitis and acute lymphyadenitis and eventually also chronic inflammation, chronic lymphangitis and chronic lymphadenitis. After a long time the lymph vessels and glands become so scarred that lymph cannot flow through them.

Symptoms and signs

Attacks of acute lymphangitis caused by filaria cause acute inflammation of a part of a limb, a joint, or a testis. Attacks of acute lymphadenitis caused by filaria cause swelling and tenderness of the lymph nodes. Severe general symptoms and signs of infection can also occur. Usually you cannot tell if the inflammation is caused by filaria or bacteria. These conditions do not improve

Figure 22.5 Diagram to illustrate the life cycle of filarial worms.

Wuchereria
bancrofti

Brugia malayi

B. timori

Figure 22.6 The distribution of filarisis.
(Source: based on WHO Technical Report Series No. 702, 1984 (Fourth report of the WHO Expert Committee on Filariasis))

much with antibiotics; but they usually get better without treatment after some days or weeks.

Attacks of 'tropical arthritis' can occur (see Chapter 29 page 321).

If there are repeated or heavy infestations with filarial worms for some years, which cause repeated attacks of acute lymphangitis and lymphadenitis, then lymphoedema of legs, scrotum, vulva, arms and breasts etc. may develop. The nearby lymph nodes are usually large and hard.

After many years of lymphoedema severe chronic oedema of the part can develop, with thick folded skin, called elephantiasis (see Figure 22.7).

Test

The test for filarial worm infestation is to look for microfilaria in blood. Collect thick blood smears (as for malaria) between 10 p.m. and 2 a.m. on 3 nights. (See Chapter 6 page 22.) Microfilaria are often not present when the patient has developed elephantiasis.

Note that the causes of lymphoedema and elephantiasis include:

1. chronic infective (bacterial) lymphadenitis,
2. tuberculous lymphadenitis,
3. chronic chemical lymphadenitis,
4. cancer of the lymph glands, as well as
5. filariasis.

However do not biospy the lymph glands as this may make the lymphoedema or elephantiasis worse. If the diagnosis of filariasis is not certain, refer the patient to the next visiting Medical Officer for advice.

Treatment

Treatment depends on the stage and severity of the disease.

During attacks of acute lymphangitis or lymphadenitis

- Rest with the affected part elevated.
- Dressings if needed.
- Aspirin 600–700 mg (2–3 tablets) 4–6 hourly.
- Anthistamines e.g. promethazine 25 mg (1 tab) 1–3 times daily.
- Antibiotics usually penicillin at first (see Chapter 11 page 42) as you cannot be sure the condition is not caused by bacterial infection.

Figure 22.7A Lymphoedema left leg early.

Figure 22.7B Lymphoedema both legs, 'Elephantiasis' left leg.

- Do not give diethylcarbamazine until the acute stage is over.

After the acute stage is over; and in the chronic stages

Give diethylcarbamazine 50 mg/kg three times a day for 3 weeks (usually 100 mg (2 tabs) three times a day). In some areas this dose causes severe allergic reactions by killing off many microfilaria quickly. In these areas therefore:

1. Start with a low dose e.g. 25 mg (½ tab) daily and double the dose daily until the usual dose (as above) is being given, and
2. Give antihistamines e.g. promethazine 25 mg (1 tab) 1–3 times a day as well for the first week.

Diethylcarbamazine kills the microfilaria easily but it does not kill the adult filaria worms as easily. You should therefore repeat the course after 6 weeks. After some months, you should examine slides for microfilaria. If microfilaria are present, treat with diethylcarbamazine again.

Lymphoedema

Give diethylcarbamazine tablets.

Tell the patient to protect the limb from more damage by bacterial infection (e.g. wear shoes or sandals; get early antibiotic treatment and dressings if infection occurs, etc.).

Tell the patient to keep the affected part higher than the rest of the body when possible.

Elephantiasis

Tell the patient to keep the affected part higher than the rest of the body when possible. He should not sit with the legs down for long periods.

Use compression dressings and bandages.

Tell the patient to wear sandals or shoes.

Give antibiotics and use dressings for any infection which occurs.

Give diethylcarbamazine tablets (see above).

Discuss with a medical officer if surgery would help (surgery is not often helpful except for the scrotum).

Control and prevention

Control and prevention on a large scale are not usually possible. Mosquito control (usually done for malaria control) helps stop the spread of the infection. Protective clothing, repellents and use of nets at night will make infection much less likely. Some countries can afford to give treatment to the whole population in severely affected areas. This reduces the reservoir of the parasite and also gives prophylactic treatment to infected people who do not yet have chronic disease.

Burkitt's lymphoma

Burkitt's lymphoma is a common cancer, especially where malaria is common and especially in children and young adults.

Usually Burkitt's lymphoma causes tumours of the jaw. At first teeth near the tumour become loose. The tumour grows in the bone and becomes very large very quickly (e.g. in one month). The tumour often pushes the eye forward. It is soft and painless. The skin over the tumour is not ulcerated. The lymph nodes are not enlarged. There is no fever. Apart from the swelling, the patient seems well at first (see Figure 22.8). Dental abscesses can look similar; but an abscess has signs of inflammation and tenderness.

Abdominal tumours may occur.

Paralysis may occur from the tumour pressing on the brain or spinal cord.

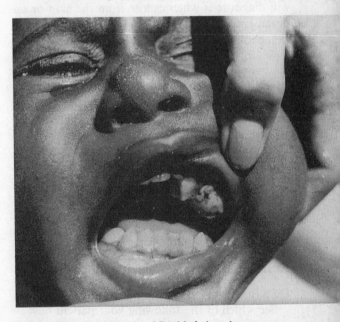

Figure 22.8 Photograph of Burkitt's lymphoma affecting the upper jaw. The teeth are loose in the swollen gum. If teeth look healthy (no holes in them) but you can very easily push the teeth back and forward in the gum with your finger, without hurting the patient, then it is likely the patient has a Burkitt's tumour.

Transfer suspected cases to a medical officer as soon as possible for diagnosis by biopsy and treatment with anti-cancer drugs as patients can get very much worse in a few days and good early treatment can cure some patients.

Cancer of the lymph nodes

There are two kinds of cancer which affect the lymph nodes.

The first kind is a primary cancer of the lymph nodes called a lymphoma. You will most often diagnose lymphoma when you biopsy a node to see if it is enlarged because of tuberculosis. Biopsy any lymph node that is enlarged and hard; but not tender, not red and not hot; especially if there is no infection on the skin etc, or the gland has not much improved after treatment with antibiotics. (See page 202.) Sometimes the biopsy report will be that the lymph node shows no tuberculosis but does show Hodgkins Disease or Non-Hodgkins Lymphoma. These are both primary cancers of the lymph glands. Sometimes they can be much improved by special treatment.

The other sort of cancer of lymph nodes you will diagnose is when cancer from the skin or an organ spreads to the lymph nodes i.e. secondary cancer of the lymph glands. One particularly common site for a primary cancer which spreads to the lymph glands of the neck, is the back of the nose or throat (naso-pharyngeal carcinoma). Often this cancer cannot be seen without special instruments or X-rays. Again this sort of cancer may be diagnosed when tuberculosis is expected. The lymph nodes in secondary cancer in most other cases are usually hard and stuck to each other or the muscles or the skin.

Refer or non-urgently transfer such patients to a Medical Officer.

Enlargement of lymph nodes

Do a full history and examination (see Chapter 6).
See which of the following your patient has:
1. Enlargement of a lymph node or some lymph nodes *and* tenderness of enlarged nodes *or* fever (see below).
2. Enlargement of a lymph node or some lymph nodes *but* no tenderness of enlarged nodes *and* no fever (see below).
3. Enlargement of *most* of the lymph nodes of the body *but* no tenderness of enlarged nodes *and* no fever (see below).

Enlargement of a lymph node or some lymph nodes and tenderness of enlarged nodes or fever

1. *Acute bacterial lymphadenitis*.
   An infected lesion of some sort in the part of the body drained by the affected lymph nodes is usually present (the lesion may be very small).
   Treat with antibiotics (see page 199 and Chapter 11 page 42).
2. *Acute filarial lymphadenitis*
   • The patient is from or in an area where filariasis occurs.
   • He has sometimes had previous attacks.
   • There are microfilaria in blood.
   Treat as for acute bacterial lymphadenitis and see page 199.
3. *Acute viral infections* such as rubella (German measles) or infectious mononucleosis.
   • Usually the patient is young.
   • Sometimes there is an epidemic.
   • Often the nodes affected are in the neck and not acutely inflamed.
   • Sometimes there are other symptoms and signs (especially a rash).
   • Usually the patient is not very sick.
   Give symptomatic treatment only and observe. (Do not give ampicillin, which may cause a rash in these patients.)
4. *Bubonic plague*
   • The patient is in or has been in an area where plague occurs.
   • Sometimes there is an epidemic; but could be first case.
   • Usually there have been recent rat deaths.
   • The nodes usually severely inflamed and soon become large, fluctuant and discharge pus (bubo).
   • The patient is very sick, with fever rigors etc.
   • Septicaemia often develops.
   • Pneumonia may develop.
   • The patient often dies within a week.
   If plague is a possible diagnosis, see Chapter 17 page 104 urgently for diagnosis and management.

Enlargement of a lymph node or some lymph nodes but no tenderness of enlarged nodes and no fever

1. *Repeated acute or chronic bacterial infection*
   - Usually in the legs of a person who does not wear shoes.
   - Often there is a history of repeated injury or infection of feet, with swelling of lymph nodes in groin.
   - Chronic infection may still be present.
   - The nodes are hard and smooth.
   - Often there is lymphoedema.

   See page 199 for management.

2. *Filariasis*
   - The patient is in or from an area where filariasis occurs and usually other people near where he lives are affected.
   - There is often a history of repeated attacks of acute lymphangitis and lymphadenitis.
   - The nodes are hard and smooth.
   - Often there is lymphoedema.
   - Microfilaria may be present in the blood (but not necessarily)

   See page 202 for management.

3. *Tuberculosis*
   - The affected patient is often young (but not always).
   - The affected nodes are often in neck (but can be anywhere).
   - A node may be joined to other nodes under the skin.
   - Sometimes there is a sinus discharging pus over the node.
   - There is no infection or other cause for the node enlargement in the area of the body drained by the node.
   - Sometimes chronic cough or other symptoms or signs of tuberculosis are present.
   - Sometimes there is a family history of tuberculosis.
   - The tuberculin test is usually positive.
   - Treatment for 3 weeks with antibiotics does not cure the disease.

   Biopsy all such glands (see page 200 and Chapter 14 page 71).

4. *Lymphogranuloma venereum*
   - There is a history of sexual intercourse with a possibly infected person.
   - The nodes in groin are affected.
   - The nodes burst and discharge milky fluid.
   - Nearby nodes are also affected and soon a number of sinuses discharging milky fluid develop.
   - Often there is fever and malaise at some stage.

   See Chapter 19 page 137 for management.

5. *Cancer of the nodes*.
   - As for tuberculosis (see 3 above) except no history suggesting tuberculosis and the tuberculin test is negative, or
   - The nodes are hard and lumpy and stuck to each other skin or the skin or the nearby muscles, or
   - There are other lesions which could be cancer in the area drained by the nodes.

   See Chapter 22 for management.

6. *Trypanosomiasis*
   Often all the nodes are affected but sometimes it is mostly in the neck nodes.
   See page 206 and Chapter 18 page 118.

7. *Visceral leishmaniasis*
   Usually all nodes are affected but sometimes it is mostly in one part.
   See below and Chapter 18 page 116.

Enlargement of most of the lymph nodes of the body but no tenderness of nodes and no fever

1. *Syphilis*
   - The patient has had sexual intercourse with a possibly affected person some weeks or months before.
   - There was a chancre (sore on genitalia) for 2–6 weeks about 6 weeks before.
   - Skin rashes are sometimes present.
   - Condylomata lata are sometimes present.
   - Mucous patches are sometimes present.
   - Malaise is sometimes present.
   - The VDRL test is positive.

   See Chapter 19 page 134 for management

2. *Cancer of lymph glands* (*lymphoma*)
   - The spleen is often enlarged.
   - The liver may be enlarged.
   - Anaemia is often present.
   - Wasting is often present.

   See page 204 for management.
   Make certain that the patient does not have severe tuberculosis.

3. *Visceral leishmaniasis* (*kala azar*)
   - The patient is in or from an area where kala azar occurs
   - There is fever at first and later.

- The spleen is enlarged (often very enlarged).
- The liver is enlarged, but not very enlarged.
- Anaemia is present.
- Repeated attacks of diarrhoea often occur.
- Wasting is often present.
- Lumps on skin are sometimes present.
- There are leishmania organisms in blood or a biopsy.
- The formaldehyde gel test is positive after a few months.

See Chapter 18 page 118 for management.

4. *Trypanosomiasis*
- The patient is in or from an area where trypanosomiasis occurs.
- There is a sore (in Africa) or a swelling (in America) at the place of the bite.
- A fever may develop later.
- The spleen is enlarged.
- The liver is enlarged.
- Anaemia is present.
- The pulse is fast.
- There may be meningitis or encephalitis or psychosis or unconsciousness (in Africa).
- There are trypanosomiasis organisms in blood or aspirated from lymph gland.

See Chapter 18 page 121 for management.

Swelling of one limb

Causes include:
1. injury,
2. infection,
3. chronic lymph vessel and lymph node disease with blocked lymph node channels (see page 119),
4. clots in the main deep vein,
5. varicose veins, and
6. snakebite or allergic reaction to sting or toxin etc.

The spleen

Anatomy, physiology, pathology

The spleen makes some of the white blood cells and also some antibodies. The spleen also takes 'worn out' red blood cells from the blood. It breaks them down and saves most of the parts for the bone marrow to make new red blood cells.

C

Figure 22.9 A, B and C. These diagrams show the normal position of the spleen (slightly enlarged). (A) Anterior or front view. (B) Posterior or back view. (C) Left lateral or side view. Note that the spleen is a posterior organ. Note that a normal spleen cannot be felt on examination of the abdomen. When a spleen enlarges it enlarges forwards, downwards and to the right. At first you can feel it right under the ribs on the left side, in the front. See Figure 22.10. Note also that the spleen is just under the ribs which protect it. If the left lower ribs are damaged (especially if they are fractured) the spleen is likely to be damaged too.

If the spleen collects and breaks down many more red blood cells than normal (e.g. in a patient with malaria which damages red blood cells), then the spleen enlarges. If the vein from the spleen (which goes through the liver) becomes blocked by disease of the liver (e.g. cirrhosis or schistosomiasis), then the spleen becomes too full of blood and enlarges.

Anytime the spleen enlarges, it can start taking normal red blood cells, normal white blood cells, and normal platelets out of the blood. The body may then not have enough of some or all of these blood cells.

An enlarged spleen is more likely to rupture (break open) and bleed than a normal spleen.

Symptoms and signs

Disease of the spleen may cause these *symptoms*.
1. Pain in the left upper abdomen. This is usually caused by trauma or inflammation.
2. Swelling of the left upper abdomen; or swelling of the whole abdomen, if the spleen is very enlarged.
3. Anaemia (and other blood disorders), if the spleen is enlarged and takes normal blood cells as well as 'worn out' red cells from the blood.
4. Shock and anaemia, if the spleen is ruptured and bleeds.

Disease of the spleen may cause these *signs*.
1. Tenderness in the left upper abdomen. (See symptoms, 1.)
2. Enlargement of the left upper abdomen or the whole abdomen. (See symptoms, 2.)
3. Anaemia (and other blood disorders). (See symptoms, 3.)
4. Shock and anaemia. (See symptoms, 4.)

Common conditions affecting the spleen

Very large spleen

A very enlarged spleen may be caused by many conditions. In some areas, some of these causes do not occur. Do not worry about causes that do not occur in your area or areas where your patients may have been.

Your patient may have more than one cause for a very enlarged spleen. It is not always possible to know what causes a patient's enlarged spleen. But you must always try to find out.

If possible do these tests on your patient (do not test if the disease does not occur where your patient has been):
1. urine for schistosome eggs (or at least for miracidia)
2. stool for schistosome eggs (or at least for miracidia)
3. blood for organisms of leishmaniasis and serum for formaldehyde gel test for kala azar
4. blood slide for malaria parasites
5. thin blood film examination sickling test and laboratory blood tests for white blood cell diseases such as leukaemia, and red blood cell

207

Figure 22.10 A and B These photographs show how to feel for a spleen. Place the left hand behind the left side of the patient's abdomen. Lift it upwards (forwards). Place the right hand with the palm flat on the patient's abdomen and the fingers pointing to the left upper abdomen. Start in the right lower abdomen (or you may not feel a very large spleen). Tell the patient to take slow deep breaths in and out. If the spleen is enlarged to where your fingers are you will feel it hit the tips of your fingers as the patient breathes in. If you do not feel the spleen, move the fingers towards the ribs and tell the patient to breathe deeply again. Keep moving the right hand up until the spleen is felt or you have felt along the edge of the ribs, and found no enlargement of the spleen.

diseases such as thalassaemia and sickle cell anaemia

Some of the causes for a very big spleen are:
1. *Schistosomiasis*
   • The patient is in or from an area where schistosomiasis occurs.
   • He has a past history of blood in the urine or dysentery.
   • There may still be urinary or intestinal symptoms and signs.
   • Late in the disease he may vomit blood or pass malena (black tarry stools).
   • Late in the disease the abdomen may be full of fluid (ascites) and there may be some swelling of legs and back (oedema).
   Diagnose and treat as soon as possible. Once late stages are reached treatment (1) is not likely to help much, (2) is likely to have severe side effects and (3) should only be given by a medical officer.
2. *Chronic liver disease usually of an unknown cause (cirrhosis)*

   • No evidence of schistosomiasis is present
   • A lot of ascites and some oedema are present with wasting of the muscles most noticeable around the shoulders.
   • Sometimes the patient may vomit blood or pass malena (black tarry stools).
   • There may sometimes be a change in behaviour or level of consciousness; sometimes jaundice; sometimes bleeding, from anywhere.
   Diuretics help the ascites and oedema; but no treatment is much help. See Chapter 24 page 245.
3. *Visceral leishmaniasis (kala azar)*
   • The patient is in or from an area where kala azar occurs.
   • There is fever early in the disease.
   • The lymph nodes are enlarged.
   • Anaemia is present.
   • Diarrhoea is present.
   • Wasting is present.
   • Sometimes skin rash is present.
   • Tests for leishmania in blood or formaldehyde gel test are positive.

Management. See Chapter 18 page 118.

4. *Tropical Splenomegaly Syndrome*
   • The patient has lived in a malarial area for some years.
   • The spleen keeps on enlarging.
   • The liver is enlarged.
   • Anaemia is present.
   • Wasting is present.
   • There are episodes of haemolysis, when there is fever, jaundice, worsening of anaemia and the spleen becomes painful and tender.
   • The malaria smear is often negative.
   • Tests for schistosomiasis and visceral leishmaniasis are negative.
   Give prophylatic antimalarial drugs for at least 2 years, and probably for life (see Chapter 13 page 59).

   In an area where malaria occurs *always think of this condition* in any patient who has a chronically enlarged spleen as tropical splenomegaly syndrome is one of the few treatable causes of very enlarged spleen. But do not treat all cases of chronic malaria as tropical splenomogaly syndrome (see Chapter 13 page 53).

5. *Chronic malaria*
   • The patient is in a malarial area; but he has not been there for long enough to have developed (semi-) immunity to malaria (which needs 4–10 years of continuous exposure).
   • He has repeated attacks of acute malaria.
   • Anaemia is present.
   • An enlarged liver is present.
   • Wasting is present.
   Treat acute attacks of malaria as soon as they start (see Chapter 13 page 51).

6. *Blood diseases*
   Leukaemia
   • The report of the blood film suggests this.
   Refer or non-urgently transfer to Medical Officer.
   Thalassaemia
   • The report of the blood film and examination for abnormal haemoglobin confirms diagnosis.
   See Chapter 21 page 190.
   Sickle cell anaemia

   • The patient is an African.
   • Anaemia is present.
   • The patient has repeated infarction crises.
   • The spleen may become smaller.
   • The report of the blood film sickling test and examination for abnormal haemoglobin confirms diagnosis.
   See Chapter 21 page 187.

Painful or tender spleen

There are many causes of an enlarged, painful or tender spleen in tropical and developing countries. You can usually use other symptoms and signs to make the diagnosis. But never forget to check for the following conditions.

Traumatic rupture of the spleen
Small injuries can cause the spleen to rupture.

Be very suspicious if there has been a left sided chest or abdominal injury.

Sometimes there is a haematoma (bruise) under the capsule (or covering) of the spleen for some hours or days after the injury before the capsule bursts and the spleen bleeds a lot.

The patient will become paler, the pulse rate faster and the blood pressure lower if the spleen is bleeding.

Generalised abdominal tenderness and later shifting dullness (See Chapter 36 pages 407 and 413) will develop.

Transfer urgently all suspicious cases to Medical Officer care after you have started an IV drip and any other necessary treatment (see Chapter 27 page 307).

Acute malaria
Always give antimalarial treatment (see Chapter 13 page 55) to any patient in a malarial area, unless you are certain he does not have malaria.

Septicaemia and typhoid fever
Always think of septicaemia in any patient who is very sick. Unless another cause for the illness can be found, treat for septicaemia. (See Chapter 12.)

23

Disorders of the Gastro-intestinal System

Anatomy, physiology and pathology

Food consists of proteins, carbohydrates, fats, salts, vitamins and water. Food is used as fuel for the muscles and other working parts of the body, and for growth and repair of the body.

Before body cells can use food, it must be crushed, digested (or broken down into simpler substances) and then absorbed into the body.

The parts of the gastro-intestinal canal in which foods are crushed, digested and absorbed are the mouth, the oesophagus, the stomach, the small intestine and the large intestine.

First the food is crushed by the teeth, and mixed with saliva, which is a lubricant that also starts digestion of the food. The saliva is made by three sets of paired salivary glands. The parotid glands are on both sides of the jaw in front of the ears. The submandibular glands are on both sides under the jaw. The sublingual glands are under the tongue. (See Figure 23.1.)

Then the food is swallowed. The oesophagus has muscles in its wall which move the food into the stomach.

The stomach is a storage bag. It lets small amounts of food into the intestine every few minutes until it is empty (a few hours). In the stomach the food is mixed with two very powerful digestive juices – hydrochloric acid and pepsin. These are made in glands in the mucous membrane of the stomach.

When the food has been partly digested by the acid and pepsin, the ring of muscle at the outlet of the stomach (which is called the pylorus), opens a little. This allows the muscular contractions of the stomach (called peristalsis) to push a little food into the first part of the small intestine (called the duodenum).

In the duodenum the food is mixed with other digestive juices. Bile made in the liver and stored in the gall bladder helps fats to be absorbed. Pancreatic juice from the pancreas contains an enzyme (trypsin) which breaks down proteins and other enzymes which break down carbohydrates and fats. (See Figure 23.2.)

The food is moved through the duodenum and the small intestine by contractions of the small intestine (also called peristalsis). The small intestine is about six to seven metres long.

As the food travels along the small intestine, more digestive juices are added from glands in the mucous membrane of the intestinal wall. All these digestive juices break down (or digest) the food into simpler compounds.

These simpler compounds are then absorbed by the special mucous membrane of the intestinal wall. The digested and absorbed food is put into the blood, which goes to the liver through the portal vein (see Figure 24.3).

When the remains of the food reaches the large intestine, it is only the fibres and hard parts which cannot be digested and absorbed by the intestine. The remains of the food has been mixed with bilirubin (which is the remains of haemoglobin from worn out red cells which is excreted in the bile). This bilirubin gives the faeces their brown colour. The food remains are also mixed with many bacteria (both dead and alive) which normally live in the intestine. There is also a lot of water from the digestive juices mixed with the food remains.

As all this material goes through the large intestine, most of the water is absorbed through the mucous membrane of the large intestine (also called the colon).

The lower part of the large intestine is called the rectum. The rectum is a storage bag for the remains of the food until it can be passed through the anus into the toilet.

The unabsorbed remains of the food and the other materials are called faeces (or stool). If the faeces stay a long time in the rectum, they be-

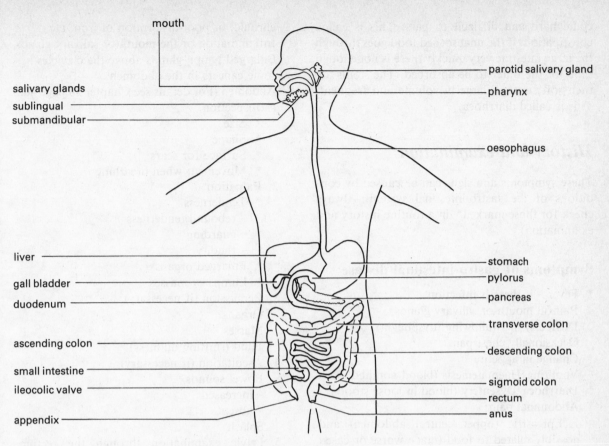

mouth

parotid salivary gland

pharynx

salivary glands
sublingual
submandibular

oesophagus

liver

stomach

gall bladder

pylorus

duodenum

pancreas

transverse colon

ascending colon

descending colon

small intestine

ileocolic valve

sigmoid colon

rectum

appendix

anus

Figure 23.1 Diagram of the main parts of the gastro-intestinal system.

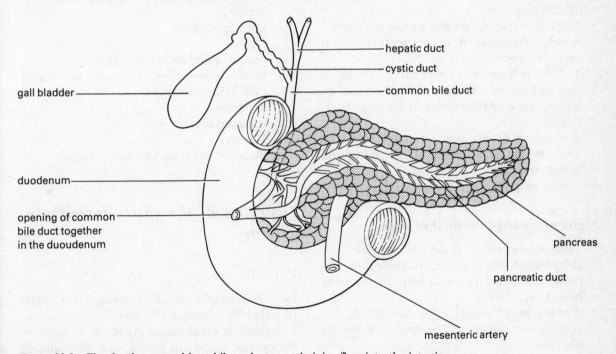

hepatic duct

cystic duct

common bile duct

gall bladder

duodenum

opening of common
bile duct together
in the duoudenum

pancreas

pancreatic duct

mesenteric artery

Figure 23.2 The duodenum and how bile and pancreatic juice flow into the intestine.

211

come hard and difficult to pass. This is called constipation. If the unabsorbed food goes through the large intestine very quickly there is not enough time for the water to be absorbed. The stools are then soft, watery, large in volume and frequent. This is called diarrhoea.

History and examination

These symptoms and signs can be caused by conditions of the gastro-intestinal system. Always check for those marked* in a routine history and examination).

Symptoms of gastro-intestinal disease

* Fever – if there is infection
  Painful mouth or salivary glands
  Difficulty in swallowing (dysphagia)
  Occasionally chest pain
* Change in appetite
* Vomiting/Haematemesis (blood vomited)
* Diarrhoea/Dysentery (blood in loose stool)
* Abdominal pain:
  1. Epigastric (upper central abdomen) and possibly related to food (made worse or eased by feed) – usually caused by stomach or duodenal disease
  2. Colic in epigastrium and around umbilicus – usually inflammation or obstruction of the small intestine
  3. Colic in the side or lower part of the abdomen and around umbilicus – usually caused by inflammation or obstruction of the large intestine
  4. Constant in any area – usually caused by inflammation or stretching of the peritoneum in that area
* Weight loss

Signs of gastro-intestinal disease

* Temperature raised – if there is infection
* Dehydration and/or shock – inelastic skin, fast pulse, low blood pressure, little or no urine passed, etc.
* Wasting/Malnutrition – if not eating; or chronic vomiting; or malabsorption; or chronic diarrhoea
* Pallor – if gastro-intestinal bleeding, acute or chronic; or poor absorption of iron, etc
  Inflammation of the mouth or salivary glands
  Enlarged lymph glands above the clavicles – some cancers in the abdomen
  Abdomen (For details see Chapter 36 page 402)
  1. Inspection
     * Size
     * Shape
     * Surface for scars
     * Movement when breathing
  2. Palpation
     * Tenderness
       – rebound tenderness
       – guarding
       – rigidity
     * Enlarged organs
     * Lumps or masses
  3. Percussion (if necessary)
     Organs
     Masses
     Fluid (shifting dullness)
  4. Ascultation (if necessary)
     Bowel sounds
     – increased
     – absent
     Splash
  5. Pelvic examination through the rectum ('PR') (if necessary) (See Figure 26.8)
     Tenderness
     Enlarged organs
     Masses
     Faeces, blood or pus in rectum
  6. Pelvic examination through the vagina ('PV') (if necessary)
     Tenderness
     Enlarged organs
     Masses
     Blood or pus from vagina or uterus

Disorders of the gastro-intestinal system

Parotitis

Parotitis is usually caused by mumps (see Chapter 16 page 100) in people who were healthy before.

Parotitis is often caused by acute bacterial infection (see below) in people who were already sick before.

Figure 23.3 Use a simple diagram like this and mark the findings of your examination on it.

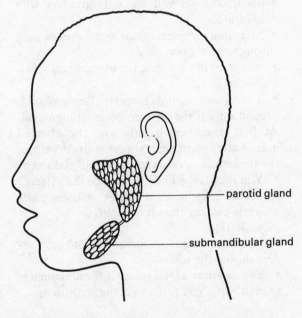

parotid gland

submandibular gland

Figure 23.4 The anatomical position of the parotid and submandibular glands.

Acute bacterial parotitis

Acute bacterial parotitis usually occurs in sick people who are not eating, drinking or caring for their mouths properly.

Symptoms include pain in the side of the face (which is made worse by movement) and swelling of the parotid area.

Signs include:

- The parotid gland at the side of the face is swollen, hard, tender, often hot and sometimes red. It is difficult for the patient to open his mouth. The swelling is sometimes very large.
- The pulse is fast and the temperature is raised.

Differential diagnosis includes: parotid tumour (which is not acute); and mumps (see Chapter 16 page 100).

Treatment includes:

- antibiotics,
- pain relief,
- mouth toilet, and
- proper hydration (intravenously, if necessary).

Prevention is by doing a mouth toilet and checking that sick patients have enough fluids.

Peritonitis

Peritonitis is an inflammation of the peritoneum (or lining of the peritonal cavity) in all parts of the abdomen. The inflammation is usually acute and is usually caused by bacterial infection. Blood in the peritonal cavity can cause similar symptoms and signs (see below). The inflammation is occasionally chronic, and is then usually caused by tuberculosis (see Chapter 14 page 64).

There may be a history or symptoms or signs of the condition which caused the peritonitis. e.g.

- inflammation of the bowel wall, e.g. appendicitis or enteritis necroticans (pigbel)
- a bowel obstruction, especially if strangulated
- an abdominal wound, e.g. spear or knife
- a peptic ulcer which has ruptured
- a genital tract infection in the female, e.g. gonorrhoea or post-partum infection
- ectopic pregnancy

Symptoms and signs

Symptoms may include:

- constant abdominal pain made worse by movement,
- vomiting, and
- constipation, usually.

213

Signs may include:
- temperature usually above normal,
- pulse usually fast,
- blood pressure low, late in the disease,
- the respiration rate may be fast late in the disease,
- dehydration may be present,
- the patient looks 'sick',
- the abdomen:
  - distension after some hours,
  - no movement on respiration,
  - tender all over with rebound tenderness, guarding and rigidity,
  - bowel sounds absent.

Tests
No tests are usually possible in a health centre.

If you do a white cell count, it is usually increased, with an increased percentage of neutrophils.

Treatment
Urgent (emergency) transfer to hospital is necessary if the patient agrees to surgery (to treat the cause; and to remove the pus, faeces or blood from the peritoneal cavity).

While waiting for transfer, treat like this:
1. IV fluids as necessary for dehydration or shock (see page 224 and Chapter 27 page 305) and then give maintenance fluids.
2. Nil orally. Insert an intro-gastric tube, and aspirate all the fluid every hour.
3. Antibiotics: chloramphenicol 1–2 g immediately and every 6 hours by IVI (or IMI).
4. Morphine 10 mg (1 ml) or pethidine 100 mg (2 ml) if necessary for pain while waiting for, and during, transfer.

Intestinal obstruction

Intestinal obstruction is present when the food and fluids in the intestine cannot go through a part of the intestine. The intestine above the part which is blocked contracts more than usual and secretes more fluids than usual, and then dilates (get bigger).

There may be a history or symptoms or signs of the disease which caused the obstruction. e.g.
- hernia
- previous abdominal operation
- enteritis necroticans ('Pigbel')
- cancer of the intestine
- previous vomiting or passing of many round-worms (ascaris) followed by a dose of (tetra-chloroethylene) (TCE)
- the swallowing of a large foreign body.

Symptoms and signs
Symptoms include:
- abdominal pain, usually central, which lasts for about half a minute and which then goes away only to come back every few minutes, often with loud intestinal sounds,
- repeated vomiting and
- constipation (no faeces or gas passed).

Signs include:
1. Dehydration occurs if the condition has been present for more than a couple of hours (fast pulse, low blood pressure, inelastic skin, little or no urine passed, etc.).
2. General signs of peritonitis (see page 213) occur if the obstruction is strangulated i.e. the blood supply to that part of the intestine is damaged. (The intestinal wall starts to die and is attacked by bacteria from inside the bowel which spread through the bowel wall into the peritoneal carity.)
3. Abdomen
   Inspection –
   - distension of the whole abdomen
   - the abdominal wall does not move well with respiration
   - intestinal movements can sometimes be seen through the abdominal wall
   - you must *always* look for hernias and scars.
   Palpation –
   - Tenderness is not present. Tenderness is present only if the obstruction is strangulated. At first tenderness is only over the affected area. Later, when general peritonitis develops, the tenderness spreads to the whole abdomen.
   - You may feel a mass. It may be the affected length of intestine or a cancer or other mass which is causing the obstruction.
   Auscultation –
   - Intestinal sounds are increased (and pain occurs during the sounds).
   - You can hear a loud splash if the abdomen is shaken while you listen with the stethoscope.

Treatment
Transfer to hospital urgently (emergency) is

necessary for operation to remove the cause of the obstruction, if the patient will agree to surgery.

Whilst waiting for transfer, treat like this:

1. Nil by mouth. Insert a tube into the stomach, and aspirate all the fluid every hour.
2. IV fluids (see: Fluid Therapy – Dehydration and Shock, page 224 and Chapter 27 page 305).
3. Treat for peritonitis if this is present (see page 213).

Peptic ulcer

A peptic ulcer is an acute or recurring acute or chronic ulcer of the wall of the stomach or duodenum caused by acid and pepsin and other factors.

Acid and pepsin are normally made by the stomach to digest food. But they do not normally digest the wall of the stomach or duodenum and so cause a peptic ulcer. A peptic ulcer can be caused by the acid and pepsin in some people at some times if other things such as drinking alcohol, smoking tobacco, taking aspirin, possibly worrying and other unknown causes are also present.

Peptic ulcer occurs everywhere; but it is common only in some areas.

Symptoms and signs
The main symptoms include:

1. Epigastric pain (i.e. in the upper central abdomen) related to food (i.e. pain made worse *or* better by food). At first the pain may occur for only a few days or weeks, and then get better. *Epigastric pain related to food is the main symptom.*
2. Later the pain may be there most of the time and may radiate (spread) to the back.
3. Sometimes there is vomiting after food (if food causes pain, the vomiting usually relieves the pain).
4. Weight loss (especially if food causes pain and there is vomiting).

The signs include:

1. 'The pointing sign'. When the patient is lying on a bed and you ask him to point with one finger to where the pain is, the patient points to one place, usually between the umbilicus and the lower end of the sternum. If the patient does this, there is usually a peptic ulcer. If the patient does not point to one place but instead rubs his hand in different parts of the abdomen, or if the pain is not between the umbilicus and the lower end of the sternum then there is usually not a peptic ulcer.
2. Epigastric tenderness. This is the main sign.
3. Weight loss (if there is pain and vomiting after food).
4. Anaemia (if the ulcer has bled).

Complications which the ulcer can cause include:

1. Penetration of the posterior (back) wall of the stomach or duodenum into the liver or back – this causes back pain which does not go away.
2. Perforation of the front wall of the stomach or duodenum – the food and acid inside the stomach or duodenum then go into the peritoneal cavity. This causes sudden severe abdominal pain and peritonitis.
3. Ulceration of a blood vessel – this causes bleeding into the stomach or duodenum with vomiting of blood (haematemesis); or digested black, tarry blood in the stool (malena); also anaemia; and sometimes shock.
4. Obstruction of the stomach outlet so that food and later fluid cannot go from the stomach into the duodenum – this causes vomiting and wasting ('pyloric stenosis').

The differential diagnosis includes all other causes of upper abdominal pain (see Chapter 36 page 402). Sometimes an infection with many hookworms in the duodenum may cause symptoms similar to a peptic ulcer.

Treatment
The treatment depends on how severe the attack is.

Mild attack:
The epigastric pain is usually made better or worse by food.
The epigastric tenderness is mild.
There are no complications.

Severe attack:
The epigastric pain may be present all the time.
The epigastric tenderness is severe.
There are no complications.

Mild attack:
Treat as an outpatient.

1. Antacids. Aluminium hydroxide compound tablet or liquid (or other antacid tablet or liquid).

   Give 2 tablets or 10–20 ml liquid 1 hour after every meal, and at night before sleeping, and at any other time if necessary for pain. Give this treatment regularly for 3 weeks.

   If the patient gets better then give 2 tablets only if necessary for pain.

   If no antacid tablets are available, give 1 cup of full cream milk (instead of 1–2 antacid tablets).

2. Tell the patient:
   • not to smoke,
   • not to drink alcohol,
   • not to drink strong coffee or tea or cola drinks,
   • not to take aspirin or codeine compound tablets or any other tablets for pain or arthritis except paracetamol, and
   • not to eat foods which he knows cause pain.

3. Tell the patient to eat at the same time every day (and, if possible, to eat 3–6 small meals every day rather than fewer larger meals).

4. Give no aspirin and as few other drugs as possible (many drugs can cause the symptoms of peptic ulcer). Give paracetamol if needed for other pain.

5. Give anti-hookworm drug (e.g. pyrantel one dose of 5 tabs. once).

6. Treat anaemia if present (see Chapter 21 page 182) but do not give oral iron while the pain is still present.

Severe attack:

Admit for inpatient treatment.

1. Rest in bed for 3 weeks. Give diazepam 5 mg (1 tab) or phenobarbitone 60 mg (2 tabs) three times a day if the patient will not rest without.

2. Give treatment as for mild attack (see above).

3. If the patient does not improve:
   (a) Check that he does not have another disease (peritonitis, amoebic liver abscess, etc.).
   (b) Increase antacid dose. Use liquid if available. Give regularly every 3–4 hours or even every 1–2 hours if necessary.

Note that rest in bed in the health centre is the most important and effective part of this treatment. The reason for this is not known.

Note also that new drugs called histamine$_2$ (H$_2$) blockers can stop the stomach making acid and cause most peptic ulcers to heal. The ulcer can come back when the drug is stopped. Also the drugs are very expensive and not usually available. They include ranitidine 150 mg b.d. and cimetidine 400 mg b.d.

Transfer

Transfer to Medical Officer care if:

1. Severe pain is not relieved by this treatment (non-urgent).
2. The pain comes back many times (non-urgent).
3. Perforation causing peritonitis occurs (urgent – emergency).
4. Haematemesis (vomiting blood) or melaena (black stool which looks and smells like tar) occurs, even if there is no shock or anaemia (urgent – emergency).
5. There is vomiting and weight loss caused by obstruction of stomach outlet (non-urgent).
6. There is constant pain in the back caused by penetration of the pancreas or back.

Prevention

Prevention is by not smoking, not drinking too much alcohol and not taking drugs (such as aspirin) when they are not needed.

Carcinoma (cancer) of the stomach

Usually old people are affected.

Early symptoms and signs include:
• epigastric pain and/or
• a feeling of fullness after only a little food and/or
• anaemia.

Later symptoms and signs include:
• all of the above, and/or
• epigastric mass, and/or
• obstruction of the stomach outlet, and/or
• weight loss, and/or
• enlarged lymph glands above the clavicle.

If cancer of the stomach is suspected, treat as an inpatient for peptic ulcer for 3 weeks. If the patient is not cured after 3 weeks, transfer him to hospital for investigation.

Roundworm (*Ascaris lumbricoides*)

Infestation (infection) with roundworms is very common everywhere.

The adult worms are about 15–25 cm long. They live inside the lumen of the small intestine.

Figure 23.5   The life cycle of the roundworm.

The female adult roundworm puts many thousands of eggs into the patient's intestine everyday. These eggs are then passed in the patient's faeces. Inside fertilised eggs, infective larvae develop after about 2 weeks. The larvae will grow best when the patient passes faeces in those places where it is cool, shady and moist; but eggs can survive in other places for years. If an infective egg from dirt or in food is swallowed, the larva hatches and travels through the small intestinal wall, portal vein, liver, right heart, lungs, bronchi, trachea and then oesophagus and stomach into the small intestine, where it develops into an adult round worm.

Symptoms, signs and complications
Symptoms, signs and complications are all uncommon.
1. Usually there are no symptoms or signs. You can only make the diagnosis if an adult worm is seen in the stool or is vomited up or if eggs are seen when the stool is examined under the microscope.
2. If there are many worms, abdominal discomfort and distension (swelling) sometimes occurs.
3. If there are many worms in children who eat a poor diet, malnutrition can occur.
4. If there are many worms in children and tetrachloroethylene is given (which irritates but does not kill the worms), a tangled mass of worms can cause intestinal obstruction (this is rare).
5. Pneumonia and asthma can be caused as the larvae travel through the lungs. (This may not be rare but the diagnosis is not often made.)

Treatment
Treat only if:
1. roundworms are vomited or passed in stool, or
2. you are giving tetrachloroethylene (TCE) to children (give roundworm treatment before giving the TCE), or
3. there is malnutrition, or
4. there is abdominal discomfort and you can find no other cause.

Treat as an outpatient.
Give piperazine or pyrantel. The dose of piperazine is 5 g (17 tablets) in one dose in the morning before eating. Repeat the same dose 2 days later. The dose of pyrantel is 625 mg (5 tablets) once.

Prevention
Tell the patient and family and village about the life cycle of the worm and that prevention is by the use of proper toilets by everyone (including children) always.

Hookworm (*Necator americanus* or *Ankylostoma duodenale*)

Infestation with hookworm is very common. The adult worms are about 1 cm in length. They live in the upper small intestine attached by their mouths to the intestine wall. They suck blood and protein from the intestine wall.

The female adult puts eggs into the patient's bowel. These eggs are then passed in the patient's faeces. In shady moist soil, fertilised eggs develop into larvae. After about 1 week the larvae can pass through the skin of a person who touches them. The larvae travel through the blood vessels, right

217

Figure 23.6 The life cycle of the hookworm.

heart, bronchi and trachea, and then the oesophagus and stomach into the small intestine where they develop into the adult worms.

Symptoms, signs and complications
1. Anaemia: This is caused by the loss of the blood which the hookworms suck from the intestine wall. The body stores of iron are soon used up by the bone marrow making new blood. When this happens the bone marrow cannot make as much blood as before.
   Anaemia is the only common and important result of hookworm.
   Anaemia occurs only if there are a large number of hookworms in the patient and the patient also has a poor diet.
2. Heart failure (if the anaemia is severe).
3. Oedema (if the anaemia and heart failure and protein loss is severe).
4. Sometimes there is epigastric pain as with a peptic ulcer. Sometimes there is just a little abdominal discomfort.
5. Sometimes a rash occurs (an itchy red rash which may be hard to see and lasts for only a few days) where larvae went through the skin (usually between the toes).

You cannot be certain of the diagnosis of hookworm in the intestine at a health centre as you cannot normally examine the stool by microscope. But if you examine the stool under a microscope, you can see the eggs if the patient has hook worm.

Assume hookworm infestation is present in all patients who have anaemia.

Treatment
1. Give pyrantel *or* tetrachloroethylene *or* bephenium hydroxynaphthoate *or* mebendazole.

(a) Pyrantel 625 mg (5 tablets) in one dose once.
No special precautions are necessary.
Pyrantel is simple and safe to use and moderately effective.
(b) Tetrachloroethylene (TCE).
Treat for roundworm first (see page 216).
The patient should not eat on the night before and on the morning of treatment for best results.
Give TCE 0.1 ml/kg (1/10 ml/kg) of body weight to a maximum dose of 4 ml. Do not give TCE to a patient who is very anaemic (Hb less than 5 g/dl) *or* jaundiced *or* sick. (Wait until these improve with other treatment. Then give the TCE.)
TCE should be repeated after two days.
(c) Bephenium hydroxynaphthoate.
Give 5 g (2.5 g base) in one dose in the morning and no food for 2 hours after the drug.
Some kinds of hookworm need 3 days of treatment.
(d) Mebendazole.
Mebendazole 100 mg (1 tab) twice a day for 3 days is very effective.
2. Give routine anaemia treatment including antimalarials usually chloroquine, iron, folic acid, good diet (containing iron, protein and vitamins) and advice on family planning if needed (see Chapter 21 page 182).

Prevention
Tell the patient, family and village about the life cycle of the worm and that prevention is by the use of proper toilets by everyone (including children) always. Wearing shoes to stop larvae going through the skin of the feet is not very important.

Threadworm (*Enterobius vermicularis*)

Threadworm infestation is very common, especially in children.

Adult worms are up to 1 cm in length. They live in the large intestine and cause no pathology.

The fertilised female comes through the anus at night, and lays eggs on the skin around the anus. This causes itching and scratching.

The eggs are taken by fingers or clothes from the skin around the anus to the mouth and are swallowed. Then they pass into the intestine where they hatch and grow into adults.

Management of the patient includes:

1. Treat the *whole family* with an anti-threadworm drug.
2. Cut the fingernails short and keep them short.
3. Wash the whole body every morning.
4. Wash clothes and bedclothes often.
5. Apply ammoniated mercury ointment to the anus every night (while taking the anti-threadworm drug).
6. Wash hands well after using the toilet.

Drugs for treatment and the *doses for adults* are piperazine 2 g (7 tablets) each day for 1 week *or* pyrantel 625 mg (5 tablets) once. (See a reference book for children's doses.)

Prevention is the same as management, especially washing the hands after using the toilet.

Whipworm (*Trichuris trichura*)

The whipworm is 0.5 cm long and lives in the small intestine.

Whipworm may cause gastro-intestinal symptoms and signs, but only if they are present in large numbers, and even then, usually only in children.

Mebendazole is needed for cure, but treatment is not usually necessary.

Strongyloides

Strongyloides is a very small worm which lives in the upper small intestine but can spread through the whole gastro-intestinal tract, and also to other parts of the body.

Symptoms are not usually caused except in certain rare conditions in adults (especially those in which normal body immunity is decreased and

which you would not normally see in a health centre) and in some small children.

Mebendazole or thiabendazole is needed for cure; but treatment is not usually given at a health centre.

Tapeworm and cysticercosis

Two large tapeworms, the beef tapeworm (*Taenia saginata*) and the pork tapeworm (*Taenia solium*), and a number of very small tapeworms affect man.

The adult taenia live in the gastro-intestinal tract of man.

They can become metres long, but the adult worms do little harm. The patient usually diagnoses the condition when a part of the worm comes out of his anus or he sees part of the worm in the stool. You can see eggs if the stool is examined under the microscope.

If the eggs in the stool are not passed into a proper toilet, the eggs may be swallowed by beef cattle or pigs. The larvae travel all through the animal but most go into the muscles. When the animal is killed you can see the larvae as little white marks in the meat. If the meat is not properly cooked (and the larvae not killed) before it is eaten, then the larvae develop into an adult worm in the intestine. (See Figure 23.7.)

The big danger to man from tapeworms is from the pork tapeworm, if the pork tapeworm eggs get into the upper gastro-intestinal tract. This occurs if a person gets some of his faeces on his food or in his mouth, or if a person eats vegetables contaminated with faeces which contain the eggs. It may also occur during vomiting when the contents of

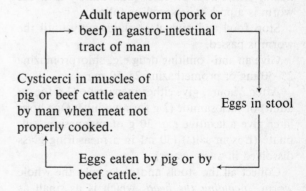

Figure 23.7 The normal life cycle of the pork and beef tapeworm.

219

the small intestine return to the stomach. If the eggs of a pork tapeworm get into the upper gastro-intestinal tract of man, then the larvae develop and travel all through the body (just as they do in pigs). The larvae cause painful muscles, fever and later muscle lumps. More importantly the larvae can also go to the brain. If very many go to the brain, then a meningo-encephalitis (see Chapter 25 page 260) develops, often with epilepsy. If only a few go to the brain, then there is often little trouble for some years. But, when the worm dies, the cyst it formed starts to swell. This causes symptoms and signs like a brain abscess or a brain tumour, with epilepsy or headaches or psychosis etc. (see Chapter 25 page 264). This condition, where pork tapeworms cause cysts in the muscle and brain, is called 'cysticercosis'.

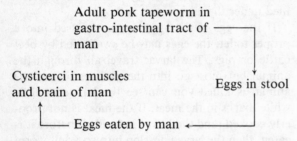

Figure 23.8 How the pork tapeworm causes cysticerci in man. The beef tapeworm cannot cause cysticerci in man.

You can diagnose the type of tapeworm infection a person has by examining the worm. But if the worm is a pig tapeworm, the worm and stools are dangerous to the patient and others. In the health centre *treat all cases immediately* as if the worm is a pork tapeworm, as follows.

Stop food and give clear fluids only until the worm is passed.

Give an anti-vomiting drug e.g. chlorpromazine 25–50 mg or promethazine 25–50 mg.

After 2 hours, give either mepacrine (1 g for an adult) or niclosamide (2 g for an adult). One hour later give a laxative e.g. 30 g of magnesium sulphate (Epsom salts) (30 ml in a measuring glass dissolved in warm water).

Collect all the stools and make sure the whole worm, *including the head*, which is as small as a pin head, has been passed. If the head is not passed, repeat the treatment.

Make sure no stools from the patient get on anyone at any time.

Prevention of tapeworm infection includes:
1. Kill the parasite in the original host. Treat all patients.
2. Stop the spread:
   (a) All people must use a proper toilet at all times.
   (b) All meat must be properly inspected for cysticerci, and not sold if cysticerci are seen.
   (c) All meat must be properly cooked. All the red colour all of the way through the meat must go before the meat is eaten.

Gastro-enteritis (or acute diarrhoeal disease)

Definition

Gastro-enteritis is a very common and sometimes serious or fatal syndrome. (It is not a specific disease with only one cause; there are many causes.)

Gastro-enteritis is diagnosed when there is:
1. diarrhoea, and
2. abdominal (intestinal) colic, and
3. usually vomiting,
4. with or without other symptoms and signs such as fever.

Causes

Causes of gastro-enteritis include:
1. '*Food poisoning*'
   Poisonous foods, especially certain fish and certain plants.
   Poisons or chemicals in food (including large volumes of alcohol).
   Drugs including antibiotics given for infections.
   Toxins in food made by organisms which have grown in the food but may be dead or cannot cause infections in the intestine (e.g. streptococci and staphlococci).
   Organisms in food which can cause infections in the bowel (see below).
2. *Infections in the intestine*
   Viruses (especially Rota virus).
   Unusual types of normal intestinal bacteria (e.g. *Escherichia coli*).
   Special bacteria, such as:
   – *Shigella* (bacillary dysentery organisms)
   – Salmonellae which cause gastro-enteritis.

– Salmonellae which cause typhoid fever.
– Clostridia which cause enteritis necroticans ('pigbel').
– *Campylobacter* which cause dysentery.
– Cholera organisms.
Amoebae (amoebic dysentery organisms).
Giardia.
Schistosoma mansoni and *Schistosoma japonicum*.
Sometimes other worms.

3. '*Medical causes*'
Any cause of fever, but especially malaria.
Any acute infections, but especially middle ear infections.
Many chronic infections, especially visceral leishmaniasis.
Malnutrition.
Malabsorption, especially lactose intolerance.
Change of diet.
Anxiety.

4. '*Surgical*' *causes*
Enteritis necroticans ('pigbel')
Intestine obstruction – early or incomplete.

Usually you cannot find the cause of gastro-enteritis at a health centre, unless there is a medical or surgical cause. But you must always look for evidence of the cause. (Details of some of the causes are found above.)

You must also ask if other people are affected, because this is the only way to diagnose 'food poisoning' in a health centre. You may need to control an epidemic.

Epidemiology

The *spread* of gastro-intestinal infections is usually:

• *From* the faeces (occasionally vomit) of an infected case or carrier.

• *To* the mouth of a susceptible person.

• *By* direct contact (personal contact) *or* vehicles (food or milk or water) into which organisms from faeces were introduced (put) by fingers or flies, or directly from improper or dirty toilets. See Figure 23.9.

Symptoms

Symptoms include:

1. diarrhoea (frequent watery stool)
   dysentery (diarrhoea with blood and pus as well), if the intestine wall is ulcerated

2. Abdominal pain
   This is colicky, i.e. it comes for some seconds and then goes away for some minutes. The pain is usually in the centre of the abdomen, but large intestinal colic can be at the side low down.
   Constant abdominal pain is NOT usually caused by gastro-enteritis.

3. Vomiting
   This is not always present; but it can be frequent.
   You must find out how often vomiting and diarrhoea are occurring and how much fluid is being lost in the vomit or the stool each time. This helps you to know if dehydration will occur.

4. Symptoms of an underlying disease may be present.

Past history
Ask if the patient has eaten possibly poisonous foods, 'bad' foods, pig meat or other high protein food (when this is not usually in the diet), food that was cooked a long time before it was eaten; or if he has taken drugs, etc.

Family and contact history
Ask about contacts with similar disease.

You can usually only diagnose 'food poisoning' at a health centre if a group of people develop gastro-enteritis together.
Always ask if other people are affected. You may need to control an epidemic. Think of cholera if there is an epidemic in which there are some cases of very rapid dehydration and death.

Signs
Signs may include:

1. *Signs of dehydration* (these develop if a large volume of fluid is lost and not replaced quickly enough):
   • the number of times the patient has had vomiting and diarrhoea and the volume of the vomitus and stool; each time you check a patient ask about these during the last 6 and the last 24 hours,

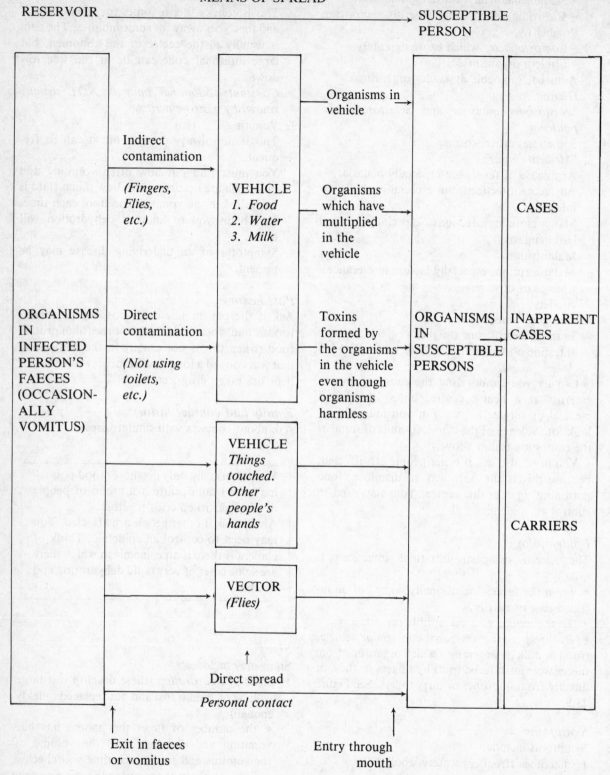

Figure 23.9 The epidemiology of most cases of gastro-enteritis.

- urine volume small and urine of dark colour (concentrated urine),
- rapid loss of weight,
- loss of full consciousness,
- decreased elasticity of skin, especially the skin of the neck (but do not mistake the inelastic skin of old age or of malnutrition or wasting for the inelastic skin of dehydration),
- sunken fontanelle (children only),
- sunken eyes,
- dry mouth,
- fast pulse,
- low blood pressure,
- cyanosis,
- fever.

> PR, BP, skin elasticity and urine volume and colour are the best signs for dehydration in adults.

2. *Signs of gastro-enteritis*:
The abdomen
- is normal in shape and moves normally on respiration;
- has no marked tenderness and definitely no guarding or rigidity;
- has increased intestinal sounds (which can be heard at the same time as the patient gets pain).
3. *Signs of cause of gastro-enteritis*
You must look for all medical causes, especially malaria, other infections and malnutrition.
You must look for all surgical causes, especially the signs of intestinal obstruction and peritonitis.

Complications
Look for these especially in the old, children, those with malnutrition, and certain virulent infections.
Complications include:
1. dehydration which can cause shock and death – *dehydration is the usual cause of death*;
2. dysentery, with the loss of large amount of blood, causing anaemia or shock;
3. septicaemia which can cause infections in other organs or shock or death;
4. paralytic ileus – because of loss of potassium the intestinal muscles become paralysed, this causes vomiting, abdominal distension, constipation but not colic;
5. continuing diarrhoea, because of lactose intolerance caused by the gastro-enteritis and milk with lactose still in the diet;
6. malnutrition;
7. anaemia.

Diagnostic features
1. diarrhoea or dysentery,
2. colicky (not constant) pain, usually in the centre of the abdomen,
3. vomiting,
4. no significant signs in the abdomen except increased intestinal sounds,
5. sometimes an underlying cause not in the gastro-intestinal tract,
6. dehydration (if vomiting or diarrhoea is often or is of large volumes or goes on for a long time).

Treatment
In all cases, look carefully for dehydration:
fast pulse (if severe),
blood pressure low if severe
inelastic skin,
sunken eyes,
dry mouth, and
urine volume small and colour dark.

Mild case, with no or mild dehydration:
- treat as an outpatient;
- tell the patient to return if he does not improve and especially if vomiting is repeated.
Severe case, with definite signs of dehydration:
- treat as an inpatient.

> Treatment includes 4 things:
> 1. Treat dehydration by oral fluids OR by IV then oral fluids (page 224)
> 2. Treat any underlying surgical or medical disease (page 224)
>   Always give antimalarial drugs.
> 3. If necessary treat any infection in the intestine (page 224)
>   Most cases do NOT need chloramphenicol or metronidazole.
> 4. Treat symptoms; but only if necessary and only after you have done the other three things. (page 225)

1. *Treat dehydration*
Oral rehydration. If
- there is no clinical dehydration, or
- only mild clinical dehydration, or
- moderate clinical dehydration but the vomiting is not repeated, and
- the abdomen is not distended (swollen),

then give oral rehydration fluid (see page 225).

Give the patient 2–4 large cups (400–800 ml) of fluid to drink. Tell the patient to drink it immediately if he has no nausea or vomiting. Tell the patient to sip it slowly over the next hour if he has nausea or vomiting.

If the patient has moderate dehydration, he must continue to drink till the signs of dehydration are gone (100 ml/kg or 3–6 litres). The patient can do this as quickly as he can if he has no nausea or vomiting. He should do it slowly over 6 hours (i.e. sip 2–4 cups during each hour for 6 hours) if he has nausea or some vomiting.

When the patient has no (or only mild) clinical signs of dehydration and does not vomit (or only vomits a little), the patient can then go home. Tell the patient to drink at least 2–4 cups of fluid in every 3-hour period (i.e. 3–6 litres/day) until the diarrhoea and/or vomiting stops.

If most of the oral fluids are refused or vomited or they are not effective, or abdominal distension (swelling) develops or there is severe dehydration, *then* admit for IV fluids.

Intravenous rehydration. If
- there is shock, or
- severe dehydration, or
- repeated vomiting, or
- abdominal distension (swelling), or
- the patient does not improve after oral fluids, or
- oral fluids are vomited or refused,

then give IV rehydration. The method for IV rehydration is as follows:
1. *Give 0.9% sodium chloride solution[1] 'fast'*
   Give 40 ml/kg (2 litres) as fast as possible (e.g. in 1 hour).
2. *Review the hydration of the patient after (1).*
   If he has improved, start (3).

   If he is still shocked or very dehydrated, give another 40 ml/kg (2 litres) 0.9% sodium chloride solution[1] as fast as possible. Then review the hydration of the patient again.

   If he still has shock, see Chapter 27 page 305.
   If he has improved, start (3).

3. *Give 0.9% sodium chloride solution[1] more slowly to complete rehydration in 6 hours.*
   Give 60 ml/kg (3 litres) over the next 4–5 hours. When the signs of dehydration have gone, start (4).
4. *Give 0.18% sodium chloride in 4.3% dextrose solution.*
   Give 1 litre every 6 hours.
5. *Start oral rehydration solution.*
   When you have done (1) to (4) and the patient has stopped vomiting start oral rehydration fluids 400–800 ml every 3 hours.
6. *Stop IV fluids.* When the patient can take enough oral fluids (400–800 ml every 3 hours) to maintain hydration stop IV fluids.

> If the patient has cholera, use Hartmanns solution (see page 228 and a reference book for details).

2. *Treat any underlying medical or surgical disease*
Antimalarial drugs must *always* be given, unless you are certain that the patient does not have malaria.
Give at least the first dose by injection.
See malaria (Chapter 13 page 55)

3. *If necessary treat any infection of the intestine*
If the patient has
- severe dehydration with shock, *or*
- severe toxaemia which continues after correction of dehydration and injection of antimalarials (i.e. after 6 hours), *or*
- more than mild abdominal tenderness, *or*
- severe dysentery (blood and/or pus in the stools which does not improve after a few days or returns),

then give chloramphenicol 25 mg/kg every 6 hours
either
- 1 g (1 bottle) every 6 hours for 14 days by
  – IVI if there is shock *or* by
  – IVI or IMI if there is vomiting, or severe diarrhoea, or the patient is very sick, *or*

---

1 Hartman's solution (Lactated Ringers Solution) is better than 0.9% sodium chloride solution; but it is not usually available. But 0.9% sodium chloride solution is not good for cholera. If the patient has cholera you must try to get Hartman's solution or an other special IV fluid for cholera.

• 1 g (4 caps) every 6 hours orally if there is no shock, no vomiting and diarrhoea not severe and the patient is not very sick
for 14 days.

> Note that **most** cases do **not** need chloramphenicol

If:
• dysentery does not get better during the course of chloramphenicol, *or*
• dysentery returns after the course of chloramphenicol, *or*
• dysentery has occurred a number of times before the present attack, *or*
• dysentery has been present for 5–7 days already, *or*
• diarrhoea does not stop after 2 weeks,

then give metronidazole 800 mg (4 tabs) t.i.d. for 5 days (possible amoebic or giardia infection).

If there is another infection or infestation especially schistosomiasis (see Chapter 18 page 122) shown by tests then give the necessary treatment.

4. Treat symptoms if necessary
Only treat symptoms after you have done rehydration, given antimalarial injection and excluded surgical conditions especially peritonitis and intestinal obstruction.

If there is severe colic, cease oral food and fluids, and give IV fluids only.

If there is severe abdominal colic or severe diarrhoea (and also vomiting), you can give morphine 10 mg (1 ml) and atropine 0.6 mg (3/5th mg) (1 ml) IMI once.

If there is abdominal colic or diarrhoea (but no vomiting), give codeine phosphate 30 mg (1 tab) every 4–6 hours if necessary.

If there is repeated vomiting, give chlorpromazine 0.5 mg/kg (½ mg/kg) but not more than 25 mg (1 ml) IMI every 6 hours if necessary. Do not give more than 2 doses. Look for the cause of the repeated vomiting.

Transfer these cases to medical officer care
1. If a surgical condition is possible – peritonitis, enteritis necroticans ('pigbel'), intestinal obstruction, etc. (urgent).
2. If vomiting continues for more than 2 days after you give IV fluids and IV or IM treatment and stop oral food, drugs and fluids (urgent).
3. If abdominal distension develops especially if there is also constipation and repeated vomiting (paralytic ileus) (urgent).
4. Diarrhoea which does not improve after the proper treatment (non-urgent).
5. Dysentery which does not stop after treatment with chloramphenicol and then metronidazole (non-urgent).

Oral rehydration solution
You can make oral rehydration solution in 5 ways.
1. Oral Rehydration Salts: 1 packet dissolved in 1 litre of clean water (boiled, if possible)
   or
2. Oral Rehydration Salts: 2 packets dissolved in 2 litres of clean water (boiled, if possible)
   Use the special bottle from the Medical Store to mix it.
   Throw away any you have not used after 24 hours.
   Wash the bottle carefully before using it again.
   or
3. 1 pinch of salt (only what you can hold between *one* finger and the thumb) and
   1 teaspoon sugar and
   1 cup clean water (boiled, if possible) or tea and
   a little lemon juice (if possible)
   or
4. Sodium chloride (common salt)   3.5 g
   Sodium bicarbonate   2.5 g
   Potassium chloride (each tablet of   1.5 g
   potassium chloride is 0.5 g)
   Glucose   20 g
   Clean water (boiled, if possible)   1 litre
   or
5. Coconut water

Control and prevention
Control and prevention includes giving health education about hygiene, food handling, water supply and toilets to the patient, his family and his village.

It is important to recognise any epidemic of gastro-enteritis. An epidemic is usually caused by a common source of the disease. This is usually food or water. You must discover the cause of any epidemic so that you can stop it.

You must think of cholera if there is an epidemic of very rapid dehydration and early deaths. Special treatment and control methods are necessary (see page 228).

Methods of control and prevention of gastro-enteritis caused by infections include:
1. Kill the organism in the body of the original host or reservoir (e.g. treat infected persons with antibiotics).
   You cannot usually do this. If you treat all cases and carriers with antibiotics, then soon many of the organisms become resistant to the antibiotics.
2. Stop the spread of the organism.
   Cases and carriers
   • do not allow them to handle food,
   • they must wash their hands after using the toilet.
   Proper disposal of faeces
   • proper toilets so that faeces do not contaminate water,
   • proper toilets so flies, etc. cannot walk on faeces and later walk on food.
   Provide a large supply of safe water.
   Cook food properly. Keep food covered and cool after cooking; but it is best to eat it immediately.
3. Raise the resistance of susceptible persons.
   Improve nutrition and health.
   • People with good nutrition usually have mild attacks.
   • People with malnutrition often have severe attacks.
   Immunisation against cholera and typhoid are available; but these immunisations are not very effective.
4. Prophylactic treatment.
   Do not give prophylaxis, except to special groups of people in a cholera epidemic.

For details of descriptions of special kinds of gastro-enteritis, see pages 226–233 and a reference book.

Cholera

Definition and cause
Cholera is an acute illness caused by the cholera bacterium *Vibrio cholerae*. There are a number of different types of this bacterium, including the El tor type. If the organism grows in the small in-testine, it can cause severe diarrhoea and vomiting, with rapid dehydration and often shock and death.

Frequency
Cholera is endemic in the Ganges basin but has now spread to many other parts of the world. In many of these places it has caused very large epidemics.

Epidemiology
Man is the only host. The reservoir includes cases, inapparent cases and carriers. The cholera organism is passed from the gastro-intestinal tract in the faeces or in the vomit. The organism then spreads to the mouths of other people. The usual way this happens is when the faeces or vomit contaminate drinking water. Contamination of food by contaminated water, hands and flies, can also occur. Direct spread from person to person can occur; but is not common.

All people are susceptible if there is an epidemic in a new area. But many infected people do not develop the clinical disease. And many people who do develop clinical disease have only mild disease. In endemic areas, most of the clinical cases are children.

A person can be a carrier for months.

Immunity after an attack only lasts for a short time.

The disease occurs mostly in countries where there is poor sanitation and the water supplies are not safe.

Pathology
There are no pathological changes in the structure of the gastro-intestinal tract. The organism does not get into the blood or other parts of the body. The toxin from the cholera organism makes the gastro-intestinal tract secrete very large volumes of salt and water. These are then lost by continuous vomiting and diarrhoea. This causes rapid dehydration (within hours), shock and death. If the lost salt and water is replaced quickly enough in the right quantity, the patient will get better.

Symptoms
If cholera comes to an area where it is not endemic, the first thing you will notice is a *group* of people with gastro-enteritis. Some of the people will develop significant symptoms.

At first there is usually watery diarrhoea. Large amounts of watery stool are passed repeatedly, or almost continuously. Several litres may be passed in the first few hours. The stools often look like the water in which rice has been boiled; but sometimes they are different.

There is usually little abdominal pain or colic.

Vomiting usually occurs after the diarrhoea, but sometimes occurs first. There is little nausea. Large volumes of fluid are vomited.

Signs

When you see a patient with these symptoms, he is usually severely dehydrated, shocked and cyanosed and often unable to speak.

Signs may include:

1. The patient is conscious, but very weak.
2. The temperature is not raised; it may be lower than normal.
3. The pulse is very fast and weak; or you cannot feel it.
4. The BP is very low; or you cannot record it.
5. The respiration rate is fast.
6. The weight is decreased.
7. Severe signs of dehydration are present with wrinkled skin with no elasticity sunken eyes and cheeks, etc.
8. There is cyanosis.
9. The abdomen
   • is sunken,
   • is not tender, guarded or rigid
   • has bowel sounds which are loud,
   • is usually soft; but sometimes there is spasm of all of the muscles of the body which may seem like guarding of the abdomen.
10. Spasm (tightening) of muscles, with cramps in the hands and feet and the calves of legs is quite common.
11. No urine is passed.

Course and complications

The disease has a course of 2–7 days.

Without treatment, over 50% of severely affected cases will die. Death can occur within a few hours.

With proper treatment, less than 1% of these cases will die.

After proper rehydration, vomiting usually stops.

Diarrhoea (of up to 60 litres) may continue for some days before it stops.

Miscarriage is common if the patient is pregnant.

Affected children may not be fully conscious, fits may occur and the temperature may be raised.

Without antibiotic treatment, many patients become carriers for some days or weeks or months.

Many mild cases and many unnoticed cases occur for every severe case.

Tests

There is no test for the disease that you can do at the health centre.

If you suspect cholera, you must do laboratory examination of the stools, rectal swabs and vomitus urgently, to confirm the diagnosis. Antibiotics, given before the laboratory tests are collected, reduce the chance of a positive culture; so you must collect at least one specimen before you start the antibiotic treatment.

Collect faeces in a sterile pan which is free from disinfectant or antiseptic. Avoid contamination with urine if possible. Use a sterile wooden spatula or a spoon to put 10–15 ml of faeces (two or three spoonfuls), containing blood and mucus, if present, into a sterile screw-topped glass or plastic container and send this to the laboratory. Put the spoon into antiseptic. When the patient is incontinent, put a sterile stiff-walled half-inch rubber tube (six inches long, cut at an angle at the end, and well lubricated) into the rectum, (with the lubricated angled end in the rectum), and drain the faeces into a sterile container. If you take swabs, take them from the rectum, not only the anus.

Send the specimen to the laboratory *immediately*. If the laboratory is not close to the place of collection, send for a suitable transport medium such as alkaline peptone water. Put 1–3 grams of faeces (½ spoonful) into 10 ml of the medium in a screw topped bottle and mix it thoroughly.

Send a letter with the specimen which gives all the details of the specimen, full clinical notes, and a request for examination for cholera organisms. If you could not collect a specimen before you gave antibiotics, then the request form must give the name of the antibiotic, the dosage and how long the patient has been having it.

You must also make a request for a microscopic examination and culture of the specimen for all other organisms which could cause a similar disease.

227

Differential diagnosis

This is the same as for gastro-enteritis (see page 220).

Diagnostic features

Suspect cholera if:

1. a single patient who has returned from a cholera area within the last week develops gastro-enteritis of *any* type; but especially if it has the typical signs and symptoms; *or*
2. there is an epidemic of gastro-enteritis with some cases with the typical signs and symptoms.

Treatment

> Treatment includes three things:
> 1. Treat and prevent dehydration and shock.
>   - Correct the dehydration and loss of salts.
>   - Replace continuing loss of water and salts.
>   - Give maintenance fluids.
> 2. Treat the infection in the intestine.
> 3. Treat symptoms if necessary; and give good nursing care.

1. Treat and prevent dehydration and shock

First you should correct the dehydration (loss of water and salts).

For severe dehydration use IV Hartmann's solution (also called Lactated Ringers solution).

For moderate or mild dehydration, use Oral Rehydration Solution (see page 225).

Table 23.1 Treatment of dehydration

Dehydration	Route	Adult	Child
Severe	IV	40 ml/kg *very fast* Then 60 ml/kg *over 2 hours*	40 ml/kg *very fast* Then 60 ml/kg *over 4 hours*
Moderate	Oral	25 ml/kg/hour *for 4 hours*	25 ml/kg/hour *for 4 hours*
Mild	Oral	15 ml/kg/hour *for 4 hours*	15 ml/kg/hour *for 4 hours*

Note about children. Hartmann's solution does not contain enough potassium or sugar or water for children. As soon as they can drink at all, give children as much Oral Rehydration Solution (see page 225, but not just salt and glucose and water) as they can drink *and* the IV Hartmann's solution.

Note: *If you have no Hartmann's solution* – use dextrose 2.5% in half strength Darrow's Solution; or if you do not have this, use 0.9% sodium chloride. If you do not have Hartmann's solution, start Oral Rehydration Solution (see page 225, but not just salt, glucose and water) when possible, as the other IV fluids do not contain everything the patient needs. This is especially important if you give 0.9% sodium chloride.

The best signs to use to judge hydration are:
pulse volume and rate,
blood pressure,
skin elasticity,
normal fullness of neck and veins,
loss of cramps, nausea and vomiting,
weight increased,
urine passed, and
loss of thirst.

After 2 to 4 hours of intravenous hydration the patient will become alert and look well. Vomiting will stop and he will start to pass urine. But diarrhoea, will continue for one to three days; but it should become less, and the stool less watery.

After correcting the dehydration you should *replace continuing loss of salt and water, and give maintenance fluids.*

Maintain the rehydrated state during the continuing diarrhoea by oral fluid.

Check the patient's hydration every two hours (see above). Keep a record of all the fluid you give (intravenous and oral). Also record the stool volume, appearance (clear, whitish, watery, yellow-watery, faecal) and frequency and how much urine is passed.

Give oral fluids every 4 hours. Give a volume of 1½ times the stool volume passed over the previous 4 hours. Continue this until the diarrhoea stops. Give Oral Rehydration Solution (see page 225 but not just the salt and glucose and water), which is either drunk or else put down an intragastric tube. If the stool loss is not more than 500 ml per hour, further intravenous fluids are not necessary.

Only rarely will further IV fluid be necessary;

but you may continue it at 10–20 ml/kg each hour for the 4 hours after rehydration if it is really necessary, while you start oral fluids.

If you do not have much intravenous fluid, you can use oral fluids immediately for most moderately or mildly dehydrated patients, and even in severely dehydrated patients immediately after they have been rehydrated intravenously. In most cases you can replace the continuing stool loss with an oral rehydration solution.

2. Treat the infection in the intestine with antibiotics

Give either tetracycline or chloramphenicol. Start the drug only when the patient has been rehydrated and is taking oral fluids, so that the antibiotic will not be vomited.

The dose of tetracycline for adults is 500 mg (2 caps) every 6 hours for 2 days.

Children under 10 kg are given chloramphenicol 125 mg (½ cap) (do not use the suspension) every 6 hours for 2 days.

Children weighing over 10 kg are given chloramphenicol 250 mg (1 cap) (do not use the suspension) every 6 hours for 2 days.

Antibiotics help to reduce the time and volume of diarrhoea, and the time the patient passes the bacteria.

3. Treat symptoms if necessary

This is not usually necessary.

The above treatment will usually cure the symptoms.

Do not give diuretics – rapid rehydration will make the patient pass urine.

Do not give chlorpromazine for vomiting – rapid rehydration will stop the vomiting.

Do not give morphine or analgesics for muscle cramps – rehydrate (and then if necessary give calcium gluconate 10% solution, 10 ml IV slowly).

Do not use stimulants like adrenaline.

Do not use adreno-corticosteroids.

Do not use plasma volume expanders.

Do not use oxygen to try to correct cyanosis.

These complications all improve with rapid IV rehydration.

Nurse patients on a bed with the mattress made of a sheet or mat with a nine inch hole in it. Place his buttocks over the hole, with a bucket under the hole. Measurement of stool volume is then easy.

The patient can start to eat when the vomiting stops.

> 1. In an epidemic, check that the patient has cholera and not another disease.
> 2. Repeated vomiting is usually caused by not enough of the right IV fluid.
> 3. Watch for overhydration and heart failure in children.

Control of epidemic

> You must immediately find out how the disease started and how it has spread so that you can use the correct methods of control. The usual means of spread is water.

Kill the organism in the body of the original hosts and the reservoir.

Admit patients. Isolate patients. Start treatment with tetracycline (or chloramphenicol) when vomiting stops. This will make the patient non-infectious and stop him becoming a carrier.

Close contacts of patients (i.e. family and others who may have been infected by the same reservoir (usually water)), may develop the disease or be mild cases or carriers. Treat them also with tetracycline (or chloramphenicol) for 2–3 days.

The usual reservoir is contaminated water. Chlorinate all water supplies and boil all water used for drinking, cooking, preparing food, washing dishes, etc.

Stop the means of spread.

Use all usual methods of stopping faecal-oral spread.

Disinfect the faeces and vomit and articles used by patients.

Staff must practice good hygiene, especially removing gowns before leaving the ward and washing hands after nursing patients and before eating or drinking. (No eating or drinking by staff is allowed in the ward.)

Check that everyone uses proper toilets.

Tell everyone to wash their hands after using the toilet.

Protect and chlorinate all water supplies.

Tell people to boil all water used for drinking or cooking or putting on food or washing dishes, etc.

Tell everyone about hygiene, cooking, handling, storing, serving and eating of food.

Try to reduce the number of flies, and keep flies away from all toilets and food.

Raise the resistance of susceptible persons
Immunise with cholera vaccine, 0.5 ml (½ ml) immediately, and then 1 ml 7–28 days later by subcutaneous injection.

Mass immunisation is not usually helpful in an epidemic. It does not give good protection to some people and is slow acting. But, you may be told to give it.

Staff of health centres should be immunised because of their possible repeated exposure.

Prophylactic treatment
During an epidemic, staff at the health centre should take regular doses of tetracycline to kill any cholera organisms which enter their gastro-intestinal tracts.

Prevention
Quarantine procedures are carried out at border posts, ports and airports to try to stop cholera entering a country.

Good sanitation and a plentiful supply of safe water and good general hygiene would stop any case which did enter a country causing an epidemic.

Immunisation may give some personal protection.

Notification
You should report all suspected cases of cholera *immediately* to the health officer, by telephone or radio or fast transport.

Cholera is one of the diseases subject to International Health Regulations. The Government will immediately report to the WHO and neighbouring countries if any case occurs.

Enteritis necroticans (pigbel)
Pigbel is common in the Highlands of Papua New Guinea if the diet is poor in protein and high in sweet potato, especially in children. Cases have also been reported from Uganda and Ghana and no doubt occur in other places.

The cause is a special type of special bacteria (*Clostridium*).

These organisms live in the intestines of animals or man or in the soil, and if they
1. contaminate food, and
2. are not all killed by proper cooking, and are eaten,
then they
1. grow in any protein food in the intestine, and
2. produce a toxin in the intestine.

If the toxin (which is a protein) is not destroyed because there is
1. little of the digestive juice (trypsin) which digests protein (because of little protein normally in diet) and
2. sweet potato present in the intestine which stops what little protein digestive juice there is from working,
then the toxin attacks the bowel wall causing inflammation or even necrosis (death) of the bowel wall.

History
The history is of a person who:
- is usually a child; most often in the Highlands of Papua New Guinea;
- usually does not have much protein in the diet;
- has eaten pig meat or other high protein food ½-4 days before;
- then develops one of the four syndromes listed below.

Symptoms, signs, course and complications
1. As for gastro-enteritis (see page 221) (diagnosis of pigbel is not made)
   or
2. (a) Severe upper abdominal pain which is constant, but there is also colic.
   (b) Vomiting; and vomitus soon becomes dark fluid (from blood) with flecks or spots in it (dead mucous membrane).
   (c) Blood in the stool sometimes with diarrhoea; (this has often stopped when the patient comes to the Health Centre).
   (d) Raised temperature, fast pulse and dehydration.
   (e) Upper abdominal distension, with parts of the intestine visible.
   (f) Upper abdominal tenderness, often with guarding and rigidity.

(g) You may feel intestinal masses.

(h) Intestinal sounds are decreased, though occasionally increased.

(i) Death occurs in a few days if the patient does not get proper treatment.

or

3. Soon after the start there is rapid development of severe general symptoms and signs of infection (septicaemia) and death.

also

4. Patients who get better may have an incomplete intestinal obstruction or malnutrition, caused by a narrowing of the affected intestine.

Treatment

Treat as for acute gastro-enteritis (see page 223 if there is no definite abdominal tenderness or distension.

Treat as for peritonitis if there are definite signs of 'pigbel' (nothing by mouth, IV fluids, IV penicillin (or chloramphenicol), IM pethidine, see page 214).

Transfer

You should arrange transfer *to medical officer care* when:

1. The patient has a severe case: i.e. his abdomen is very swollen, and he has black flecked vomit and marked general symptoms and signs (urgent – emergency).
2. The patient has only a mild case (only some abdominal swelling, not toxic, no black flecked vomit), but does not improve after 2 days of treatment.

Control and prevention

1. Kill the organism in the reservoir.
   This is not possible.
2. Stop the means of transmission.
   Proper cooking of *all* foods to kill all organisms helps. It is difficult to make people do this.
3. Raise the resistance of susceptible persons.
   More protein in the diet and not eating sweet potato can increase the activity of the digestive juices from the pancreas. But it is also difficult to make people do this.

   People can be immunised against the disease. You should give immunisation if you work in a place where the disease is common, (e.g. in PNG in the Highlands). Give a dose of 0.5 ml of vaccine by IMI at the same time as each dose of triple antigen, (i.e. at 2 months of age, 2 months after the first dose and again 2 months after the second dose).

Amoebiasis

Amoebiasis is an infection with special amoebae (*Entamoeba histolytica*). These amoebae are protozoal organisms which usually live in the large intestine.

The amoebae in the large intestine make cysts, which are passed in the stool. These cysts are infective if swallowed. Direct faecal-oral spread can occur, but much more commonly, faeces with cysts contaminate food or water. When the food or water is swallowed, the cysts develop into amoebae in the intestine.

Most infected people have no symptoms or signs. The amoebae eat only bacteria and surface cells of the mucous membrane. But, these persons are infective to others.

Sometimes the amoebae eat into the intestinal wall and form ulcers. This can cause any or all of the following:

1. short periods of diarrhoea over many years; but examination shows nothing abnormal; *or*
2. more severe attacks with malaise, fever, severe bowel colic and dysentery (frequent bloody stools). Examination shows general abdominal tenderness and an enlarged liver. Chloramphenicol does not cure the dysentery.
3. Sometimes very severe attacks with complications.

Chloramphenicol does not cure these conditions.

Sometimes large masses of chronic granulation tissue form in the intestinal wall. Symptoms and signs similar to cancer or obstruction of the intestine can occur. You can often feel the mass made by the amoebae in the abdomen, or on pelvic examination PR.

The amoebae can travel up the portal vein to the liver and cause liver abscesses (see Chapter 24 page 245).

The amoebae can live on the skin and produce ulcers around the anus, or on the genitalia (see Chapter 19 page 136).

Treatment to kill amoebae in all parts of the body is metronidazole 800 mg (4 tabs) three times a day for 5 days (400 mg three times a day for 10 days if nausea present). Tell the patient not to drink alcohol while taking metronidazole.

You can also use chloroquine, tetracycline and emetine but only in certain circumstances (see Chapter 24 page 246 or a reference book for special doses of these).

Give treatment for gastro-enteritis (see page 223) if present.

Control and prevention is the same as for all gastro-intestinal infections. See page 225.

Bacillary dysentery (shigellosis)

Bacillary dysentery is an acute inflammation of the intestine caused by infection with *Shigella* – the dysentery bacteria. It causes diarrhoea or dysentery (frequent stools with blood and mucus), abdominal pain and fever. Sometimes mild cases with just diarrhoea occur and many infected persons have no symptoms. But, severe cases with complications can also occur.

The usual reservoir is man. Spread is from infected faeces to the mouth of another person. This spread is direct or in contaminated food or by flies.

In a health centre, there is no way that bacillary dysentery can be distinguished with certainty from other causes of acute diarrhoeal disease or gastro-enteritis which have caused dysentery. However, if the dysentery does not need metronidazole to cure it (if metronidazole is needed it was probably due to amoebae) it is assumed that the cause was the bacillary dysentery organism.

For symptoms and signs, course and complications, treatment, control and prevention, see page 221 or a reference book. Antibiotics should not be given unless the bacteria (1) invade deeply into the intestinal wall and cause severe disease with abdominal tenderness or (2) spread into the blood stream and cause symptoms and signs of septicaemia.

Salmonella causing typhoid

Typhoid is caused by only very special *Salmonella* organisms.

Infection with these organisms causes malaise, fever, abdominal pain and constipation with a slow pulse for the first week. During the second week the patient gets worse and diarrhoea, en-

largement of the spleen and rash occur. In the third week intestinal haemorrhage or perforation and severe general symptoms and signs of infection may occur and the patient may die. (See Chapter 18 page 112 for details.)

You are not likely to mistake typhoid for one of the usual or undiagnosable forms of gastro-enteritis.

Salmonella food poisoning

Salmonellae are bacteria which very often cause gastro-enteritis. They can cause a mild or moderate or severe attack of acute diarrhoea and sometimes dysentery. The patient usually has a fever. There are no specific symptoms and signs which you can use to make the diagnosis in the health centre.

The reservoir of the salmonellae is the gastro-intestinal tract of man and many other animals. Spread can be direct, but it is usually by food or drink which is contaminated with the faeces of an infected man or animal. The organisms multiply in the food (especially milk, meat, eggs, fish, etc.), especially if it is stored for a time before eating. If there are enough organisms in the food when it is eaten, acute diarrhoeal disease with fever occurs, after an incubation period of 4–48 hours.

If group of people eat the infected food, there will be an epidemic of acute diarrhoeal disease with fever 4–48 hours later.

Treatment is as described for gastro-enteritis (see page 223). Do not give antibiotics unless the conditions described on page 224 developed.

Toxin type of food poisoning

If staphlococci or streptococci get into food or drink (especially milk), they grow in it and produce a toxin.

If the food or drink is swallowed, the bacteria do not cause disease; but the toxin causes acute gastro-enteritis. There is usually the sudden onset of severe vomiting only. There is no fever. The other usual symptoms and signs of gastro-enteritis can be present. The gastro-enteritis usually gets better after a few hours, even without treatment.

The reservoir is the infected respiratory tract or skin of patients or carriers. These people contaminate food or drink with the organisms. Enough toxin can form to cause disease, especially if the food is milk, and especially if it is kept warm before eating. The incubation period is 1–6 hours. There is no infection of the patient by the organisms.

If a group of people eat the infected food there will be an epidemic of acute gastro-enteritis without fever 1–6 hours later.

Treatment is the same as for gastro-enteritis (see page 223). Do not give antibiotics.

Schistosomiasis

See Chapter 18 page 122 for details if *Schistosoma mansoni* or *S. japonicum* affect people in your area.

Intestinal symptoms and signs start between 2 months and 2 years after infection.

There is often diarrhoea with blood and mucus in the stools and intestinal colic. All of these can be severe. These conditions can improve after some days or weeks; but they return some weeks later. On examination you can often feel the large intestine and it may be tender.

After some time, masses of infected tissue can form inside the intestine. You can often feel these masses on abdominal examination and they can prolapse (come out) through the anus.

It is difficult to tell the difference between amoebic infection and cancer of the large intestine and schistosomiasis, without tests.

Later, the eggs travel to the liver and damage the liver blood vessels causing portal hypertension with ascites and a large spleen (see Chapter 24 page 244).

If patients have only a few worms or if they do not have repeated infections, they may not have these symptoms and signs.

See Chapter 18 page 126 for diagnosis and treatment and control.

Appendicitis

Appendicitis is an acute inflammation of the appendix. The inflamed appendix may burst and cause a localised abscess or general peritonitis if it is not treated. (See a specialist surgery book for details.)

The patient usually complains of a central abdominal pain at first. After some hours the pain moves to the right iliac fossa and is constant. The patient loses his appetite from the start of the disease.

On examination there is usually:
mild fever,
pulse faster than normal,
abdomen
- not distended,
- may not move well on respiration,
- tenderness and rebound tenderness and guarding in the right iliac fossa, and tenderness on the right side on pelvic examination through the rectum.

Later, if it is not treated, an abscess with a tender mass in the right iliac fossa, or general peritonitis, develops.

Treatment is urgent transfer to Medical Officer care, if patient agrees to surgery, to remove the appendix.

Meanwhile give:
- nil by mouth;
- IVI fluids, 1 litre of 4% dextrose in 0.18% sodium chloride each 8 hours;
- IVI or IMI chloramphenicol 1 g (1 bottle) each 6 hours;
- pethidine 100 mg (2 ml) IMI before transfer.

Cancer (carcinoma) of the intestine

See a specialist surgery book for details.

Cancer of the intestine occurs more often in old people.

Cancer of the intestine may cause:
- anaemia from bleeding into the bowel;
- attacks of constipation and diarrhoea, often with blood in the stool;
- intestinal colic and later obstruction of the intestine;
- a palpable abdominal mass; and
- weight loss and malaise.

It may be difficult to distinguish cancer of the intestine from amoebic dysentry and amoeboma and schistosomiasis, which can have similar chronic histories and similar signs.

If cancer of the intestine is suspected, give the patient a full course of anti-amoebic treatment (metronidazole 400 mg (2 tabs) three times a day for 10 days preferably with tetracycline (500 mg 6th hourly). If the disease does not improve rapidly and get completely better after some weeks, transfer the patient non-urgently to hospital.

Pain or difficulty swallowing (dysphagia)

Do a full history and examination (see Chapter 6).

Weigh the patient, test the urine and do the haemoglobin estimation.

Look for evidence of these conditions:

1. *Foreign body in throat or oesophagus*
   - sudden pain when swallowing
   - feeling of something stuck in the neck or chest
   - vomiting at first
   - no fever or other abnormal signs at first

   Urgently transfer to medical officer if you cannot see and remove the foreign body as severe, usually fatal, neck or chest infections can develop.

2. *Snake bite*
   - cannot swallow
   - cannot open eyes, talk or cough properly
   - history of snake bite
   - sometimes pain near the bite or abnormal bleeding from many places

   See Chapter 33 page 374 urgently and give antivenom.

3. *Infection in the mouth or throat*
   - pain on swallowing
   - acute start
   - inflamed mucous membrane with patches of *Monilla* (thrush) or ulcers in the mouth or pus on the tonsils or tender swelling of abscess in throat or neck
   - sometimes fever
   - lymph nodes in neck often enlarged

   See page 163 and Chapter 20 page 163.

4. *Tetanus*
   - starts over a few days
   - cannot open mouth widely
   - spasms of rest of body may be present
   - recent wound often
   - no tetanus immunisation

   See Chapter 25 page 263.

5. *Diseases of the oesophagus including cancer, Chagas Disease, achalasia, stenosis etc*
   - slow start of difficulty in swallowing – at first only solid food; but later also soft food, then fluids
   - may vomit food and fluid eaten, but no bile in vomitus
   - weight loss

   Transfer all such cases to a medical officer at a hospital.

6. *Acting out*
   - The patient has a big problem.
   - The patient has no abnormal signs on examination.
   - The condition gets better if you discover his problem and solve it.

   Discover and help solve the patient's problem.

Transfer

Transfer patients to medical officer care when there is:

1. a foreign body (urgent),
2. tetanus (urgent),
3. no improvement after treatment of the suspected cause (non-urgent), or
4. you cannot find the cause after observing the patient for a week (non-urgent).

Nausea or vomiting

Causes include:

1. Irritation of the gastro-intestinal tract.
   (a) All causes of gastro-enteritis (see page 220).
   (b) Alcohol. Some foods. Some drugs.
   (c) Peptic ulcer (see page 215).
2. Block or paralysis of the gastro-intestinal tract.
   (a) Intestinal or 'pyloric' obstruction (see pages 214 and 406).
   (b) Paralytic ileus
   - after abdominal operation for 1–3 days
   - water and salt problems after prolonged gastro-enteritis
   - pus or blood in the peritoneal cavity
   (c) Peritonitis (see page 213).
   (d) Haemorrhage into peritoneum (e.g. ectopic pregnancy or ruptured spleen) (see page 406).
3. Irritation of vomiting centre in brain.
   (a) From disease of brain:
   - cerebral tumour or tuberculoma or abscess, etc. (see Chapter 25 page 264)
   - meningitis (see Chapter 25 page 256)
   - encephalitis (see Chapter 25 page 260)
   (b) From changes in blood going to the brain:
   - any fever (including malaria)
   - any infection (especially middle ear inflammation)
   - pregnancy (and hormone change)
   - chemicals – drugs, poisons, toxins
   - kidney (renal) failure
   - hepatitis

(c) From 'higher' centre in the brain:
- fear
- worry
- severe pain of any cause

Diagnosis

Do a full history and examination (see Chapter 6). Test the urine for protein, sugar, bile and pus. Diagnose the cause by the other symptoms and signs the patient has. Then treat the cause.

Which of these seven groups of symptoms and signs does your patient have?

1. *Vomiting and*
   constipation and
   abdominal pain which is colic and
   abdominal swelling (distension).
   Then: intestinal obstruction. See page 214.
   If he *also* has constant abdominal pain or a tender area in the abdomen especially over a hernia. *Then*: strangulated obstruction. See page 406.

2. *Vomiting and*
   constipation and
   abdominal pain which is constant and
   abdominal swelling (distension) and
   abdominal tenderness all over.
   Then: paralysis of the intestine because of pus or blood in the peritoneal cavity (peritonitis or haemoperitoneum).
   See page 213.

3. *Vomiting and*
   diarrhoea and
   abdominal pain which is colic but
   no abdominal tenderness.
   Then: gastro-enteritis. See page 220.

4. *Vomiting after food*
   abdominal pain: $\begin{cases} in\ epigastrium \\ worse\ after\ food \\ relieved\ by\ vomiting \end{cases}$
   abdominal tenderness only in epigastrium.
   Then: peptic ulcer. See page 215.

5. *Vomiting and*
   headache or
   stiff neck or
   confusion or
   fitting or
   paralysis or
   unconsciousness.
   Then: meningitis, *or*
   cerebral malaria, *or*
   encephalitis, *or*

head injury, *or*
brain tumour, etc.
If the condition is acute and the patient is very 'sick' (but not if he has a head injury), do a malaria smear, give IMI quinine, do a lumbar puncture and see Chapter 25 page 271.
If the condition is chronic and the patient is not acutely 'sick' or if he has a head injury and is not improving, transfer to the Medical Officer.

6. *Vomiting and*
   conditions found which could affect blood going to brain.
   Then:
   - fever of any cause (especially malaria (see Chapter 13 page 51)), *or*
   - infection of any type (especially middle ear infection (see Chapter 20 page 159)), *or*
   - if menstrual period/s have been missed: pregnancy (see an obstetrics book), *or*
   - if jaundice: hepatitis, (see Chapter 24 page 242, *or*
   - if wasted, anaemic, BP high, protein in urine: kidney failure (see Chapter 26 page 289 and a medical reference book).

7. *Vomiting and*
   pain or
   fear or
   worry but
   no other abnormalities found on physical examination.
   Then:
   pain (see Chapter 7 page 28), *or*
   fear (see Chapter 35), *or*
   worry (see Chapter 35).

Vomiting blood (haematemesis)

If a patient has recently vomited blood, then:
1. Immediately start an IV drip (before doing 2).
2. Do a full history and examination and test the urine (see Chapter 6).
3. Find out the answers to these four questions.

1. *Did the patient really VOMIT the blood?*
   Check that the patient vomited blood and did not:
   (a) cough up the blood, or
   (b) vomit up blood swallowed after coughing up blood (haemoptysis) or bleeding from the upper respiratory tract (e.g. bleeding nose).

Look at the blood.

(a) If it is brown it is from the stomach (the acid turns it brown).

(b) If it is bright red it is more likely to be from haemoptysis or the upper respiratory tract; but if there is a lot of gastro-intestinal bleeding the blood can be bright red.

If the patient has blood in the gastro-intestinal tract he will later pass melaena (black, smelly stools like tar).

2. *How much blood has been vomited up?*

If more than 300 ml (1 cup), it is an emergency. Put an IV drip up *immediately*, in case the patient bleeds again and needs resuscitation.

3. *Is the patient shocked?*

If he is shocked, start intravenous resuscitation immediately (see Chapter 27 page 307) and make arrangements for emergency transfer or blood transfusion.

4. *What is the cause of the bleeding?*

(a) Stomach and duodenal diseases.

• Peptic ulcer.

History of epigastric pain related to food.

Tenderness in the epigastrium.

• Peptic ulcer caused by aspirin or alcohol.

The recent taking of aspirin (even only a few) or alcohol (usually a lot).

• Cancer of the stomach.

Older person.

Feeling of fullness soon after eating.

Weight loss.

Not cured by proper treatment for severe peptic ulcer.

(b) Oesophageal diseases.

• Cirrhosis of the liver with varicose veins in the oesophagus.

Ascites.

Some oedema.

Wasting and other signs of liver failure.

• Tear in the oesophagus after vomiting from any cause.

Bleeding started AFTER vomiting.

(c) Bleeding disease.

• Snake bite.

History of being bitten by a snake.

• Rare blood diseases.

If the patient:

1. has vomited more than 1 cup of blood and/or
2. has vomited blood more than once and/or
3. has melaena too and/or

4. is anaemic and/or
5. is shocked;

then manage as follows:

1. Set up an IV drip. Give IV fluids/plasma volume expanders/blood as necessary (see Chapter 27 page 305).
2. Give sedation – diazepam 5–10 mg (1–2 ml) IMI; or if you are certain the patient does not have cirrhosis, morphine 10 mg (1 ml) IMI.
3. Insert an intragastric tube and aspirate till the stomach is empty; then aspirate hourly. When there is no bleeding, give antacids every hour.
4. Transfer the patient to Medical Officer care in case he bleeds again and needs blood transfusion.
5. See index for other treatment of the diagnosed condition.

Diarrhoea or dysentery

Diarrhoea (frequent soft or watery stools) is a symptom – not a disease. You must always find out the cause. Diarrhoea can cause dehydration and death.

Dysentery (diarrhoea with blood and often mucus) is a symptom – not a disease. You must always find out the cause. Dysentery can cause: dehydration and death; but also anaemia and shock from blood loss; and also allow infection into blood (septicaemia).

Diarrhoea and dysentery usually occur with intestinal colic (often), vomiting (sometimes) and other symptoms and signs (sometimes) i.e. gastroenteritis.

Often you cannot find the cause in a health centre.

But it is always important to do the following 3 things:

1. Try to find the cause (see below).

Treat any cause you find.

2. Look for dehydration of the patient (see page 221).

Prevent or treat dehydration (see page 223).

3. Find out if others are also affected (i.e. an epidemic).

Control and prevention may be necessary.

Do these things by doing a full history and examination (see Chapter 6).

Causes to look for include:

1. 'Food poisoning'

Often there is a history of others who ate the

same food also being affected (i.e. an epidemic).

Sometimes there is a history of eating food which may be poisonous (certain fish or plants); or food which did not look, smell and taste as it should; or food which was not eaten soon after it was cooked.

Sometimes there is a history of taking drugs.

2. Infections in the intestine.

These include viruses, bacteria (*Escherichia coli*, *Shigella*, *Campylobacter*, *Salmonella typhi*, *Clostridium*, cholera), amoebae, *Giardia* and *Schistosoma*.

Dysentry is caused by some of these infections. Fever is often caused by infections.

3. 'Medical' causes include:
   - any cause of fever, especially malaria,
   - any acute infection, especially middle ear infection,
   - any chronic infection, especially visceral leishmaniasis,
   - malnutrition,
   - lactose intolerance (if the patient has drunk milk),
   - change in diet, and
   - anxiety.

4. 'Surgical' causes:

Intestinal obstruction, early or incomplete.
Enteritis necroticans

Management includes:

1. Prevent or treat dehydration (see page 223).
2. Treat any underlying cause you find (see above).
   Always give antimalarial drugs (see Chapter 13 page 55 unless you are certain that the patient does not have malaria.
3. Give chloramphenicol or metronidazole only if necessary (see page 224).
4. Transfer to medical officer care if necessary (see page 231).
5. Do any control and prevention that is necessary (see page 231).

Blood in stools

Always look at stools:
1. to check there is blood in the stools and
2. to see what kind of blood there is and
3. to see where the blood is.

If fresh blood is on the outside of the stool, then it is probably due to:
- haemorrhoids (see a surgery book), or
- anal fissure (see a surgery book).

If blood is mixed with diarrhoeal stool, then it is:
- dysentery, see gastro-enteritis (page 220) for cause, (note especially – bacterial dysentry especially *Shigella,* amoebic dysentery, and schistosomiasis); or
- cancer of the intestine (see page 233).

If blood is mixed with solid stool, then it is most likely to be:
- cancer of lower large intestine (see page 233).

If black smelly stools (like tar), then it is:
- upper gastro-intestinal tract bleeding (see haematemesis, page 235).

Constipation

Constipation is present when the patient does not pass faeces for longer than is normal for that person.

Complete constipation
- no faeces or gas passed.
- usually serious and important.
- causes – bowel obstruction (see page 214) or paralytic ileus (see page 234).

Incomplete constipation
- less frequent bowel movements than normal.
- usually it is not serious.
- causes – not eating much, dehydration (see page 221), incomplete bowel obstruction (page 214), drugs, e.g. codeine or morphine.

Abdominal pain – tenderness – guarding – rigidity

See Chapter 36 page 402.

Abdominal swellings

See Chapter 36 page 412.

Loss of weight

See Chapter 36 page 401.

24

Disorders of the Liver and Bile Ducts

Figure 24.1 A and B (below)   The normal position of the normal liver (A) on the front of the body and (B) on the right side of the body. Note that most of the normal liver is under the right ribs. In the mid-clavicular line at the right side the liver is almost as high as the nipple and is only about 1 cm below the edge of the ribs.

Figure 24.2 (opposite)   The anatomy of the bile ducts, pancreas and duodenum.

Figure 24.3 (opposite below)   The anatomy of the liver portal venous system. Blood is carried from the stomach, intestines, spleen and pancreas into the liver by the portal vein. Hepatic veins then carry the blood from the liver to the the inferior vena cava. The liver also has its own supply of arterial blood from the hepatic artery.

cystic duct joins gall bladder to common bile duct

common hepatic duct - bile from the liver comes down this duct   most goes into the gall bladder for concentration and storage

gall bladder where bile is concentrated and stored

common bile duct - bile from the gall bladder passes through this duct on the way to the duodenum during a meal

duodenum

opening of the bile and pancreatic ducts together into the duodenum

pancreas

pancreatic duct

superior mesenteric artery

inferior vena cava

oesophagus

right and left hepatic veins

liver

stomach

portal vein

splenic vein

spleen

duodenum

gastro-epiploic vein

superior mesenteric vein

pancreas

small intestine (start of)

colon

inferior mesenteric vein

colon

small intestine (end of)

rectum

Physiology and pathology

The liver has many functions including:

1. manufacturing and storing bile;
2. storing sugar and controlling the amount of sugar in the blood;
3. manufacturing proteins and other substances; and
4. removing toxins, poisons, drugs and hormones, etc. from the blood.

Manufacturing and storing bile

The liver cells make bile. Small ducts take the bile from the liver cells. These join to form larger tubes, until they all join into one large tube called the common hepatic duct. The cystic duct goes from this to the gall bladder (see Figure 24.2) where the bile is concentrated and stored. When a person eats, the gall bladder squeezes the bile back through the cystic duct to the common bile duct which takes the bile into the duodenum. In the duodenum the bile mixes with the food.

Bile contains bile salts which help the fat in the food to be digested. Bile salts are re-absorbed further down the intestine so that they can be used again.

Bile also contains bilirubin. Bilirubin is a yellow waste product from worn out or damaged red blood cells. Red blood cells are usually destroyed in the spleen. The spleen then puts the bilirubin into the blood. This bilirubin is insoluble and cannot get into the urine from the blood. So, the liver cells take it out of the blood, change it (to make it soluble), and then put it into the bile. When the bilirubin in the bile reaches the intestine it becomes brown, and makes the faeces brown. If any of this changed bilirubin in the bile gets back into the blood, it is dissolved and passed in the urine. The urine then looks brown or black (like tea or coffee without milk or like 'cola' drinks), though many patients say it looks 'red'. (Also the colour of the froth on the urine is yellow – normally urine froth is white, even if the urine is yellow.)

In haemolytic conditions, when many red cells are destroyed, much bilirubin goes into the blood. If the amount of bilirubin in the blood is more than the liver can take out, the amount of bilirubin in the blood rises. The patient therefore looks yellow; he is jaundiced. But the urine colour and the faeces colour remain normal (as the bilirubin cannot get into the urine and the faeces cannot be any more brown).

In conditions which obstruct (or block) the bile ducts, the bile is reabsorbed into the blood. The bile salts cause itch. The bilirubin, which is the sort changed by the liver, is dissolved and passed in the urine, which becomes dark. No bile reaches the intestine so the faeces become light or even white.

In hepatitis, the liver cells are damaged and cannot take all the bile out of the blood. The small bile ducts are also damaged, and bile with changed bilirubin goes back into the blood. The patient becomes jaundiced. The urine becomes dark. The faeces may become lighter; but they do not become white.

Storing sugar and controlling the amount of sugar in the blood

The blood which comes to the liver through the portal vein (see Figure 24.3) after eating is often full of sugar absorbed from the intestine. The concentration of sugar is often far more than the body needs. The liver cells receive messages from the pancreas (through a hormone called insulin) to remove much of the sugar and store it. When the concentration of sugar in the blood falls, the pancreas makes less insulin and the liver puts some of the sugar back into the blood. So the body does not have too much sugar after eating and not enough between meals.

Manufacturing proteins and other substances

The liver is the main place for building up the proteins the body needs. These proteins are built up from the substances which the intestine absorbs from the food, and which come to the liver in the portal vein (see Figure 24.3). Some of these proteins stay in the blood to hold water inside the blood vessels, and stop it going out of the blood vessels and causing oedema and ascites. Other proteins made in the liver have other functions, including helping blood to clot.

If the liver does not work properly, the person may develop oedema and ascites, wasting of muscles and bleeding.

Removing toxins, poisons, drugs and hormones etc. from the blood

The liver also destroys many poisons, toxins, drugs and hormones etc. which enter the blood. If the liver is not working properly, ordinary doses of some drugs may be dangerous; hormones may stay in the blood and cause enlargement of the breasts in men; and toxins from the intestines which come to the liver through the portal vein (see Figure 24.3) may damage the brain causing mental disturbance or unconsciousness.

History and examination

If you suspect liver disease or jaundice, try to find out if there is:

1. Liver structure abnormality
   - pain or tenderness of the liver
   - swelling of or lumps in the liver
2. Obstruction of the bile ducts
   - jaundice
   - dark urine
   - pale stools
3. Liver cell failure (failure of the liver cells to their work)
   - jaundice
   - fluid in the body tissues – oedema and ascites
   - wasting of muscles
   - bleeding
   - loss of full consciousness or abnormal mental state
4. Haemolysis, if jaundice is present
   - anaemia
   - enlarged spleen, etc
5. Infection in the liver or other parts of the body
   - fever, malaise, etc ⎱ general symptoms and
   - temperature raised ⎰ signs of infection
   - fast pulse
   - symptoms and signs of pneumonia, malaria or septicaemia
6. Signs of high pressure in the portal vein
   - ascites
   - gastro-intestinal bleeding

In the routine clinical examination of a patient, you may find these things in liver disease or jaundice:
- Loss of full consciousness ⎱ if there is liver
- Mental abnormally ⎰ failure

- Temperature raised, if there is infection
- Pulse fast, if there is infection; but sometimes the pulse is slow in deep jaundice
- Wasting, if there is liver failure (usually chronic)
- Oedema, if there is liver failure (usually chronic)
- Pallor, if there is haemolysis
- Jaundice if there is haemolysis or liver cell disease, or obstruction of the bile ducts
- Bleeding if there is liver failure (as especially gastro-intestinal bleeding if there is high portal venous pressure)
- Ascites if there is liver failure (especially if there is high portal venous pressure)
- Liver enlargement (see page 247 for causes)
- Liver tenderness (see page 248 for causes)
- Splenomegaly if there is haemolysis or high portal venous pressure (but the spleen is often enlarged because of malaria or kala azar)
- Enlarged veins on the abdomen which suggest high pressure in or obstruction of the portal vein
- Urine – dark (like tea) and bile present on testing, which suggests liver cell disease or obstruction of the bile ducts (urine is normal in haemolysis)
- Faeces – light or white if there is obstruction of the bile ducts.

Method of examination of the liver

Gently put the right hand with the fingers pointing to the patient's head flat on the right lateral abdomen. Place the hand outside the rectus muscle

Figure 24.4 Method of palpating for the edge (size) of the liver. See text for description of the method.

241

(the long strong muscle which runs down the middle 1/3rd of the abdomen). Put the other hand either on top of the right hand or at the back of the patient to hold the liver forward. Ask the patient to take a deep breath. As the patient breathes in, gently press the hand inwards and upwards.

Start low down in the abdomen (in the right iliac fossa). Move the hand up a little each time the patient breathes out until the fingers reach the edge of the liver, on the edge of the ribs. The edge of the liver hits the ends of the fingers as the patient breathes in.

Feel the surface of the liver for tenderness and lumps.

If you are not sure about the size of the liver, percuss in the mid-clavicular line from high up in the chest down to the dullness of the liver. (Just below the right nipple.) Check how far down the dullness of the liver goes.

Disorders of the liver and bile ducts

Acute viral hepatitis

Viral hepatitis is a viral infection of the whole body, but which mainly causes inflammation of the liver.

The cause is one of several viruses. Hepatitis A (infectious hepatitis) virus spreads mainly by faecal-oral means. Hepatitis B (serum hepatitis) virus spreads mainly by injection of blood from an infected person. But both viruses may spread by both ways. Hepatitis non A non B virus is a more recently discovered virus which is spread mainly by blood like hepatitis B.

Other viruses can cause acute hepatitis (e.g. Yellow Fever virus). But these diseases cause much more acute disease than clinical 'acute viral hepatitis' (see Chapter 17 page 108).

The incubation period for Hepatitis A is long (2 – 6 weeks) and for Hepatitis B very long (6 weeks to 6 months).

Symptoms and signs
For the first week the patient complains of
- mild fever (a high fever is not common),
- malaise,
- loss of appetite, nausea, vomiting, etc.,

- mild right upper abdominal pain (over the liver).

After
- dark urine (like tea – test for bilirubin positive),
- jaundice,
- liver smooth enlarged and tender (but not very enlarged or very tender).

The patient feels much better soon after the jaundice appears; but he may not feel completely well for months.

The jaundice usually gets worse for about 2 weeks and then slowly (sometimes very slowly) gets better.

Hepatitis B is a more serious disease. The patient may die from severe acute hepatitis with liver failure. After months or years some patients develop chronic liver disease (see page 243). After some years, some patients develop hepatoma or primary cancer of the liver (see page 246).

Some patients with Hepatitis B infection cannot destroy all the virus in their body even when they become well. The virus stays in their blood. They are then 'carriers' of Hepatitis B. This may also occur with Hepatitis non A non B.

Differential diagnosis
See jaundice page 248, tender liver page 248, or fever with jaundice Chapter 17 page 110 if the patient is very sick.

The condition you are most likely to confuse with viral hepatitis is hepatitis caused by drugs, especially drugs for leprosy, tuberculosis or schistosomiasis. If a patient becomes jaundiced or develops hepatitis always stop all drugs and discuss the problem with a medical officer.

Treatment
There is no cure.

Admission is not normally necessary.

If he is 'sick', the patient must rest in bed.

If he has repeated vomiting, give IV fluids for dehydration and maintenance fluids (see gastro-enteritis Chapter 23 page 223).

Encourage the patient to drink as much sugary fluid and eat as much good food as possible. Tell him not to drink beer or alcohol.

Give antimalarial drugs as indicated, usually chloroquine 450–600 mg (3–4 tabs) daily for three days and 300 mg (2 tabs) weekly until he is well.

Do not give drugs which could affect the liver, especially chlorpromazine or TCE (tetrachloroethylene). Stop all drugs the patient is taking, including oral contraceptives. If the patient is taking tuberculosis or leprosy drugs, stop these drugs and transfer the patient to a Medical Officer urgently. (Do *not* just stop tuberculosis or leprosy drugs and take no other action.)

Control and prevention
1. Kill the organism in the body of the original host and reservoir. This is not possible (even with the people who are carries of Hepatitis B virus).
2. Stop the means of spread.
    (a) Good personal hygiene for patient, family and staff. (Everyone must wash their hands after using the toilet. Patients should not handle other people's foods, etc.)
    (b) Supply and use proper toilets.
    Supply and use safe water.
    Check toilets and water supply if an epidemic occurs.
    (c) Proper sterilisation of needles and syringes. Check that your staff are doing proper sterilisation if an epidemic occurs.
    (d) Give blood transfusions only if they are really necessary. In hospitals all blood is tested for Hepatitis B before it is transfused.
    (e) Isolation of the patient does not help. The patient is infectious before the jaundice appears but for only a few days (not more than 1 week) after it appears.
3. Raise the resistance of susceptible people.
    (a) An injection of normal human immunoglobulin (gamma globulin) has antibodies against Hepatitis A virus in it. You can give it to increase the resistance of contacts if necessary (e.g. a case in a school or institution).
    (b) You can give special Hepatitis B immunoglobulin to people who have been exposed to Hepatitis B (e.g. staff who have contact with an Hepatitis B patient's blood) and who have no resistance to Hepatitis B infection as they have no anti-hepatitis B antibodies when these are tested for in the laboratory. In many tropical and developing countries a large number of people do have resistance to Hepatitis B as they have anti-hepatitis B antibodies probably from a mild infection when they were children, and were still protected by their mothers' antibodies.
    (c) A live virus vaccine which will cause the immunised person to develop anti-hepatitis B antibodies, and therefore protect against Hepatitis B infection, has now been produced. As yet it is very expensive and not usually available in developing countries. At present it could be given to those who have no anti-hepatitis B antibodies but who are exposed to infection (e.g. health workers, teachers etc.). If the vaccine becomes freely available and cheap, it could be given to all babies to prevent Hepatitis B infection and most cases of hepatoma.

Cirrhosis of the liver (chronic liver disease)

Cirrhosis of the liver is a disease which slowly destroys liver cells in all parts of the liver. Fibrous scar tissues and some, but not enough, new liver cells grow. All this slowly destroys the structure and function of the liver.

Cirrhosis is a common disease. It usually affects middle aged adults; but it can also affect the young and the old.

Pathology and clinical features:
When a patient has cirrhosis, liver cells die. After a long time there are not enough liver cells for the liver to function properly. (See page 240.)

Very importantly the following effects of liver failure occur:
1. it does not make enough serum proteins, and fluid goes out of blood vessels, causing oedema;
2. it does not metabolise hormones, and changes in the sex characteristics of the patient occur;
3. it does not metabolise drugs and the effects of some drugs last a very long time;
4. and it does not metabolise toxins from the intestines and the brain may not work properly.

The new fibrous scar tissue presses on the portal veins (see Figure 24.3). The pressure in the portal vein is more than normal and the vein becomes overfilled and stretched. So fluid from the vein goes into the peritoneum causing ascites. Sometimes the vein bursts and the blood goes into the gastro-intestinal tract causing vomiting of blood (haematemesis) or passing of faeces which are made of digested blood and so are black tarry and smelly (melaena).

You cannot find out the cause of cirrhosis in a health centre. Previous infection with Hepatitis B virus is the most common and important cause in a health centre. Drinking a lot of alcohol every day for a long time can cause cirrhosis. Toxins which form in badly stored grains or groundnuts can cause cirrhosis. In parts of the world where schistosomiasis occurs, schistosomiasis is the common cause of liver damage; especially if the damage is mostly to the portal vein.

Symptoms usually include:
1. swelling of the abdomen (usually the first symptom),
2. swelling of the legs,
3. malaise, weakness, etc.
4. haematemesis (vomiting blood) or melaena (black tarry smelly bowel motions made of digested blood).

Signs usually include:
1. Wasting. This is not marked at first; but later it is very severe. You can see it most in the arms and shoulders (as the legs are swollen with oedema). (This is caused by liver cell failure.)
2. Oedema of the legs and back. (This is caused by low protein in the blood from liver cell failure.)
3. Very swollen abdomen caused by ascites. (This is caused by both low protein in the blood from liver cell failure and high portal vein pressure.)
4. The spleen is enlarged (This is caused by high portal vein pressure; but there are often other causes for an enlarged spleen as well.)

Note two things.
1. The liver is often not enlarged.
2. Jaundice is not common until late in the disease.

Check the patient does not have one of the other common causes of these symptoms or signs.

Oedema see Chapter 36 page 398.
Wasting see Chapter 36 page 400.
Splenomegaly see Chapter 22 page 207.
Ascites see Chapter 36 page 412.

Check the patient does not have abdominal tuberculosis which causes ascites *but*:

Figure 24.5 A typical patient with cirrhosis: an adult, very swollen abdomen (ascites), some swelling of the legs (muscle wasting but hidden by oedema), very thin arms and shoulders (muscle wasting).

- little or no oedema,
- abdominal pain or tenderness (sometimes),
- abdominal masses (sometimes), and
- no help from diuretic treatment.

Test the stools and the urine for schistosomiasis to see if this is the cause (see Chapter 18 page 122).

Complications may develop:
1. Gastro-intestinal bleeding
   This comes from burst varicose veins in the oesophagus or stomach caused by high portal pressure. Haematemesis, melaena, anaemia or shock may develop. In most places there is nothing a medical officer can do to help, so do not transfer the patient. Find out what you

should do in your area. Treatment at the health centre is with IV fluids. See Chapter 23 page 224 and Chapter 27 page 307 but do not give morphine. Treat also for peptic ulcer in case the patient has bled from an ulcer. Be ready to treat for brain disturbance (see 2 below).

2. Brain function disturbance

If there is high protein food or blood in the gastro-intestinal tract, toxins from this may go past the liver (as there are not enough liver cells left to take the toxins out of the blood) and these toxins can stop the brain working properly. The patient may become psychotic or unconscious. If this happens, give proper nursing care, give streptomycin powder for injection *orally* or down an intragastric tube (not by injection), 1 g every 6 hours until the patient improves. Give enough magnesium sulphate to make the patient pass faeces 2–3 times every day.

Treatment

Cure is not possible.

If the cause is schistosomiasis, the drugs for treatment of schistosomiasis are usually more dangerous if the patient has liver disease. Do not give these drugs until you have discussed the case with the medical officer.

Manage complications as described above.

Routine treatment is for the ascites and oedema to make the patient feel better for the rest of his life.

1. Diuretics – hydrochlorothiazide 50–100 mg (1–2 tabs) should be given every morning.
   • You can also give frusemide 40–160 mg (1–4 tabs) every morning if hydrochlorothiazide alone is not effective.
   • You can give frusemide 20–60 mg (2–6 ml) by IVI every morning for some days if the tablets are not effective.
   • Always give a small dose of each drug first. If the drug is not effective after 3–4 days, increase the dose.
2. If the patient is not eating a tuber diet (i.e. sweet potato, yam, taro, etc.) or if you have given him frusemide, then add potassium chloride 1200 mg (2 tabs) three times a day.
3. The patient must eat food with high protein but no added salt. He should not eat tinned meat or fish as these contain a lot of salt. He should eat fresh foods if possible.

4. Usually you should *not* drain the ascitic fluid through a needle. See a medical reference book.

Check the effect of the treatment every time you see the patient by measuring his:
1. weight
2. amount of oedema of legs and back; and also,
3. the abdominal circumference, at the level of the umbilicus.

After some months or years, even increased doses of diuretics will not help the oedema, and the patient will die.

Note that if you give large doses of diuretics quickly this may damage the brain function and cause death.

If the patient only has ascites, or if intravenous diuretics do not cure the ascites, refer or transfer (non-urgently) the patient to a medical officer to check if he or she has another disease (e.g. tuberculosis of the abdomen or ovarian cyst).

Prevention is impossible, except prevention of schistosomsisis (see Chapter 18 page 126) and Hepatitis B (see page 242). Dry storage of grains and groundnuts (so that toxins cannot form in them) may help.

Liver abscess

Liver abscess is an acute (but sometimes chronic) infective inflammation of the liver. It is usually caused by ameobae. Acute abscesses are occasionally caused by bacteria. The infecting organism causes inflamation, then pus and then an abscess forms in the liver.

A liver abscess is not very common; but it is important. If it is treated, it is cured. If it is not treated, the patient dies.

The amoebae spread to the liver from the intestine through the portal vein. The patient often does not have symptoms or signs of amoebic infection in the intestine (or a history of these).

Symptoms include:
1. Pain and swelling of the abdomen, especially the right upper part.
2. The general symptoms of infection – malaise, weight loss, fever, etc.
Signs include:
1. The liver is tender and enlarged. Sometimes

Figure 24.6 Method of examining for tenderness of the liver (which is under the ribs) by percussing over the ribs. It is usual for the liver to be tender if a liver abscess is present. Sometimes you can find the tender area in the liver caused by an abscess by palpating with the fingers between the patient's right ribs, low down at the side or the back.

you can feel a soft area. Percussion of the right lower ribs causes pain. (See Figure 24.6.)

2. Fever, fast pulse, anaemia, weight loss, etc. may be present. Jaundice is not common.
3. A right pleural effusion of right sided pneumonia may develop.

The patient gets progressively worse and dies.

Hepatoma causes a similar clinical appearance. *Management* includes:

1. Check there is not another cause for the enlarged, tender liver, (e.g. malaria, acute heart failure, hepatitis).
2. Admit for inpatient treatment.
3. Take 10 ml of venous blood and send the serum to the hospital laboratory with a request for examination for alpha feto-protein (AFP). (AFP is positive if it is hepatoma.)
4. Give treatment for abcess while waiting for the result of the AFP. Note the effect of the treatment.
   (a) Metronidazole 800 mg (4 tabs) three times a day for 10 days. If this dose causes nausea, reduce the dose to 400 mg, 2 tablets, three

times a day. Advise the patient not to drink alcohol until the treatment is finished.
   (b) Chloroquine 150 mg (1 tab) three times a day until cured, transferred, diagnosed as hepatoma, or finished 3 weeks' treatment.
   (c) Chloramphenicol 1 g (4 caps) four times a day until cured, transferred, diagnosed as hepatoma, or finished 2 weeks' treatment.
5. If AFP is positive, stop this treatment. Inform the patient's relatives of the diagnosis (hepatoma) and prognosis. (See below.) Allow the patient to go home if he wants to. Give analgesics (see Chapter 7) as necessary at home, or in the hospital, or health centre.
6. Transfer these cases to Medical Officer care:
   (a) High fever, toxicity, etc. (i.e. general symptoms and signs of severe infection) which do not improve after 2 days or are not cured after 5 days (?pyogenic liver abscess). (Urgent.)
   (b) If signs develop suggesting the abscess is about to burst, i.e. fluctuant area in liver (urgent).
   (c) Not cured by treatment and AFP is negative. This is especially important in the first 4 months of pregnancy. In other cases a liver biopsy will probably be necessary. (Non-urgent.)

Hepatoma

Hepatoma is a primary cancer of the liver cells themselves. It is common in many tropical countries. It affects young people and older adults.

The cause is now known to be infection with the Hepatitis B virus, usually many years before. Some cases may be caused by toxins in badly stored groundnuts or grains.

Symptoms usually appear and get slowly worse over weeks or months and include:
1. pain in the right upper abdomen,
2. abdominal swelling, and
3. weight loss and weakness and malaise.

Signs include:
1. wasting, and
2. an enlarged hard lumpy liver, which is usually very tender.

Late in the disease liver failure with oedema, ascites and jaundice may occur.

The alpha feto-protein (AFP) test is positive. Send the serum from 10 ml of clotted blood to the hospital laboratory for this test immediately if you suspect hepatoma.

The patient usually gets quickly worse and dies in a few months.

Check the patient does not have amoebic abscess.

1. Send blood for AFP
2. Meanwhile treat for amoebic abscess
3. If AFP comes back positive, stop anti-amoebic treatment
4. If AFP comes back negative and the anti-amoebic drugs have not cured the patient, transfer him to hospital for liver aspiration or biopsy.

See page 245 for details of the above.

No cure is possible. But, aspirin, codeine co., pethidine or morphine can be given for pain as necessary (but only if the diagnosis is confirmed by AFP). (See Chapter 7 page 28.) Arrange for care and analgesics with the relatives at home; or, if the patient prefers, in the health centre.

Biliary colic, acute cholecystitis and obstructive jaundice

If something suddenly blocks the bile duct (which goes from the liver to the duodenum) or the cystic duct (which goes to and from the gall bladder), the patient feels severe pain called *biliary colic*. If the obstruction remains, infection may occur behind the obstruction. *Obstructive jaundice* may also occur. The patient will become yellow, the stools will become pale and the urine will become dark. These conditions are uncommon. But they can, sometimes be caused by gall stones or by a roundworm going from the duodenum into the bile ducts.

The patient feels *biliary colic* as a sudden upper central abdominal paint that gradually increases in waves and usually moves to the right upper abdomen. He may feel it in the back, the right side and the right shoulder. The pain is extremely severe and may cause vomiting. The pain usually lasts several hours and then suddenly stops, leaving a feeling of soreness in the right upper part of the abdomen. During the attack, there is some muscle spasm and guarding in the right upper part of the abdomen, but no fever.

Give an injection of pethidine 100 mg (2 ml) and atropine 0.6 mg (1 ml) for biliary colic. If the pain

stops, the patient needs non-urgent transfer to a hospital for investigation. If the pain does not stop after one or two injections, you must refer the patient to the medical officer urgently.

If obstruction and infection of the gall bladder occurs it is called *acute cholecystitis*. In acute cholecystitis following an attack of biliary colic, some pain remains. The patient develops both the general symptoms and signs of infection and the localised symptoms and signs of infection over the gall bladder in the right upper part of the abdomen. There is fever and a fast pulse. There is tenderness and guarding over the gall bladder.

Transfer a patient with acute cholecystitis urgently to hospital. Meanwhile manage like a case of peritonitis – nil by mouth, intravenous fluids, pethidine and chloramphenicol if necessary. (See Chapter 23 page 213.)

Slow obstruction of the bile duct which finally becomes complete occurs when a cancer presses on the main bile duct. This does not usually cause pain or infection. It causes *painless obstructive jaundice* with marked jaundice with itching, very dark urine and pale or almost white faeces. The liver may be enlarged. If the obstruction is in the common bile duct past the gall bladder (see Figure 24.3), the gall bladder may be enlarged: you can feel it as a soft lump underneath the front of the liver.

You should transfer the patient non-urgently to hospital to confirm the diagnosis, and for surgery if necessary.

Diagnosis of liver symptoms and signs

Enlargement of the liver

The normal liver is not more than 1 cm below the ribs of the right side of the chest.

Causes of enlarged liver include:

1. Malaria. Where malaria is common 70% of the normal population has an enlarged smooth non-tender liver. The liver functions normally. No treatment is needed for this liver enlargement.
2. Unknown. Up to 20% of normal people in tropical developing countries have an enlarged smooth non-tender liver even in areas where malaria is not common. The liver functions

normally. The cause is not known. No treatment is possible.

3. Other diseases.
   Viral hepatitis
   Amoebic hepatitis or abscess
   Hepatoma
   Secondary cancer
   Hydatid cyst
   Heart failure
   Kala azar
   Brucellosis
   Schistosomiasis
   Sickle cell disease
   Rare blood diseases
   Others – see a specialist reference book.

Tenderness of liver

The liver may be tender for any of these reasons:
1. Enlargement which happened quickly e.g. acute heart failure;
2. Acute inflammation e.g. amoebic abscess, viral hepatitis, infarction in sickle cell anaemia;
3. Hepatoma (tenderness is unusual if it is a secondary cancer);
4. Others – see a specialist reference book.

Jaundice

There are 3 types of jaundice (see page 241). There may be more than one type at the same time in a patient (see below, 4 groups).

Do a full history and examination (see Chapter 6).

Test the urine for protein and bile.

Look at the colour of the stools.

Diagnose and treat the cause.

Find out which of the 4 groups of symptoms and signs your patient has.

1. *Acute severe infections with red blood cell and liver cell damage* (i.e. acute haemolysis and acute hepatitis in varying degrees)
   The symptoms and signs are:
   fever, often high;
   'sick';
   sometimes diagnostic symptoms and signs;
   sometimes diagnostic tests if available;
   jaundice;
   dark urine with bile;
   stools not white.

Causes include:
malaria,
relapsing fever,
yellow fever,
pneumonia,
septicaemia, etc.
See Chapter 17 page 110.
Treat with antimalarials and antibiotics if diagnosis is not possible (see Chapter 17 page 110).

2. *Hepatitis caused by a virus or a drug*
   The symptoms and signs are:
   feels sick with nausea or vomiting;
   right upper abdominal pain;
   dark urine;
   stools not pale;
   fever (not high);
   tender enlarged liver (not severe);
   bile in urine.
   Treat like this:
   (a) If he feels 'sick', the patient must rest in bed.
   (b) If he has repeated vomiting, give IV fluids for dehydration and maintenance fluids (see Chapter 23 page 224).
   (c) Encourage him to drink as much sweet fluid and to eat as much good food as possible.
   (d) Give an antimalarial drug as indicated (see Chapter 13 page 55).
   (e) Stop all drugs including oral contraceptives.
   If the patient is on tuberculosis or leprosy treatment, stop all drugs and urgently transfer the patient to medical officer care.
   Give no drugs which could affect the liver, especially not chlorpromazine or TCE (tetrachloroethylene).
   (f) Check the patient's home and village sanitation and water supply.
   Check sterilisation procedures of the patient's health workers if the disease could be hepatitis B. Give health education about these things if required.
   (g) If a case of viral hepatitis occurs in a closed community (e.g. college) consult with the Medical Officer about using immunoglobulin to prevent an epidemic.

3. *Obstructive jaundice*
   The symptoms and signs are:
   jaundice,
   urine dark and test for bile positive,

stool light colour or white,
often an itch.

Causes include:

cancer,
enlarged lymph
nodes
} pressing on and blocking the bile duct,

gall stone or liver fluke or roundworm in the bile ducts, and some drugs including chlorpromazine.

Treat like this:

(a) Stop all drugs except antimalarials.

(b) Transfer to medical officer care – urgent if the patient has a fever or is sick, non-urgent if he has no fever and is not sick.

4. *Haemolytic jaundice*

The symptoms and signs are:
jaundice,

stools normal colour,
urine normal colour and test for bile negative.

Causes include chronic haemolytic anaemias including:
tropical splenomegaly syndrome,
sickle cell anaemia and
thalassaemia.

Causes also include acute haemolysis in tropical splenomegaly syndrome or sickle cell anaemia.

Find and teat the cause if possible.

Transfer to medical officer if a blood transfusion is necessary.

25

Disorders of the Nervous System

The nervous system consists of 3 parts:
1. the brain and spinal cord – the central nervous system;
2. the peripheral nervous system; and
3. the special sense organs (organs of sight, hearing, smell, taste).

The nervous system is made of nerve cells and some other cells which support and help the nerve cells. The nerve cells have a body, and some have very long extensions (like tails) called axons (see Figure 25.2). These axons conduct (or carry) messages from one part of the nervous system to other parts of the nervous system, or to other systems (in a way similar to the wires which carry electrical messages in a telephone system).

cerebellum

cervical nerves

thoracic nerves

spinal cord

lumbar nerves

cauda equina

sacral nerves

siatic nerve

cerebrum

brachial plexus

radial nerve

median nerve

ulnar nerve

lumbosacral plexus

femoral nerve

Figure 25.1 Two parts of the nervous system. 1. The central nervous system, i.e. brain (cerebrum and cerebellum etc.) and the spinal cord. 2. The peripheral nervous system i.e. the peripheral and cutaneous nerves.

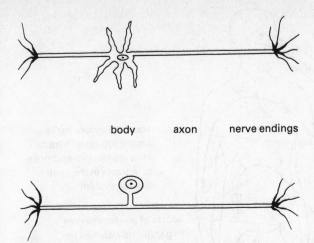

body   axon   nerve endings

Figure 25.2 The microscopic structure of two types of nerve cell.

The nerve cells in the nervous system which have the same function are grouped together in one or more areas.

In the brain the bodies of the nerve cells which deal with speech or movement or sensation etc. are grouped together in special areas on the surface (or cortex) of the brain, and these areas are called the speech area, motor (movement) area, sensory area, etc. (see Figure 25.3).

In the *spinal cord* the bodies of nerve cells which deal with movement are in the front of the cord, and those which deal with sensation are in special extensions of the spinal cord, called 'dorsal root ganglia', attached to the back of the cord (see Figures 25.4, 25.5 and 25.10).

The *axons* of nerve cells which run from one part of the nervous system to another are also grouped together (like the wires of a telephone system, which run in a cable). These groups of axons are called '*tracts*' if they are in the central nervous system. They are called '*nerves*' if they are in the peripheral nervous system (see Figures 25.4, 25.5 and 25.6).

The central nervous system

The central nervous system consists of the brain and spinal cord.

The central nervous system is like a telephone exchange. Messages about sensation travel from many parts of the body through nerves (called 'sensory nerves') to the central nervous system. These messages are then sent to other parts of the central nervous system and/or to the nerves which go from the central nervous system to other parts of the body. The nerves which go from the central

Figure 25.3 The anatomy of the cortex or the outer layer of the brain. Note the positions of the groups of bodies of nerve cells which have the same special function (e.g. hearing).

251

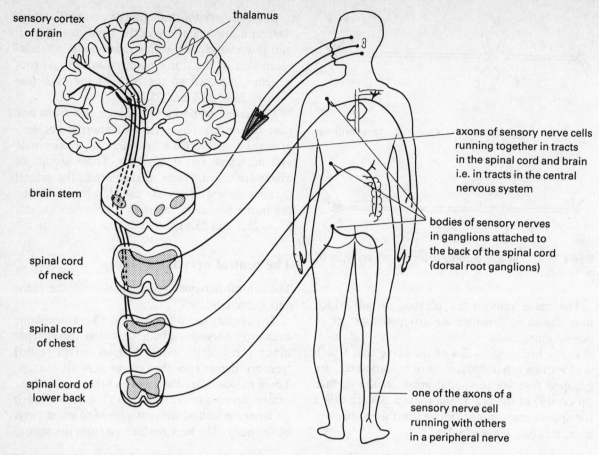

Figure 25.4 This diagram shows how one of the sensations of the body (pain) is taken from the skin to the cerebral cortex of the brain where the person can feel it. Pain nerve cell axons are all grouped together in one tract after they enter the central nervous system. Other sensations have other tracts. Note that tracts also go to the cerebellum (not shown).

Figure 25.5 Diagram showing the spinal cord and a reflex arc. Pain sensation from sensory nerve endings in the skin goes along the axon of the sensory nerve and into a connecting nerve cell. The message then goes into the motor nerve cell. The motor nerve cell then sends a message to the muscle to move that part of the body away from what is causing the pain. The sensation of pain is also sent up to the cerebral cortex of the brain (see Figure 25.4) and the cerebellum.

parts of the motor area
of the cerebral cortex

the cerebral
cortex of brain

leg

arm

face

upper motor neurone
nerve cell axons in
the pyramidal tracts
to the brain stem and
spinal cord

crossing over
('decussation')
of pyramidal
tracts in brain
stem

a lower motor neurone
(nerve cell) with an axon
in the nerve to the
muscles of face

a lower motor neurone
(nerve cell) with an axon
in the nerve to the
muscles of arms

the spinal cord

a lower motor neurone
(nerve cell) with an axon
in the nerve to the
muscles of legs

Figure 25.6 Diagram to show the axons of the nerves in the motor area of the cerebral cortex which go in tracts to the brain stem and spinal cord. Note that the motor tracts cross to the other side of the body in the brain stem.

nervous system are called 'motor nerves' because they carry messages to make parts of the body move.

The sensory system
Sensory messages coming into the central nervous system can go to three different places.
1. Sensory messages can go up the spinal cord to the cerebral cortex of the brain. The person then knows what is happening and can decide to do something or not.
2. Sensory messages from joints and muscles, about the position of limbs, can go to the cerebellum. The cerebellum then sends messages back to the muscles to help the person stand or move properly (the way he has decided in the cerebral cortex).
3. Sensory messages coming into the spinal cord do not all go up the spinal cord (to the cerebral

cortex or cerebellum). Some go to other nerves in the spinal cord and may cause reflex action. For example, if a sensory message comes into the cord that says the hand is being burned by fire, the message immediately goes to the right nerve in the spinal cord to pull the hand away from the fire. This reflex action pulls the hand away without the person thinking.

Usually, when a sensory message comes into the central nervous system, it causes all these things as necessary:
• reflex action,
• control of movement by the cerebellum, and
• decision about action by the cerebral cortex.

The motor system
The cerebral cortex controls movement through motor nerve cells whose fibres go from the cortex through the brain to the spinal cord. In the spinal cord, they join other motor nerves which go to muscles. Motor messages travel in tracts and nerves to the muscles in the same way that sensory nerve cells take sensation to the brain from the body.

Note that *movement and sensation of one side of the body are controlled by the opposite side of the brain.* This is because the nerve axons cross over to the other side of the body where the cerebellum and spinal cord meet (at the brain stem) or in the spinal cord. See Figures 25.4 and 25.6.

Note also that the *control of the body in the brain is upside down* i.e. the sensation and movement of feet are at the top of the brain, and the face at the lower part. See Figures 25.7 and 25.8.

Note also that there are large areas of the brain connected to the parts of the body which have many sensations and many complicated movements (e.g. face and hands). See Figures 25.7 and 25.8.

Damage to the special motor or sensory parts of the cerebral cortex will cause loss of sensation or movement on *the opposite* side of the body. Damage to the spinal cord will cause loss of movement and loss of joint and touch sensations on *the same* side of the body, but pain sensation on *the opposite* side of the body, below the lesion. Damage to the brain stem (where the cross-over of nerve fibres occurs,) may cause a mixture of motor and sensory losses on different sides of the body and face.

253

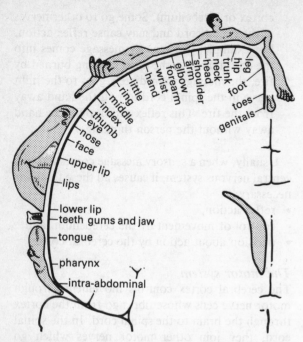

Figure 25.7 A diagram of a section cut through one half of the brain at the level of the sensory cortex (see Figure 25.3). This diagram shows which parts of the sensory cortex make the person aware of sensation in various parts of the body.

Figure 25.8 A diagram of a section cut through one half of the brain at the level of the motor cortex (see Figure 25.3). This diagram shows which parts of the motor cortex move the various parts of the body.

The meninges

The *meninges* surround the whole of the central nervous system. The meninges are three layers of membranes (see Figures 25.9 and 25.10). In the middle layer, there is a mesh-work of fibres in which circulates a fluid called the cerebro-spinal fluid (CSF). The meninges and CSF protect and give food to the central nervous system.

vertebrae with bodies in front and spinal canal enclosed by plates of bone behind - the spinal cord runs through the spinal canal

Figure 25.10 Diagram showing the three layers of the meninges surrounding the spinal cord in the vertebral canal. The structure of the meninges which surround the cord is the same as the structure of the meninges which surround the brain (see Figure 25.9).

CSF circulates through the mesh-work of the fibres of the arachnoid

bone of skull

brain or spinal cord

dura mater   arachnoid   pia mater

meninges

Figure 25.9 Diagram showing the structure of the meninges around the brain.

The peripheral nervous system

Nerves are the white cords which take messages between parts of the body and the central nervous system. They go to and from the spinal cord and brain through gaps between the vertebrae of the spine or holes in the skull. They consist of very many axons (thin fibres which are the tails of nerve cells which are in the spinal cord or in ganglia). (Ganglia are special groups of nerves cells attached to the spinal cord.)

Most nerves contain both sensory and motor fibres. Most nerves therefore both take sensation to the central nervous system and take motor messages back to parts of the body. The small nerves in the skin are called *cutaneous nerves* and contain only sensory nerve fibres.

Symptoms and signs of disease of the nervous system

Note that you will find only those symptoms and signs marked with an asterisk (*) in a routine history and examination. If you have a special reason to suspect nervous system disease, then check for the other symptoms and signs too.

Symptoms

Headache
Fits or convulsions
Change or loss of sight, hearing, smell or taste
Weakness or paralysis of arm/s and/or leg/s
Weakness of the bladder
- retention of urine
  (the patient cannot pass urine)
- incontinence of urine
  (the patient cannot stop the passing of urine)
Change or loss of sensation
Clumsiness
*Fever and general symptoms (if there is infection)

Signs

- *Change in level of consciousness.
- *Confusion. Poor memory. Disorientation. Not thinking properly, sometimes with mixed up thoughts, hallucinations or delusions (organic psychosis).
- *Meningeal irritation (Stiff neck. Stiff back.

Positive Kernig's sign. Bulging fontanelle but only in infants.)
- *Fitting.
- Change or loss of sight, hearing, smell or taste.
- Change or loss of speech.
- Stiffness or weakness or paralysis of eye/s and/or face, and/or arm/s, and/or leg/s.
- Paralysis of the bladder, with retention or incontinence of urine.
- Change or loss of sensation of the face, and/or arm/s, and/or trunk and/or leg/s.
- Shaking or clumsiness.
- Reflexes
  plantar – if abnormal, the big toe goes up if you stratch the outside of underneath the foot
  tendon – decreased or increased⎫
       – right side not equal to⎪
        left side   ⎬if abnormal
       – arm not equal to leg⎪
        on same side⎭
- *Fever, fast pulse, etc, if there is infection.

Pathology tests in diseases of the nervous system

You can get CSF for naked eye and laboratory examination by doing a lumbar puncture (LP). (For the proper method of doing a lumbar puncture and for the laboratory examination of CSF, see Appendix 1, at the end of this chapter.)

Naked eye examination of the CSF

Normal CSF should look clear like clean water.

If CSF does not look clear, assume that it contains pus, and treat for bacterial meningitis. In viral meningitis and encephalitis the CSF usually looks clear (because there are not enough mononuclear cells for you to see with the naked eye). The same is true for some early cases of tuberculous meningitis.

Sometimes a few red cells can make the CSF look cloudy and you may treat some patients for meningitis who do not have it. But this is better than not treating some patients with meningitis.

Sometimes the CSF is red and obviously has red blood cells in it. Find out if this is caused by a 'traumatic tap' or if there is blood in all the CSF (see page 277).

Sometimes the CSF is clear but yellow. This is called 'xanthochromia'. Xanthochromia is caused by red blood cells that are destroyed and release their haemoglobin and other pigments into the CSF, i.e. there has been a haemorrhage into the CSF. Xanthochromia appears 4 hours after the haemorrhage. There are also other causes of yellow CSF including tuberculous meningitis, cerebral tumours, etc. So, unless the patient has clinical evidence of a haemorrhage, transfer him for tests to find the cause of the 'xanthochromia'.

If you leave the CSF for a day in a cool area, a clot (sometimes like a spider's web) may form. This is not normal. There are various causes for this, including tuberculous meningitis.

Common conditions affecting the nervous system

Acute bacterial ('purulent') meningitis

Acute bacterial meningitis is an acute bacterial infection of the meninges (the coverings) of the brain and spinal cord. This infection causes:
1. acute inflammation with pus in the meninges, and
2. damage to the brain, and
3. toxaemia or septicaemia.

It is a common disease and often causes death.

The cause is one of many bacteria. Meningococci and pneumococci are very common causes. These bacteria can spread to the brain:—
1. from the upper respiratory tract in the blood, or
2. directly from an ear infection or through a compound fracture of the skull.

Symptoms and signs

Symptoms may include:
Headache
Fever
Photophobia (pain in the eyes and head, if the eyes are open in the light)
Pains in the back, neck and other parts of the body.
Nausea and vomiting.
(In children there may be few symptoms.)

Signs (see Figure 25.11) include any of these:
1. Signs of damage to the brain.
   Any loss of full consciousness, e.g. sleepiness, drowsiness, unconscious, etc.
   Any irritation of the brain, e.g. restlessness, irritability, confusion, delirium, psychotic behaviour, muscle twitching, fitting, etc.
2. Signs of inflammation of the meninges.
   Full or bulging fontanelle (infants only)

Figure 25.11 This patient has meningitis. Not only does he have a stiff neck but he also lies with his neck bent backwards (sometimes called 'neck retraction'). This is a sign of severe meningeal irritation.

Stiff neck
Stiff back
Positive Kernig's signs
(In children these signs may not be present.)
3. General signs of infection are usually present, e.g. fever, fast pulse, fast respiration, dehydration.
Signs of septicaemia may be present, e.g. haemorrhagic rash, shock, etc.

Tests
You must do a lumbar puncture on *every* person who has symptoms or signs which could be caused by meningitis.

Do a lumbar puncture for anyone who:
1. is not fully conscious or is unconscious, or
2. has fitted (and is not known to be epileptic), or
3. who is not mentally normal (and is not known to suffer from a mental disease), or
4. who has signs of meningeal irritation (neck stiffness, back stiffness, etc.), or
5. who has a severe illness with a fever which you cannot diagnose.

If the CSF is cloudy or like pus, treat as bacterial meningitis.

If the CSF is blood-stained, treat as bacterial meningitis.

If you do not get any CSF (lumbar puncture failed), treat as bacterial meningitis.

If the CSF is clear but the patient has the clinical signs of meningitis, he must have:
cerebral malaria, or
viral meningitis, or
encephalitis, or
tuberculosis meningitis, or ⎫ Sometimes the
very early bacterial meningitis ⎬ CSF may look
(before much pus has formed). ⎭ clear.

If it is possible keep the CSF cool and send it to the hospital laboratory for examination for cells, bacteria, protein, sugar and culture with sensitivity testing (see Table 25.1 page 278).

If you strongly suspect acute bacterial meningitis in a very sick patient, give an extra dose of chloramphenicol or penicillin by IMI immediately (while you are doing the lumbar puncture and starting the IV drip).

Management
Treat for meningitis if:

CSF is not clear (cloudy)
CSF is bloody
You cannot get CSF (LP failed)

Treat all cases of meningitis also for cerebral malaria with quinine (or chloroquine) (see Chapter 13 page 56) unless you are sure that the patient does not have malaria.

If the CSF is clear, treat only for cerebral malaria with quinine. But, if there is no improvement after 24 hours, repeat the lumbar puncture.

> Treatment includes 5 things
> 1. An antibiotic, preferably chloramphenicol, in a large dose, for at least 2 weeks (see below)
> 2. IV fluids; but only if necessary (see below)
> 3. Anti-convulsants if necessary (see below)
> 4. Antimalarial drugs, usually quinine (see below)
> 5. Care of unconscious patient if necessary (see below)

1. ANTIBIOTICS
Give chloramphenicol *or* penicillin

Chloramphenicol – (25 mg/kg each 6 hours
For an adult of average weight give 2 g immediately then 1 g every 6 hours.
Give it by IVI *if*:
• there is shock (essential), or
• an IV drip is needed for another reason and is running.
Give by IMI to *all other cases* until they can take oral doses.
Give orally (4 caps) *only if* the patient:
• is not shocked, and
• is not very sick or after he improves (when oral drugs are reliable enough), and
• can swallow, and
• has no vomiting or severe diarrhoea.

Benzyl (crystalline) penicillin
You can give penicillin *instead of* chloramphenicol. It is usually effective in adults. However chloramphenicol is better.
Give 2,000,000 units (4 ml) by IVI immediately.
Give 2,000,000 units (4 ml) by IVI every 3 hours after the first dose.

Give by IMI if a drip is not running. However IVI is essential if the patient is in shock.

If you cannot give injections every 3 hours then give 4,000,000 units (8 ml) *slowly* (at 1 ml/minute) by IVI or by IMI every 6 hours instead.

Continue the antibiotic for at least 2 weeks or for 1 week after the fever stops – whichever is longer.

Do *not* reduce the dose of chloramphenicol unless the patient appears to be cured very quickly (see Chapter 12).

You can reduce the dose of penicillin to 2,000,000 units (4 ml) every 6 hours when the patient appears to be cured.

2. *IV FLUIDS* if necessary
Do not give more IV fluids than necessary. Too much IV fluid can cause cerebral oedema with convulsions and death.
If shock is present, see Chapter 27 page 305.
If dehydration is present, see Chapter 23 page 224.
If only maintenance is needed, or if there is a drip to allow repeated IV instead of IM injections, give 0.18% sodium chloride in 4.3% dextrose solution – 1 litre each 8–12 hours.

3. *ANTICONVULSANT DRUG* if necessary for fitting or restlessness
Give paraldehyde 0.2 ml/kg (1/5 ml/kg) (5–10 ml) IMI immediately. Repeat after 10 minutes if necessary; if further fits occur, repeat every 6–12 hours until the patient improves (usually 2–3 days).
Give diazepam by slow IVI if paraldehyde (every 6 hours) is not effective. But also continue the regular paraldehyde.
See Convulsions (page 266).
Do not use phenobarbitone if you are giving the patient chloramphenicol (because it may reduce the concentration of chloramphenicol in the body).

4. *ANTIMALARIAL DRUG* as for cerebral malaria
Give IMI quinine 10 mg/kg. If you cannot weigh the patient, give 10 ml for a large adult (>50 kg) or 7.5 ml (7½ ml) for a small adult (<50 kg). (See Malaria Chapter 13 page 56.)

5. *ROUTINE CARE OF UNCONSCIOUS PATIENT* if necessary
See page 264.

Transfer
Transfer the patient to Medical Officer care if:
1. He is still inconscious after 24 hours of full treatment (urgent).
2. He is not improving after 2 days of full treatment (urgent).
3. He still has a fever after 1 week of full treatment (urgent – but not an emergency).
4. He is not cured after 2 weeks of full treatment (urgent – but not emergency).
5. Any complications develop which you cannot manage the health centre (urgent).

Prevention
This is not usually possible.

Give prophylactic antibiotics (e.g. procaine penicillin or tetracycline for 5 days to people in closed communities (e.g. boarding schools) if one member develops bacterial meningitis.

Also give prophylactic antibiotics to staff who have close personal contract with an untreated patient (e.g. who do mouth to mouth ventilation).

There are effective vaccines; but these are not usually available when needed.

Cerebral malaria
Cerebral malaria is the acute damage of the brain (encephalitis) and meninges caused by falciparum malaria parasites and their toxins in the blood vessels of the brain.

Cerebral malaria is clinically similar to acute bacterial meningitis (see page 256) but there are some differences.

The history is similar *but* the history may also suggest malaria, e.g.
- the patient is a non-immune person recently in a malarial area,
- he has had recent attacks of fever.
  The signs of brain damage are similar, i.e.
- loss of full consciousness,
  e.g. the patient may be sleepy, drowsy, unconscious, etc.
- irritation of the brain,
  e.g. the patient may be restless, irritable, confused, delirious, psychotic, twitching, fitting, etc.

The signs of inflammation of the meninges are similar e.g. stiff neck, stiff back, etc.

The general signs of infection are similar, e.g. fast pulse, fast respiration, dehydration, etc. *but* there are no signs of septicaemia.

There may be other signs of acute or chronic malaria, e.g. anaemia and/or jaundice, enlarged tender spleen, or enlarged liver.

But you cannot tell the difference between acute bacterial meningitis and cerebral malaria without a lumbar puncture.

> Always do a lumbar puncture if you suspect cerebral malaria OR meningitis.

In cerebral malaria the CSF will be normal and look clear. The CSF will also look clear in:
- viral meningitis,
- encephalitis,
- tuberculous meningitis (sometimes), and
- very early acute bacterial meningitis (rarely).

Treatment

Treatment includes five things:
1. Antimalarial drugs by injection (See Malaria, Chapter 13 page 57)
   Give quinine 10 mg/kg by *slow* IV drip or by IMI
   - immediately, *and*
   - 6–8 hours later, *and*
   - 24 hours after first dose, *and*
   - then repeat every 12 hours until the patient can take oral antimalarial drugs.

   Quinine should be given by slow IV drip. But, if you are not successful in having the drip running in 15 minutes or you are not certain that the staff can care for the drip, give IMI quinine instead of IVI quinine.
   Give chloroquine by IMI if you cannot get quinine.
   Quinine takes effect faster than chloroquine, and quinine is essential if there is any chance of the patient having chloroquine resistant malaria.
   See Chapter 13 page 56 for details of giving these drugs.

2. Anticonvulsants if there is fitting.
   Give paraldehyde 0.2 ml/kg (1/5 ml/kg) (10 ml usually) by IMI immediately. Repeat in ten minutes if necessary. If further fits occur repeat every 6–12 hours until the patient improves (usually 1–2 days).
   Give diazepam by IVI slowly for fitting that is not controlled by paraldehyde.
   See Convulsions page 266 for details of giving these drugs.

3. If the patient is unconscious, give routine care for unconsciousness.
   See page 264 for details. Patients may be unconscious for some days and still make a complete recovery.

4. Reduce temperature if 40°C or above.
   See Chapter 13 page 57 for details.

5. IV fluids if necessary.
   Do not give more fluid than necessary. Too much fluid can cause cerebral oedema and death. See meningitis page 258.

Transfer patients to medical officer care:
1. if they are unconscious of more than 1 day;
2. if they are not greatly improved after 2 days; or
3. if they are not cured in 2 weeks.

Tuberculous meningitis

See also Chapter 14 page 68.

Tuberculous meningitis is a sub-acute or chronic infection of the meninges with tuberculosis organisms.

Tuberculous meningitis is clinically similar to acute bacterial meningitis (see page 256).

Symptoms and signs include:
- headache, and other symptoms and signs of brain damage;
- signs of meningeal irritation, with stiff neck, stiff back etc;
- general symptoms and signs of infection;
- abnormal CSF (but sometimes you cannot see this without a microscope).

But there are differences to acute bacterial meningitis:
- The history is often longer (days or weeks, not hours or days).
- The patient is often not as 'sick' at first.
- Evidence of tuberculous infection is sometimes present in other parts of the body.

- The CSF may only be yellow; or, when left standing for some hours, form a spider's web type clot; or be almost clear.
- Proper antibacterial meningitis treatment causes no improvement in 2 days, no loss of fever in 1 week and no cure in 2 weeks.

The tuberculin test is usually negative.

Suspect tuberculous meningitis if any of these things occur and transfer all suspected cases urgently to a medical officer for diagnosis and treatment with special drugs.

In areas where African trypanosomiasis (sleeping sickness) occurs, this may cause similar signs and symptoms. This patient needs urgent transfer to a medical officer for diagnosis and treatment.

Virus meningitis

Virus meningitis is an inflammation of the meninges caused by infection with one of many viruses.

It is clinically similar to acute bacterial or tuberculous meningitis (see above) *but*
1. The CSF looks clear.
2. Most cases get better with no treatment. Antibiotics do not help.

You will diagnose most cases in a health centre (where laboratory tests are not available) incorrectly as cerebral malaria. This does not matter as the management is as for cerebral malaria.

Treat as for cerebral malaria (see page 57).

Transfer to medical officer care if the patient is unconscious for more than one day, *or* not improving after 2 days, *or* not cured after 2 weeks.

Encephalitis

Encephalitis is inflammation of the brain itself, usually caused by one of many viruses. Often the meninges are also inflamed (i.e. it is a meningo-encephalitis).

It is similar to acute bacterial or tuberculous meningitis (see pages 256 and 259), *but*:
1. The CSF looks clear.
2. Many cases get better with no treatment. Some cases may have permanent brain damage. A few cases (and any case due to rabies) die. Antibiotics do not help.

You will diagnose most cases incorrectly as cerebral malaria; but this does not matter because management is as for cerebral malaria (see page 259). If you could be certain that the patient did not have malaria, you would not give the antimalarial drugs.

However, always think of rabies (see below) if you are in an area where rabies occurs.

A chronic meningo-encephalitis may also be caused by African trypanosomiasis (see below).

Transfer to medical officer care if the patient is: unconscious for more than one day, *or* not improving after 2 days, *or* not cured after 2 weeks.

African trypanosomiasis (Sleeping Sickness)

See Chapter 18 page 118 for details.

The patient is in (or from) an area where African trypanosomiasis occurs.

Early signs may be:
1. fast pulse, and perhaps heart failure,
2. anaemia,
3. enlarged lymph glands,
4. enlarged spleen, and
5. proteinurea.

Chronic meningo-encephalitis follows and causes:
1. headache;
2. tiredness, sleepiness and no interest in anything (the patient may not even eat);
3. sleeping in the day, but sometimes not at night;
4. changes in personality, confusion, and development of organic psychosis (see Chapter 35 page 384);
5. shaking, weakness, pains, difficulty in walking;
6. coma and death.

Transfer all such cases for diagnosis and treatment by a medical officer.

Rabies

Rabies is an acute viral disease of the brain (encephalitis) and the salivary glands of animals, which sometimes affects man.

It is spread from one animal to another animal by infected secretions (usually saliva). The means of spread is usually a bite by an infected animal. All animals can be infected with rabies.

Rabies occurs in most countries. Find out if it occurs in your area.

Symptoms and signs of rabies in man include:
1. There is a history of an animal bite, usually from a dog which was behaving abnormally.
2. The disease has a long incubation period (1 week to 1 year), before the first signs appear.
3. The patient becomes 'sick' for a few days with fever, headache, etc.
4. The patient then has a period of encephalitis. Some patients become very anxious. Sudden noises and lights, etc. cause strange behaviour. There are episodes of wild behaviour and muscle spasms and fear. The patient cannot swallow. The sight of water causes spasms of the throat. This also causes 'foaming at the mouth'. Other patients become very depressed and quiet, and become paralysed. But, they also get spasms of the throat and cannot swallow.
5. The patient dies, usually within 10 days (but it can be shorter or longer).
6. Cases which are not typical may be common. Suspect rabies in any unusual disease of the nervous system in an area where rabies occurs.

Signs of rabies in the dog or other animals are similar to those in man.

Confirmation of the diagnosis is by special tests.

If you strongly suspect rabies in a patient or an animal, notify the nearest medical and veterinary officer urgently.

No treatment can cure rabies once it has developed.

Prevention of rabies includes:
1. Kill the organism in the body of the original hosts (reservoir).
   In areas where rabies occurs:
   (a) all dogs without owners should be killed, and
   (b) all dogs with owners should be immunised against rabies.
2. Stop the means of spread.
   Control dogs.

3. Raise the resistance of persons who are bitten. Treat local wounds.
   Give passive immunisation with anti-rabies serum.
   Give active immunisation.

If a person is bitten by an animal, manage as follows:
1. *Give proper treatment for the bite*
   Wash the wound with a lot of soap and water.
   Rinse with a lot of water.
   Then apply iodine in spirit.
   Then do the necessary surgical toilet.
   Do not stitch the wound.
   Dress the wound and apply a compression bandage to stop bleeding.
   Give tetanus prophylaxis (see page 263).
2. *Try to find out if the animal has rabies and transfer the patient for immunisation if necessary.*
   (a) If the animal looks healthy, lock it up for ten days. It is still alive and well after 10 days, the animal did not have rabies and no immunisation of the patient is necessary. If the animal shows any sign of sickness before the 10 days is finished, transfer the patient immediately for immunisation.
   (b) If the animal has disappeared, transfer the patient for immunisation.
   (c) If the animal has been caught and looks sick, lock up the animal carefully (make sure that it does not bite anyone) and inform the local veterinary officer. Transfer the patient for immunisation.
   (d) If the animal has been killed leave the body for the veterinary officer. If the veterinary officer cannot come and you do not have special ways of removing animal brains, bury the animal carefully. Immediately transfer the patient for immunisation.

Poliomyelitis

Polymyelitis is an acute inflammation of parts of the brain and spinal cord caused by one of the polio viruses. It can cause the sudden paralysis of groups of muscles in 1–2 days. Other groups may then be paralysed in the next week or so. Often a number of limbs are partly paralysed. This is different from a stroke or injury where usually the whole of one limb or the whole of one side of the body is paralysed.

Poliomyelitis also causes:

1. severe pain and aching of the affected muscles,
2. no loss of sensation,
3. clinical virus meningitis before the paralytic disease (and most cases of polio meningitis do not go on to cause any paralysis),
4. A non-specific viral gastro-enteritis or febrile illness before polio meningitis (and most cases of this polio infection do not even go on to cause polio meningitis).

If you have a patient who could have poliomyelitis contact the Medical Officer urgently about care and transfer of the patient and the need for vaccine for contacts.

You can prevent an epidemic by using Sabin vaccine. You can prevent individual cases by giving 3 doses of Sabin vaccine.

Polio can cripple people so that they cannot care for themselves (see Figure 25.12). Many people who have suffered from polio become beggars. You can make cheap surgical aids to help these people care for themselves again. (See Huckstep, R.L, 'Orthopaedic appliances for developing countries' *Tropical Doctor* 1971; **1**: 64–7.)

Cerebro-vascular disease (stroke)

A stroke is a sudden paralysis or loss of one of the other functions of the body controlled by the brain. This is caused by disease of the blood vessels which bring blood to the brain.

When people get old, their blood vessels get narrower; and the blood in them may clot. If a person has high blood pressure, it can damage the blood vessels; one of these damaged blood vessels may burst or the blood in one of them clot. Some people are born with weakness in part of a blood vessel (called an aneurysm); the weak blood vessel can burst. Diseases, especially meningitis and syphilis, can damage blood vessels; and then the blood in these blood vessels can clot. A clot of blood from a diseased heart can break off and suddenly block a normal blood vessel. All of these blood vessel conditions can stop the flow of the blood to a part of the brain which then does not work and then dies, i.e. they can cause strokes.

The symptoms and signs depend on which

Figure 25.12 A boy who had polio affecting both legs and could not walk – he could only crawl. Calipers were made for him in a health centre at a cost of about US$1. He can now walk without help.

blood vessel disease is the cause and what part of the brain is affected.

If a haemorrhage occurs the stroke usually starts suddenly. If the blood goes into the subarachnoid space, it will cause symptoms and signs of meningeal irritation like meningitis (see page 256) i.e. severe headache, stiff neck, etc. A lumbar puncture will show blood in the CSF which does not decrease in each bottle of CSF.

If a blood vessel clots then the stroke will start slowly over a few hours; and there will be no signs of meningeal irritation.

If the part of the brain which controls movement is affected, then the patient will have paralysis. The patient will have loss of sensation, blindness, loss of speech, etc, if other parts of the brain are involved.

Do a lumbar puncture to check that the patient does not have meningitis. If the patient is young, do a VDRL test (see Chapter 19 page 129) to check that the patient does not have syphilis.

The patient often dies in the first two days. If the patient lives for the first 2 days, he will often greatly improve for 6 months or more (sometimes even 24 months).

Treatment includes:
1. Nursing care as necessary. If the patient is unconscious, see page 264.
2. Physiotherapy. All limb joints must be moved 10–20 times each, twice daily. If the patient cannot do this, the nurse or orderly must do it.
3. Early mobilisation. The patient must get out of bed as soon as possible after the first 2 days. Help the patient to walk as well as he can. The patient must not stay in bed all the time. If he does, many complications will develop, and he will not get better.
4. If the patient improves, but his blood pressure stays high (more than 160–200/100–110), then refer the case to a medical officer for treatment of the high blood pressure.

Tetanus

Tetanus is an acute disease of the nervous system caused by tetanus toxin. Tetanus toxin is made if tetanus bacteria grow in the body.

Tetanus bacteria normally live in the intestines of animals and in dirt. They can get into a person's body when dirt gets into the body e.g. through wounds or burns, the female genital tract at delivery, and the cut end of a baby's umbilical cord at birth. Usually the tetanus bacteria grow and make the toxin in special types of wounds: puncture wounds, wounds or burns which get dirt in them and wounds infected by other bacteria.

The first *symptoms* are usually pain and stiffness of the jaw, difficulty in opening the mouth wide and difficulty in swallowing. The pain and stiffness then spread to the whole body. Several days later, spasms of the whole body usually occur. The spasms last from a few to several sec-

Figure 25.13 Tetanus. Note the muscles of the body are all in spasm, the head is bent backwards and the lips are pulled back (as in a smile). The patient is in great pain.

onds. Movement of the patient's body or a sudden noise can sometimes start the spasms. During the spasms the patient is conscious and in great pain (this is different from 'fits').

There are *no tests* to make the diagnosis. If you have real doubt about meningitis or cerebral malaria, do a lumbar puncture and a blood slide, and start treatment as on page 257. Spasms can sometimes be caused by drugs such as chlorpromazine. If you suspect this, see Chapter 35 page 392. You can only diagnose tetanus from the history of the wound, the symptoms of jaw stiffness and the signs – the mouth will not open wide, general body stiffness and later spasms.

Treatment at a health centre is not usually possible. If you make as the diagnosis, immediately arrange urgent transfer of the patient to hospital. Management before transfer includes:

1. Give IMI chlorpromazine 100 mg (4 ml) immediately.
2. Give IMI phenobarbitone 100–200 mg (½–1 ml) *or* IMI paraldehyde 10 ml immediately.
3. Set up an intravenous drip.
4. Also give IVI diazepam 10 mg (2 ml) slowly when necessary to control the spasms.
5. Give IMI tetanus immunoglobulin 1,000 units (4 of the 250 unit vials used for prevention of tetanus) immediately.
6. Give benzyl penicillin 2,000,000 units (4 ml) immediately.
7. Nurse the patient on his side with the head lower than the feet. Gently suck out the patient's airway if it is blocked, or he is breathing noisily. Do not disturb the patient if possible.
8. Give nothing to eat or drink by mouth.
9. Clean and dress any wound.
10. A good health worker must go with the patient to the hospital. This person will care for the patient's airway, suck out the airway if necessary and give further drugs for spasms if necessary.

Prevention includes:

1. Immunise everyone with triple antigen or tetanus toxoid three times. See Chapter 10 page 37.
2. Treat wounds and burns properly. Clean them all well, and remove all dead tissue from wounds.
3. If the wound is:
   (a) a deep wound, a puncture wound or a compound fracture:
   (b) a wound which has a lot of dead tissue in it;
   (c) a wound which has foreign bodies especially wood, dirt or manure (animal faeces) in it;
   (d) many hours old before you treat it, or is already clinically, infected:
   then (a) give antibiotics, (b) give tetanus immunoglobulin if not immunised against tetanus (c) start tetanus immunisation with tetanus toxoid if not immunised.

Diagnosis and management of common symptoms and signs

Unconsciousness (coma)

Causes of unconsciousness include:

1. Disease of the brain and meninges.
   (a) head injury,
   (b) meningitis – bacterial, viral, tuberculous,
   (c) cerebral malaria,
   (d) encephalitis,
   (e) African trypanosomiasis (sleeping sickness),
   (f) cerebro-vascular disease,
   (g) tuberculoma, abscess, tumour,
   (h) malnutrition with beriberi, and
   (i) others – see a medical reference book.
2. Abnormality of the blood going to brain.
   (a) alcohol, drugs, poisons,
   (b) toxins from infections, especially septicaemia and pneumonia and typhoid,
   (c) toxins, etc. from the body – chronic kidney failure, chronic liver disease,
   (d) low oxygen from anaemia, shock, heart failure, lung diseases,
   (e) high sugar from diabetes; low sugar from too much insulin,
   (f) eclampsia, and
   (g) small volume of blood circulation because of severe dehydration, especially cholera.
3. Non-organic mental illness.
   acting out.

Management of the unconscious patient

Management includes 4 things:

1. Give routine nursing care to the unconscious patient.
2. Record the level of consciousness hourly.
3. Diagnose and treat the cause.
   Take a full history from the patient's relatives or friends.
   Do a full physical examination.
   Make a malaria smear and give quinine.
   Do a LP. Treat for meningitis if necessary.
   Test the urine.
4. Transfer to medical officer care if the level of consciousness gets worse, if complications develop or if the patient is still unconscious after 24 hours.

Figure 25.14 Diagram showing the position in which you should nurse an unconscious patient (the recovery position).

1. *Routine nursing care of the unconscious patient*

Maintain the airway (check that the patient can breathe):

- lay patient on his side (never on his back) (see Figure 25.14),
- bend his head back,
- pull his jaw forward,
- suck out his pharynx every hour or when there is noisy or blocked breathing (noisy breathing or snorting means blocked breathing),
- raise the foot of the bed to let secretions run out of his mouth,
- insert 'airway' if necessary, and
- give artificial ventilation if the patient stops breathing because of something you can treat. (e.g. snake-bite, poisoning by drugs, etc.)

Care of pressure areas – turn every two hours. Give intravenous fluids if necessary. If you give intragastric fluids nurse the patient with his head down and on the side, and maintain his airway carefully.

Use an indwelling catheter if the bladder becomes distended and cannot be emptied by gentle pressure every 2–4 hours (bladder distention is one of the common causes of restlessness in an unconscious patient).

2. *Record the level of consciousness*

You should also record the size of the pupils of the eyes. Repeat these observations every hour to see if the patient is improving or getting worse. Observations will show it the patient:

- is fully conscious, or
- answers only simple questions, or
- obeys only simple commands, or
- responds only if hurt
- does not respond if hurt, or
- is dead.

3. *Diagnose and treat the cause*

Always take a full *medical history* from the patient's relatives or friends (see Chapter 6). Ask about the possibility of drug overdose or poisons (including alcohol) or if he has had recent treatment for an illness (including insulin) or a head injury.

Always do a full, careful *physical examination* of the patient. (See Chapter 6.)

- Smell the breath for alcohol, diabetes and kidney failure.
- Look carefully for a head injury.
- Check the BP (especially if pregnant (eclampsia)).
- Check for shock, especially from bleeding or severe dehydration (cholera), and treat if pres-

ent (See Chapter 27 page 305).
- Check for severe infection (e.g. septi-caemia), and treat if present (See Chapter 12).
- Check for chronic conditions (e.g. cirrhosis, kidney failure African trypanosomiasis).

Always do a malaria smear and *give antima-larials* for cerebral malaria (see page 258). Unless you are certain that the patient does not have ma-laria give quinine 10 mg/kg by IMI immediately or by SLOW IV drip (if you cannot weigh the patient, give 10 ml for large adult and 7.5 ml (7½ ml) for small adult).

Always do a *lumbar puncture*. Treat for menin-gitis if:
- the CSF is cloudy, or
- the CSF is blood stained, or
- the CSF is not obtained (failed LP).

Always *test urine* for sugar, protein and bile (diabetes, eclampsia and chronic kidney failure).

Try to find out if patient has a psychiatric con-dition ('acting out') (see Chapter 35 page 390). But do not diagnose this until the patient is fully conscious again.

4. *Transfer*

Transfer to Medical Officer care:
(a) if the level of consciousness gets worse every hour for 4 hours (urgent-emergency) (especially important if the cause can be treated); or
(b) if the size of one pupil does not stay the same as the size of the other pupil (urgent); or
(c) if another complication develops which you cannot treat at the health centre (e.g. the patient is not breathing enough) (urgent); or
(d) if the patient is still unconscious after 24 hours and not obviously improving (urgent).

Do not transfer if the cause cannot be treated.

Simple faint (syncope)

In a faint (or attack of syncope), the patient feels light headed, not able to see properly and muscle weakness, he cannot stand, and he loses full consciousness.

If you lay the patient down, he will recover quickly – 1–3 minutes.

Check that the patient does not have another condition, especially a fit.

Look for and treat the cause:
1. diseases of the brain,
2. abnormality of the blood going to the brain, or
3. mental disturbances.
See Unconsciousness page 264 for list of causes.

Most cases are caused by:
1. standing still for a long time (blood stays in the legs and not enough goes back to the heart to go to the brain);
2. anaemia (not enough oxygen in blood going to the brain); and
3. fear, worry, disgust and pain.

Dizziness (vertigo)

This is a feeling of movement (e.g. things going around) often with faintness and nausea or vomit-ing.

Causes include:
1. diseases of brain (see Unconsciousness page 264 for list);
2. abnormalities of blood going to brain (see Unconsciousness page 264 for list);
3. some eye conditions; and
4. some ear conditions.

Convulsions (fits) and epilepsy

Convulsion (fit)

In a convulsion or a fit, the patient suddenly loses consciousness, and falls. All the muscles of his body suddenly contract and stay contracted. The face and the limbs become stiff. The patient can-not breathe and so goes blue. He may pass urine and faeces. Usually after about 30 seconds, the muscles relax. Then the muscles start to contract and then relax again and again quickly. This makes the patient's limbs jerk, and his mouth and eyes open and close. Often the patient bites his tongue. Breathing starts again but it may be very noisy. This period can last a very short or very long time; but it usually stops without treatment. Then the patient usually sleeps deeply for about half an hour. When the patient wakes, he cannot remember anything about the convulsion. Sometimes he is confused and has a headache. This is a general convulsion (grand mal).

These symptoms and signs are caused by the patient losing control of all of his brain. Without control the brain makes the body act abnormally.

You can easily see the loss of control and the abnormal working of the area of the brain which makes the muscles move. All the other parts of the brain are also without control and also working abnormally during a general convulsion (or fit).

Some convulsions (fits) are different from these general convulsions. The patient may have a feeling which tells him that the fit is about to start. If only one part of the area of the brain which controls muscles is affected, only one part of the body may jerk (e.g. the face or one limb or one side of the body), and the patient may stay conscious. If only one part of the area of the brain which controls sensations is affected, the patient may only have abnormal sensations in one part of his body. If only another part of the brain is affected, the patient may have only abnormal (often violent) behaviour.

But any of these other types of fit may develop into a general convulsion if the abnormal working of part of the brain spreads to all of the brain, including all the areas which control the muscles.

Sometimes convulsions do not stop but continue for hours or longer. This is a very dangerous condition that often results in death. This is called 'status epilepticus'.

The causes of convulsions or fits are the same as the causes for unconsciousness. See page 264.

A convulsion (or a fit) is not a disease and is never the only diagnosis. A convulsion is caused by something which upsets the normal working of the brain. The cause of the convulsion must always be diagnosed too.

Epilepsy

Epilepsy is diagnosed if there are *repeated convulsions* over weeks, months or years. The *causes of epilepsy* are the same as the cause of a single fit. See page 266. Often it is not possible to find the cause of epilepsy. But this does not mean that there is no cause.

Epilepsy is not a disease and is never the only diagnosis. Epilepsy is caused by something which affects the normal working of the brain. You must diagnose the cause of the epilepsy if possible. Epilepsy is not infectious.

Management of a patient with convulsions (fits) or epilepsy

Management includes 6 things:
1. When the patient is fitting, check that he does not hurt himself.
2. When the patient is unconscious, give the necessary nursing care.
3. Stop the fit with anticonvulsant drugs: give IMI paraldehyde; if not successful give IVI diazepam.
4. Find and treat the cause.
   Take a full history from the patient's relatives or friends.
   Do a full clinical examination.
   Make a malaria smear and give quinine.
   Do an LP. Treat for meningitis if necessary.
   Test the urine.
5. Give phenobarbitone when the patient can swallow, until you cure the cause of the fits (if possible).
6. Transfer if you cannot stop the fits or if you cannot find or treat the cause of the fits in the health centre.

---

1. *When the patient is fitting*
   Check that he does not hurt himself, e.g. fall off a bed, fall into a fire, etc. Do not try to stop the movements as this is not possible and you may injure the patient. When the mouth is opening and closing, put something between the teeth so that the patient does not bite his tongue.

2. *If the patient is unconscious*
   Give nursing care (see page 264). Check that the airway is clear (i.e. the patient can breathe) – keep on his side, keep his neck bent back, keep his jaw forward, clear his airway and suck out his throat if necessary.

3. *Give anticonvulsant drugs*
   Paraldehyde 0.2 ml/kg (1/5 ml/kg) or 10 ml for the average adult, immediately, by IMI. Repeat in 5 minutes if the patient is still fitting. After this give it once every 4–6 hours if necessary.

   If paraldehyde does not stop the fitting, give diazepam when necessary; but continue paraldehyde regularly every 6 hours.

Diazepam 0.1 ml/kg (1/10 ml/kg) by slow IVI. The usual dose needed is only 2–4 ml or 10–20 mg. The maximum dose for a large adult is 6 ml. Give slowly by IV at 1 ml/minute.

Stop the injection when the fitting stops.

If this does not stop the fitting, you can repeat the dose after 20 minutes.

Give artificial ventilation if breathing stops (see Chapter 37 page 416).

You can give diazepam IMI; but this is slow acting.

4. *Find and treat the cause* (if the patient is not a known epileptic). (See page 267.)
Always take a full medical *history* from the patients relatives or friends (see Chapter 6). Ask about the possibility of drug overdose or poisons (including alcohol) or if he has had recent treatment for any illness (including insulin).

Always do a full careful *physical examination* (see Chapter 6)
• Smell the breath for alcohol.
• Look for head injury.
• Check the BP, if pregnant.
• Check for shock and treat if present.
• Check for severe infection (e.g. septicaemia) and treat if present.
• Check for chronic conditions (e.g. cirrhosis, kidney failure, African trypanosomiasis).
Always do a *lumbar puncture*.

Treat for meningitis if:
the CSF is cloudy, or
the CSF is blood stained, or
the CSF is not obtained (failed LP).

Always do a *malaria smear* and give *antimalarials* for cerebral malaria unless you are certain that the patient does not have malaria. (See page 258.) Give the patient quinine 10 mg/kg by IMI immediately or by SLOW IV drip. If it not possible to weigh the patient give 10 ml for large adult and 7.5 ml (7½ ml) for small adult.

Always test the urine for protein, sugar and bile.

Always check that the patient did have a fit and does not have another condition e.g. tetanus, rigor, rabies, or psychiatric condition ('acting out').

5. *Give phenobarbitone*
Give phenobarbitone 90 mg (3 of the 30 mg tabs) twice daily *or* 180 mg (6 of the 30 mg tabs) daily when the patient can swallow (and then stop paraldehyde) until the cause of the fits is found treated and cured (if possible). But do not give phenobarbitone if the patient is taking chloramphenicol; use paraldehyde instead. Other drugs such as phenytoin are very effective; but are more expensive and usually not available in health centres.

6. *Transfer*
Transfer to Medical Officer care:
(a) if you cannot stop the fitting by treatment in the health centre (urgent);
(b) if patient has his first fit or has only recently become epileptic and you cannot find the cause (non-urgent);
(c) if patient has another abnormal sign in the nervous system which has recently developed or is getting worse (non-urgent);
(d) if phenobarbitone alone will not control the fits (first check that the patient is taking the phenobarbitone) (non-urgent).

Paralysis

Paralysis is when the patient cannot make a muscle or group of muscles work.

The cause is not usually in the muscle although check that the patient does not have a *muscle* injury or infection (pyomyositis) or a *bone* injury (fracture) or infection (osteomyelitis) which makes it too painful to move the muscle. The cause is usually a disease of the *nerves* which normally make the muscle move. Common diseases which cause paralysis include:
in the limbs –
1. leprosy,
2. trauma, when a nerve is cut or pressed on,
3. nerve damage from drugs, especially INAH without pyridoxine;
in the spinal cord –
1. poliomyelitis,
2. fracture of the spine,
3. tuberculosis of the spine,
4. encephalitis or African trypanosomiasis;
in the brain –
1. cerebro-vascular disease (stroke),
2. trauma,

3. brain abscess or tuberculosis or tumour, etc;
mental disturbance –
1. acting out.

There are other causes in all of these places. See a specialist medical reference book if it is not one of the above.

Paraplegia and quadriplegia

Paraplegia is paralysis of both legs.

Quadriplegia is paralysis of both legs and both arms.

The usual causes are:
1. injury to spinal bones, or
2. tuberculosis of spinal bones
pressing on the spinal cord.

Transfer all cases for medical officer investigation and treatment.

If the paralysis started recently take great care not to make it worse. Do not bend or twist the patient's spine in any direction (especially the neck). Transfer the patient lying flat with sandbags or pillows packed around him so that he cannot bend or move the spine.

Headache

Headache is common. It occurs with many different kinds of illness.

Unless headache is the only symptom, use another symptom for diagnosis, e.g. headache and cough – find out and treat the cause of the cough, and the headache will probably go away.

If headache is the only symptom, think of all the structures in the head and neck. Take a history and do the examinations and tests to find if there is disease of one of them. Start with the structures on the inside of the head and neck, and work out towards the skin (see below).

If there is no evidence of disease, remember that anxiety is the most common cause of headache.

But do not miss the common curable causes – meningitis (especially the chronic meningitis of tuberculosis) and cerebral malaria.

Causes include diseases in the following structures:
Brain (*acute* diseases)
• cerebral malaria
• encephalitis
Do a lumbar puncture if necessary. Take a malaria slide and give quinine if necessary.

Brain (*chronic* diseases)
• African trypanosomiasis (sleeping sickness)
• tuberculoma (a 'lump' of tuberculosis)
• brain abscess
• brain tumour (cancer)
Ask about epilepsy and other nervous symptoms.
Look for weakness or change in reflexes or other nervous system signs.
Look for other symptoms and signs of these diseases.
Do not do a lumbar puncture.
Transfer to a Medical Officer.
Meninges
• meningitis – bacterial and tuberculous
• cerebral haemorrhage
Do lumbar puncture if necessary
See pages 256, 259, 262 and 271.
Skull
• trauma
History of trauma
Haematoma or tenderness under scalp.
Muscles
• tension from work, worry or habit
Feel for tenderness of muscles.
Move neck in all directions for stiffness and painful movements of muscles.
Ears
• infection
Examine ears with auriscope.
Nose
• sinusitis
Press over the sinuses for tenderness.
Look for pus in nose.
Mouth
• tooth decay and dental abscess
Tap each tooth gently for tenderness.
Eyes
• doing close work if long sighted
Test eyesight with small print.
• iritis or glaucoma
Pupil too large or small and irregular (see Chapter 31 pages 343 and 346)
Blood vessels
• hypertension
• pre-eclamptic toxaemia
Take BP.
Look for oedema.
Test urine for protein.
• migraine
History of changes in sight and/or nausea and vomiting with pain on one side of the head.

Blood coming to head
- other diseases especially those causing fever

Take temperature.

Do examination of the rest of the body.

Neck stiffness

There are four common causes of neck stiffness:

1. *Real 'neck stiffness'*, i.e. meningeal irritation.
   The patient cannot move his head forwards and the head is often held backwards (See Figure 25.11 page 256).

   If you try to bend the neck forward, this causes pain and the patient will stop you.

   Other signs of meningeal irritation may be present and are helpful if you are not certain if the neck is stiff or not (e.g. full fontanelle but only in infants, back stiffness, positive Kernig's sign).

   Very important causes include:
   - acute bacterial (purulent) meningitis,
   - cerebral malaria,
   - tuberculous meningitis, and
   - subarachnoid haemorrhage.

2. *'Meningism'* or *'Meningismus'*
   No organic disease of the meninges is present and the CSF is normal.

   This sometimes occurs with other infections, especially middle ear inflammation and pneumonia.

   You must always do a lumbar puncture and find clear CSF *before* you make this diagnosis.

3. *Tetanus*
   See page 263.

4. *Torticollis and diseases of the muscles and bones of the neck*.
   The patient cannot move his head from side to side.

   Causes include:
   - muscle spasm,
   - arthritis of the spine, and
   - infections in the neck.

   If you have any doubt about the diagnosis always do a lumbar puncture before you make this diagnosis.

Appendix 1 The proper method of doing a lumbar puncture

First you must understand the anatomy of the spine and the spinal canal. Look at Figure 25.15.

The front of a vertebra is a strong short cylinder of bone which is called 'the body' of the vertebra. It is joined to similar bodies above and below it by 'intervertebral discs' (see Figure 25.16). This column of bone and discs is called the spine. It supports the weight of the body and allows the body to bend. (See Figure 25.17.)

vertebrae with bodies in front and spinal canal enclosed by plates of bone behind - the spinal cord runs through the spinal canal

Figure 25.16 Diagram to show how vertebrae fit together and form the spine and spinal canal. The spinal cord goes through the canal, and nerves come from the through holes in the spine.

A

B

Figure 25.15 Diagram to show a single lumbar vertebra (A) from above and (B) from the side.

Behind the body of a vertebra are thinner plates of bone which have several functions.

1. They form a hole surrounded by bone. The hole in each vertebra is lined with strong ligaments. These ligaments also go inside the hole in the next vertebrae, above and below. This makes a long cylindrical space surrounded by bone and strong ligaments, behind the vertebral bodies. This space is called the spinal *canal*. The spinal *cord* goes out of a hole at the bottom of the skull and down the spinal canal to the level of the 1st lumbar vertebra.
2. They have joints with the vertebrae above and below which make the spine stronger.
3. They have pieces of bone on each side and at the back called 'spinous processes'. These spinous processes are joined by strong ligaments and muscles to the spinous processes of vertebrae above and below them. These ligaments and muscles make the spine stronger and also move (bend and straighten etc.) the spine.
4. They fit together with the vertebrae above and below leaving holes at the sides. Nerves pass through these holes from the spinal cord to the body. (See Figure 25.16.)

271

atlas   axis

1
2
3
4
5
6
7
1
2
3
4
5
6
7
8
9
10
11
12
1
2
3
4
5

lumbosacral

lateral (side) view

occipital bone

cranium

atlas
axis

mandible

transverse process

intervertebral disc

vertebral body

rib

spinous process

cervical vertebrae

thoracic

lumbar

sacral

coccygeal

Posterior (back) view

coccyx

Anterior (front) view

Figure 25.17   Diagram to show the vertebrae (or the spinal bones). The spinal cord goes from the brain through the spinal canal and ends at about L1. Lumbar puncture is done at L3–4. Note how flexion (bending forward) of the spine will open up the space the lumbar puncture needle must go through into the spinal canal.

272

Figure 25.18 Diagram to show the ligaments through which you must push the lumbar puncture needle to get into the spinal canal. The ligaments join the bones of the spine. The diagram shows the 2nd, 3rd and 4th lumbar vertebrae in section from the front to the back.

In a lumbar puncture you push a needle through the skin and ligaments between the posterior spinous process of the fourth and fifth (or the fourth and third) lumbar vertebrae, and then into the spinal canal (see Figures 25.18, 25.19 and 25.20). The needle will then go through the outer layer of the meninges (dura mater) and CSF will flow back through the needle. As the spinal cord ends at about the first lumbar vertebrae (a little lower in infants) there are only some nerves in this

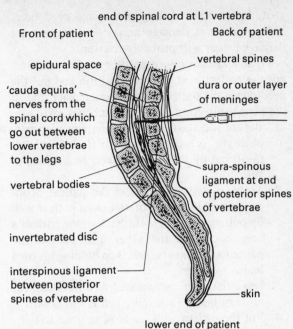

Figure 25.19 This diagram shows the lumbar and sacral spine in section from the front to the back. Note the anatomy of the spine and spinal cord. Note the structures through which the lumbar puncture needle goes to get into the spinal canal between the 3rd and 4th lumbar vertebrae. If the needle is directed too high or too low it will hit bone and not enter the spinal canal. Note that flexing (bending forward) the lumbar spine will open up the spaces between the lumbar vertebral posterior spinous processes and leave more space for the needle.

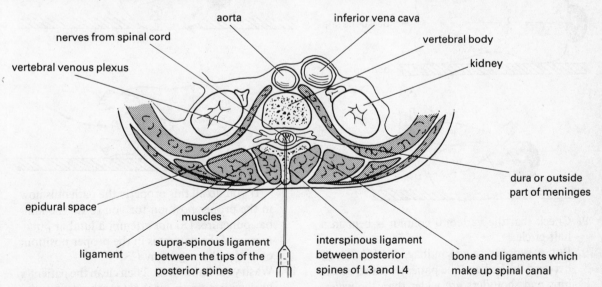

Figure 25.20 This diagram shows the third lumbar intervertebral disc (in section from side to side). Note that a lumbar puncture needle must go straight in to reach the spinal canal. If it goes to one side it will miss the spinal canal.

273

area. You cannot damage the spinal cord here. You should not damage nerves; but if they are damaged, they will probably recover.

To do a lumbar puncture successfully, you must put the patient in the proper position and put the needle into the patient in the proper place and in the proper direction. This is the proper method:

1. Before you start, sedate the patient with paraldehyde 0.1–0.2 ml/kg (1/10–1/5 ml/kg) (5–10 ml) by IMI if he is likely to be unhelpful.
2. Train an assistant to hold the patient properly. Good assistants often hold a patient well by putting one arm at the back of the patient's bent neck and the other arm behind the patient's bent knees, and then holding his own hands together.
3. Use a flat, hard surface such as a wooden bed, table or bench (a sagging bed is not good).
4. Put the patient with his head to your left.
5. The vertebral column (backbone) must be close to the edge of the bed.
6. The lumbar vertebral column must be parallel with the edge of the bed.
7. The head must be bent forward, with the chin on the chest.
8. The knees and hips must be completely bent and the knees pushed up onto the chest.

backbone line

bed top

9. Check that the vertebral column is bent in a half circle.
10. Put a support (e.g. sandbag, folded towel) between the bed and the patient's waist, as the hips and shoulders are wider than the waist. (This is not necessary in children or very fat patients).

If you do not do this, the vertebral column will be twisted.
11. When looking from above the patient, check that the right shoulder is exactly above the left shoulder.
12. When looking from above the patient, the right iliac crest (hip) must also be exactly above the left one. Put the right knee on top of the left knee, with a pillow between them.

If you do all this properly the patient is now in the proper position for you to do the lumbar puncture. Do not attempt a lumbar puncture until the patient is in the proper position; or you will not get any CSF.
13. Wash your hands well. Then clean the patient's back with iodine in alcohol (or other antiseptic).
14. Put a drape on top of the right iliac crest and waist.

this horizontally with your thumb-nail on the skin.

There will now be a cross on the skin between the vertebral spines and in the centre line of the spine. This is where you will put the lumbar puncture needle in.

Gently clean the area again with iodine (or other antiseptic).

18. In an older child or adult, give 2–5 ml of 1% lignocaine using a 26G needle. Put the needle through the skin exactly in the centre of the cross. First raise up a swelling *in* the skin (i.e. give an intradermal in injection). Then inject deeper between the spines of L4 and L5. So that you do not lose the place after injecting the local anaesthetic, disconnect the syringe but leave the needle in the skin until you are ready to put the LP needle in. Wait 3 minutes for the local anaesthetic to work.

19. Put the lumbar puncture needle in the gap between L4 and L5 where the needle for the local anaesthetic was, exactly in the centre of the cross. Check that the LP needle is in the proper position. *It must be at a right angle (90°) to the patient's back* at the L4 level *in both directions*. Check that this is so by looking *both* from above the patient and from the end of the patient along his spine. Then push the needle in, always checking that it is at right angles to the patient in both directions.

15. With your right hand, move a finger from the top of the right iliac crest straight down to the backbone. This will show you the position of the vertebral spine (bony lump) of the 4th lumbar vertebra.

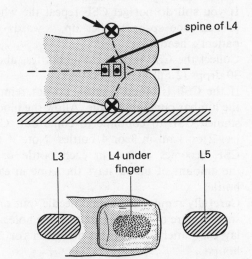

spine of L4

L3   L4 under finger   L5

16. Move the finger which is on the spine of L4, straight down towards the patient's buttocks to find the space between L4 and L5 – this is where you will put the spinal needle in. Mark the skin vertically in the centre of this space by pressing firmly with your thumb-nail for half a minute.

17. Now you must find the centre line of the spine from the head to the buttocks. It is the line which joins the centre (highest parts) of the bony spines. It almost always is *not* the same place as the hollow of the skin along the spine. You must feel the bony spines to find it. Mark

Check by looking from the end of the patient and from above the patient to see if the needle is straight.

20. In children you can use a needle from an IV drip set or a disposable needle.

    In adults, use a size 20 or 18 spinal needle with the proper fitting inner part (stilette or trochar) (as the disposable and drip set needles are often not long enough for adults).

21. The layers you push the needle through are in order
    (a) the skin
    (b) subcutaneous fat
    (c) spinal ligament
    (d) meninges (dura mater) – this is the last layer and you often feel the needle suddenly go through into the space where the CSF is.

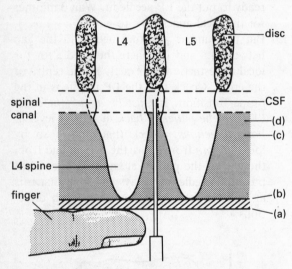

Push the needle in *very* slowly. Stop several times and remove the stilette and look to see if CSF comes out especially after you feel the needle has gone through something. Turn the needle round if you think the needle is in the proper position but no CSF comes out when you remove the stilette.

25. If you do not get CSF when you cannot push the needle in any further check that the needle:
    (a) is exactly in between two vertebral spines; and that it

(b) is in the centre of the spine lengthways (and not in the centre of the skin fold in the back which often does not lie over the the centre of the spine); and that it
(c) has gone in the right direction (at right angles to the patient at L4 in both directions).

If all these are so, remove the stilette, continue to turn the needle around slowly, and slowly pull it out looking to see if CSF comes as you start to pull the needle out.

If you get no CSF put the needle in again in a slightly different direction – usually more towards the patient's head. Pull the needle right out to the surface of the skin before trying again.

If you still get no CSF after several changes of position (including pushing the needle towards the feet), take the needle right out.

26. Check that the needle was in fact in the centre line of the spine and in the middle of the space. Then try the LP again.

27. If you still do not get CSF repeat the whole process one space further up, towards the patient's head.

28. Collect the CSF in two sterile bottles, about 30 drops (2 ml) in each bottle.

29. If the CSF is blood stained, do not remove the lumbar puncture needle. Allow the blood-stained CSF to continue to come out. Collect 2 or 3 ml in 3 or 4 bottles. Note if the CSF becomes clearer in each bottle or if the amount of blood stays the same in each bottle.

30. Carefully remove the spinal needle, put on a small square of sterile gauze over the hole and lay the patient flat on his abdomen for 2–3 hours.

31. The whole procedure must be sterile. Wash or scrub the hands well, as for an operation. If possible, wear sterile gloves. Clean the patient well with an alcoholic solution of antiseptic. Only use a sterilised LP needle. *Never* touch the part of the needle which goes into the patient (especially the needle tip) with the fingers even after scrubbing up and putting on sterile gloves (i.e. use a 'no touch' technique).

Appendix 2 Examination of the CSF

Naked eye examination of the CSF
See page 255.

Laboratory examination of the CSF
Always send the CSF for laboratory examination if possible. Ask for the first 5 of these tests on all CSF samples. Ask for a medical officer to send you a report on what the tests mean. (See Table 25.1 page 278.)

Tests on CSF samples:
1. Cells, total count. Normally less than 5/cmm are present.
2. Cells, differential count. Normally all are mononuclears (usually lymphocytes). (No red blood cells.).
3. Protein. Normally 15–45 mg%.
4. Sugar. Normally 45–100 mg% (varies with blood sugar).
5. Gram stain for organisms. Normally negative (or no organisms seen).
6. ZN stain for AFB. Normally negative (or no AFB seen).
7. Culture/Sensitivity for bacteria. Normally negative (or no growth).
8. Culture for tuberculosis organisms. Normally negative (or no growth).
9. Other tests if necessary.

Table 25.1 Typical CSF test results in the common conditions for which CSF tests are necessary
N = Neutrophils   L = Lymphocytes

	Cells		Gram stain	Protein	Sugar	ZN stain	Bact. cult.	TB cult.
	Total	Diff.						
Normal	0–5	All lymphocytes	no organisms	15–45 mg%	40–100 mg%	no AFB	no growth	no growth
Acute bacterial meningitis	increased (up to thousands)	N > L	often bacteria	increased	< 40; usually none	no AFB	often growth	no growth
Cerebral malaria	normal	L > N	no organisms	normal or increased	normal	no AFB	no growth	no growth
Viral meningitis	increased (tens or hundreds)	L > N	no organisms	increased	normal	no AFB	no growth	no growth
Encephalitis	normal or increased (tens or hundreds)	L > N	no organisms	increased or normal	normal	no AFB	no growth	no growth
Tuberculous meningitis	increased (up to hundreds)	L > N usually; N > L early	no organisms	increased	decreased or none	sometimes AFB	no growth	often growth
Cerebral haemorrhage early	many RBCs	normal	no organisms	increased	normal	no AFB	no growth	no growth
Cerebral haemorrhage late	normal or increased	L > N	no organisms	increased	normal	no AFB	no growth	no growth
Traumatic tap	many RBCs	normal	no organisms	increased	normal	no AFB	no growth	no growth
Cerebral tumour or tuberculoma or abscess	normal or increased	varies	no organisms	increased or normal	normal	no AFB	no growth	no growth

26

Disorders of the Urinary System

Anatomy and physiology

When the cells of the body do their work, they make several waste products, including urea, uric acid and carbon dioxide. The blood removes these waste products from the cells.

The carbon dioxide passes from the blood into the air in the lungs.

Each time the heart contracts (pumps), about 1/5 of the blood it pumps out goes through the kidneys. The kidneys remove most of the waste products from the blood which goes through them.

The kidneys remove the waste products from the blood so efficiently that when this 1/5 of the blood mixes with the other 4/5 of the blood which did not go through the kidneys (and still has waste products in it) the concentration (or amount) of waste products in the mixed blood is never high.

The waste products removed from the blood by the kidneys are dissolved in water, and this is called urine. The urine goes down a tube, called a ureter, from each kidney, to the bladder. The bladder is a muscular storage bag in the pelvis. The bladder can hold about ½ litre of urine before it must be emptied. The body passes the urine from the bladder out through the urethra. (See Figures 26.1 and 26.2.)

The urine also contains any salt or water which the body does not need. There is normally no protein and no sugar in the urine.

The body needs to pass about 800 ml of water in the urine everyday, in order to remove the normal amount of waste products made each day.

Figure 26.1 The anatomy of the urinary system.

279

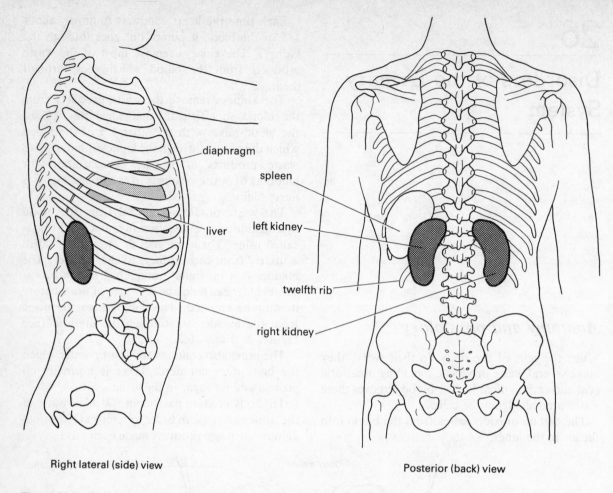

diaphragm

spleen

liver

left kidney

twelfth rib

right kidney

Right lateral (side) view

Posterior (back) view

Figure 26.2 The position of the kidneys. Note that the kidneys are both posterior (at the back) and are also high in the abdomen, partly under the ribs.

Pathology

If the body is dehydrated, there is not enough water to make 800 ml of urine each day. So all the waste products in the urine are dissolved in only a little water. The urine is concentrated. The common causes of acute dehydration are gastroenteritis (when much fluid is lost from the body in vomiting or diarrhoea) and when the patient is too sick to drink enough. Chronic dehydration can occur in hot dry places in people who drink only a little water. In some of these people the waste products are not all dissolved in the water of the urine. The waste products then make small (or even large) stones in the kidneys or bladder. Infections in the urinary tract can make stones in the kidneys or bladder even when there is no dehydration.

If the body is very dehydrated, it will make very little urine. Then the body cannot remove the waste products and salt, and the concentration of the waste products and salt rises in the blood. This is called 'kidney failure'. If this happens quickly, it is called acute kidney failure.

Some acute conditions can damage the kidney very severely – and stop the kidney working. The kidney cannot make urine, so the waste products and salt remain in the body and cause death in a few days. This is also called acute kidney failure.

Some conditions damage the kidney so that it can still work; but it cannot work properly. It cannot dissolve all the waste products in only 800 ml of water. It needs much more water to remove all the waste products. And still more waste products than normal remain in the blood. This is called chronic kidney failure. If a person with chronic kidney failure does not get enough fluid, then the concentration of waste products in his blood quickly rises, and he also gets acute kidney failure.

Infection is the most common pathological condition of the urinary tract. Infection in one part of the urinary tract easily spreads to another part (or all parts) of the urinary tract.

Urea is the main waste product of the body which you can easily measure in a laboratory. In the blood of a normal healthy person, there is less than 40 mg urea/100 ml of blood or less than 6.6 mmol urea/1 (litre) of blood. If the blood urea is more than 100 mg/100 ml or more than 16 mmol/l, then the patient has kidney failure and may die unless you give him treatment.

Symptoms and signs of disease of the urinary tract

Symptoms of urinary tract disease

1. *Urinary symptoms*
   urethral discharge of pus, or white fluid, or watery fluid
   dysuria
   urinary frequency
   change in colour of urine
   blood in urine
   pain in
   • urethra (felt in the penis)
   • prostate (felt in the perineum in front of the anus)
   • bladder (felt in the lower central abdomen)
   • kidneys (felt in the loin (or back where the lower ribs join the spine))
   • ureter (felt anywhere from one loin to the iliac fossa or genitalia or inner upper leg on the same side)
2. *Symptoms of infection*
   fever
   rigors
   malaise
   etc.
3. *Symptoms of kidney failure*
   see page 289.
4. *Symptoms of oedema*
   swelling of ankles, back, face, etc.

Always ask all patients about these urinary symptoms:
1. pain or a burning feeling when passing urine (called dysuria),
2. passing urine more often than normal (called urinary frequency),
3. abnormal colour of the urine, including blood in the urine.

Signs of urinary tract disease

1. *Urinary tract signs*
   (a) kidney tenderness (See Chapter 36 page 407 and Figure 26.3.)
   kidney enlargement (See Figure 26.4.)
   (b) bladder tenderness (See Chapter 36 page 407.)
   bladder enlargement (See Chapter 36 page 410.)
   (c) urethral discharge (See Chapter 19 page 128.)
   urethral tenderness

left   right

Posterior

Figure 26.3 Diagram showing where (marked with a cross) you *gently* hit the patient with the side of your fist, to find out if the kidneys are tender.

Figure 26.4 Photograph showing the method of palpation of the kidneys. Use both hands. Put one hand flat on the abdomen beside the long central abdominal muscle and below the edge of the ribs. Put the other hand in the angle between the ribs and the spine and gently lift the kidney upwards. Ask the patient to take a deep breath. When the patient has nearly finished breathing in, press the front hand gently down and quickly bend the fingers of the back hand upwards. If the kidney is enlarged you will feel the kidney hit the top hand. Then feel the kidney slide back between the hands as the patient breathes out. In thin people you can often feel the lower part of a normal right kidney.

(d) abnormalities of the external genitalia

(e) prostate
or
uterine
$\left\{\begin{array}{l}\text{enlargement}\\\text{lumpiness}\\\text{tenderness}\end{array}\right\}$
on pelvic
examination
through the
rectum

(See Figures 26.5, 26.6, 26.7 and 26.8.)
or

(f) vaginal, urethral, bladder or uterine abnormalities on pelvic examination through the vagina

(See Figure 26.7 and an obstetrics and gynaecology textbook.)

2. *Signs of infection*
raised temperature
fast pulse rate

3. *Signs of kidney failure*
See page 290.

4. *Signs of oedema*
Swelling of the ankles, back, face etc. If you press gently with a finger you will make a hollow in the skin and underlying tissues which only returns to normal slowly.
See Chapter 36 page 398.

5. *High blood pressure*
See Chapter 27 page 300.

Figure 26.5 The anatomy of the male pelvis. The pelvis is shown in section from front to back. Note the structures which you can feel anteriorly (in the front) on pelvic examination through the rectum (per rectum or 'PR') – anal sphincter (muscle), prostate, seminal vesicles and bladder.

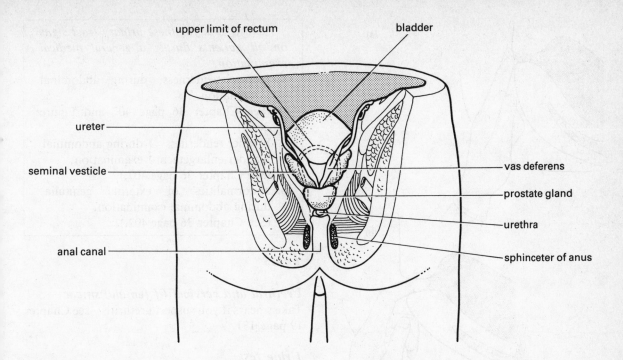

Figure 26.6 The male pelvis from the back, as if the buttocks and bones and rectum at the back had been cut away. Note again the structures which you can feel on rectal examination 'PR' – anal sphincter, prostate, seminal vesicles and bladder.

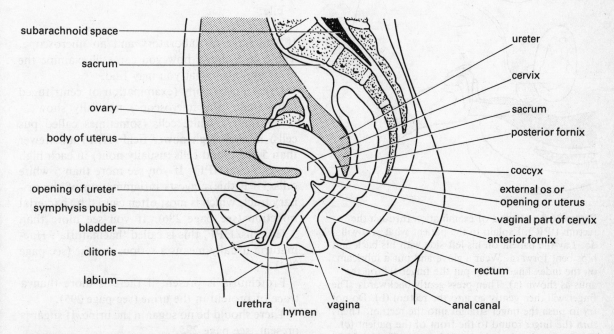

Figure 26.7 The anatomy of the female pelvis. The pelvis is shown in section from front to back. Note the structures which you can feel anteriorly (in the front). Through the rectum (per rectum or 'PR') you can feel the vagina and the cervix of the uterus. Through the vagina (per vaginum or 'PV') you can feel the urethra, bladder, cervix and uterus. For method of examination 'PV' see a specialist gynaecology/obstetrics book.

Tests

Urethral and cervical (if female) smear

Take smears if you suspect urethritis – see Chapter 19 page 131.

Urine test

Test urine for
    protein,
    sugar,
    blood,
    pus, and
    bile.

If you have no laboratory and no microscope, Table 26.1 shows how you can still examine the urine and also what you may find.

Urine microscopy (examination of centrifuged urine under the microscope) normally shows – fewer than 5 white cells (sometimes called pus cells) in each high power field (HPF) and fewer than 5 red blood cells (usually none) in each high power field (HPF). If you see more than 5 white cells/HPF this suggests inflammation of the urinary tract, which is most often caused by bacterial infection (see page 286). If you see more than 5 red cells/HPF, this is called 'haematuria'. Haematuria usually means a serious disease (see page 294).

Proteinuria is present if there is more than a trace of protein in the urine (see page 295).

There should be no sugar in the urine. If sugar is present, see page 295.

Blood urea

See page 281.

Figure 26.8 Method of examination through the rectum ('PR'). Explain to the patient what you will do. Lay the patient on his left side with his back and hips bent forward. Wear a glove and put a lubricant on the index finger. First put the finger flat on the anus as shown (a). Then press gently backwards. The finger will then gently go into the rectum (b). Do not try to push the finger straight into the rectum. Then turn the finger round to the front of the patient (c). Gently examine the structures shown in Figures 26.6, 26.7 and 26.8 for tenderness, lumpiness or enlargement. At the end of the examination gently clean any lubricant remaining outside the anus.

Table 26.1   Examination of the urine without a microscope

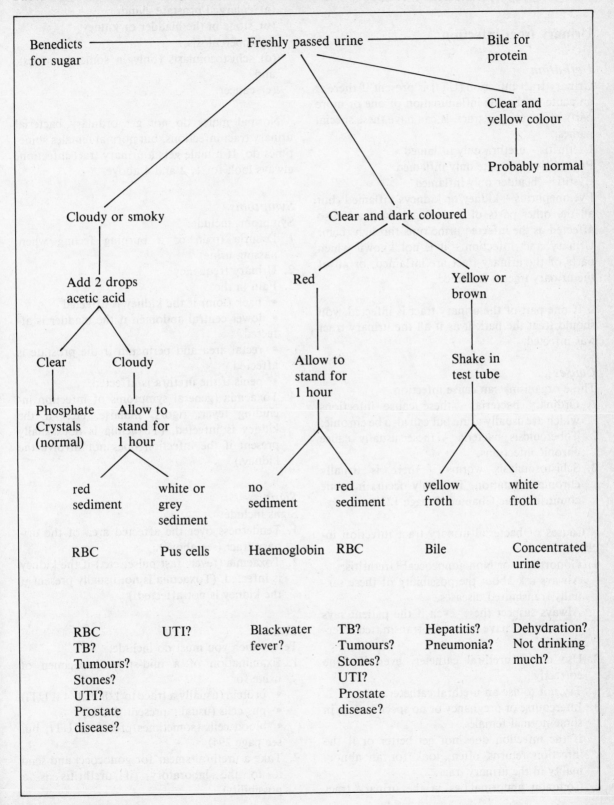

Diseases of the urinary tract

Urinary tract infection

Definition
Urinary tract infection (UTI) is present if there is an acute or chronic inflammation of one or more parts of the urinary tract. It can have these special names:

Urethritis – urethra only inflamed

Prostatitis – prostate only inflamed

Cystitis – bladder only inflamed

Pyelonephritis – kidney or kidneys inflamed (but all the other parts of the urinary tract are also affected as the infected urine runs through them.

Urinary tract infection – it is not known which parts of the urinary tract are inflamed, or all of the urinary tract is inflamed.

If one part of the urinary tract is infected, you should treat the patient as if all the urinary tract was infected.

Causes
These organisms can cause infection
1. Ordinary bacteria – these cause infections which are usually acute but can also be chronic.
2. Tuberculosis bacteria – these usually cause chronic infections.
3. Schistosomiasis worms – there is usually chronic infestation. This only occurs in some countries. (See Chapter 18 page 122.)

Causes of bacterial urinary tract infection include:
1. Gonorrhoea or Non-gonococcal Urethritis:
   Always ask about the possibility of these sexually transmitted diseases.
   Always suspect these, even if the patient says he could not have a sexually transmitted infection.
2. Use of an urethral catheter, even if done correctly.
   Try not to use an urethral catheter.
3. Intercourse or pregnancy or no special cause in some normal females.
   If the infection does not get better or if the infection returns often, look for an abnormality in the urinary tract.
4. Common abnormalities in the urinary tract

include:
   (a) enlarged prostate gland,
   (b) stone in the bladder or kidney,
   (c) tuberculosis,
   (d) schistosomiasis (only in some countries), and
   (e) cancer.

Normal males do not get ordinary bacterial urinary tract infections, but normal females sometimes do. If a male gets a urinary tract infection, always look for 1, 2 and 4 above.

Symptoms
Symptoms include:
1. Dysuria (pain or a burning feeling when passing urine)
2. Urinary frequency
3. Pain in the:
   • back (loin) if the kidney is affected
   • lower central abdomen if the bladder is affected
   • rectal area and perineum if the prostate is affected
   • penis if the urethra is affected.
4. Toxaemia (general symptoms of infection including fever, rigors, malaise, etc.) if the kidney is infected. (Toxaemia is not usually present if the infection does not involve the kidney.)

Signs
Signs include:
1. Tenderness over the affected area of the urinary tract (see above).
2. Toxaemia (fever, fast pulse, etc.) if the kidney is infected. (Toxaemia is not usually present if the kidney is not affected.)

Tests
Tests which you must do include:
1. Examination of a mid-stream specimen of urine for
   • protein (usually a trace to 1/8 or 1/4 if UTI)
   • pus cells (usually present if UTI)
   • blood cells (sometimes present if UTI; but see page 294)
2. Take a urethral smear for gonococci and send it to the laboratory (if urethritis is a possibility).

Details of management

Examine a mid-stream specimen of urine for pus, blood, protein and sugar (if there is infection, pus and usually protein are present).

Ask if urethral or vaginal discharge is present and if a sexually transmitted disease is possible. Take a urethral and (in females) cervical smear for gonococci and treat for gonorrhoea if the history or examination suggests it is possible (see Chapter 19 page 131).

Do an abdominal and pelvic examination (PV in women and PR in men) to check for genital tract disease (especially important if the infection is not quickly cured or it returns after treatment).

Check that the patient does not only have urinary frequency from normal pregnancy.

Treat as an outpatient. Admit for inpatient treatment only if sick.
1. *If* there is any possibility of gonorrhoea:
   ampicillin 3.5 g (7 of the special 500 mg caps) orally immediately, once
   or
   aqueous procaine penicillin 4,800,000 units (16 ml) (8 ml in each buttock) IMI immediately once (the patient must lie down for the injection and for 10 minutes after it)
   and
   probenecid 1 g (2 tabs) orally immediately once.
2. Sulphadimidine 1 g (2 tabs) four times a day for 10 days.
3. If the patient does not improve after 2–4 days or is not cured after 10 days of sulphadimidine, give tetracycline (if not pregnant) or ampicillin (if pregnant) 250–500 mg (1–2 caps) four times a day for 10 days.
4. If the patient does not improve after 2–4 days or is not cured after 10 days of tetracycline or ampicillin, give chloramphenicol 750 mg (3 caps) four times a day for ten days.
5. Give antimalarial drugs as indicated, if there is any fever (see Chapter 13 page 55).
6. Tell the patient to drink plenty of fluid.

Examine a mid-stream specimen of urine (for pus and protein) after the treatment is finished to check that the infection has gone.

Transfer or refer to Medical Officer care:
1. if the patient is not clinically cured and the urine tests are not clear after this treatment (non-urgent);
2. if a male has more than one attack (non-urgent);
3. if a female has an infection that returns often (e.g. 3 or more infections in less than one year) (non-urgent); or
4. if there is blood in the urine at any time which is not caused by schistosomiasis (see Chapter 18 page 122) (non-urgent).

Nephrotic syndrome

Definition
Nephrotic syndrome is a condition in which a patient has
1. oedema of the whole body (swelling caused by an abnormal amount of fluid), and
2. much protein in the urine (more than 1/8 or +), and
3. you can find no other cause for the oedema (such as malnutrition, severe anaemia, heart failure, chronic liver disease, toxaemia of pregnancy, acute glomerulonephritis, filariasis, etc.).

Nephrotic syndrome is caused by any condition which damages the kidney so that the kidney allows much of the protein in the blood to go into the urine. There is then not enough protein in the blood to keep the salt and water of the blood inside the blood-vessels. The water and salt of the blood then go into the tissues of the body and cause oedema.

Causes
Causes of damage to the kidney, which lead to nephrotic syndrome, include:
• diabetes mellitus
• unusual diseases affecting the immune system
• some kinds of glomerulonephritis
• some cases of lepromatous leprosy or other chronic infections or chronic inflammations of any sort
• some cases of malaria
• some drugs
• and many others.

In many cases it is not possible to find out what condition has led to nephrotic syndrome but this does not affect the management of the disease. You should, however, check that your patient does not have a cause you can stop.

Symptoms

Usually swelling caused by oedema is the only symptom (see Figure 26.9). Malaise may be present.

Signs

Usually oedema is the only sign.

Tests

The urine has much protein in it (more than 1/8 or +). You must test the urine in all patients who have oedema.

Differential diagnosis

See Chapter 36 page 398 for causes of oedema of the whole body. Very important causes include:
1. kidney diseases, including nephrotic syndrome,
2. malnutrition,
3. heart failure,
4. severe anaemia, especially if caused by hookworm, and
5. chronic liver disease (cirrhosis).

Details of management

Do not diagnose nephrotic syndrome unless there is generalised oedema and much protein in the urine (more than + or 1/8th).

Check that the patient does not have another cause for generalised oedema (other kidney disease, heart failure, malnutrition, severe anaemia, chronic liver disease or filariasis).

Admit for inpatient treatment to check the effect of treatment and the progress of the disease (but you can treat as an outpatient if necessary).

Give the following treatment
1. Routine diuretics.
   Hydrochlorothiazide 50–100 mg (1–2 tabs) each morning.
2. High protein diet with no added salt.
   (Tinned fish and meat are not satisfactoy as they contain much salt. Give fresh foods if possible.)
3. Antimalarial drugs as indicated, usually chloroquine 450–600 mg (3–4 tabs) daily for 3 days then 300 mg (2 tabs) weekly.
4. Treatment for intestinal worms.
   Pyrantel 625 mg (5 tabs) once (to stop any protein loss from worms in bowel).
5. Test the urine for protein every day and weigh the patient to check if he is improving.

Figure 26.9 A child with nephrotic syndrome. Note that he has swelling of *all* of his body including his face. Swelling of the face suggests (but does not prove) a kidney cause for oedema of the whole body. General oedema (though often with a different distribution can be caused by : (1) kidney disease (especially nephrotic syndrome), (2) malnutrition, (3) chronic liver disease (cirrhosis), (4) severe anaemia, (5) heart failure (6) filariasis (usually only the limbs affected), (7) other conditions (see text). Swelling of the face along may be caused by an allergic reaction and needs urgent treatment with adrenaline and antihistamine, if the allergic swelling starts to block breathing.

6. Give powerful diuretics if the patient is not improving. Start with a small dose.
   Frusemide 40–160 mg (1–4 tabs) daily. If this is not successful give frusemide 20–60 mg (2–6 ml) IVI daily for a few days.
7. Potassium chloride 1200 mg (2 tabs) three times daily *if* you give frusemide and/or the patient is not on a tuber diet.
8. Look carefully for acute bacterial infections and malaria. Give proper treatment quickly if they occur.

Transfer the patient to medical officer care, but only after discussion with the medical officer:
1. if you cannot remove the oedema after 3–6 weeks; or
2. if the proteinuria has not gone after 3–6 weeks; or
3. if a micro-urine examination shows more than the normal number of red blood cells or white blood (pus) cells;

as other drugs (e.g. prednisolone) can sometimes help special cases.

Schistosomiasis

Schistosomiasis is a very important cause of disease of the urinary tract.

Schistosomiasis only occurs in parts of Africa, the Middle East, India, South East Asia including the Philippines, and South America. (See Figure 18.13 page 123.)

Find out if you are in an area where schistosomiasis occurs. If so, see Chapter 18 page 122 for details of schistosomiasis.

Acute glomerulonephritis

Definition
Acute glomerulonephritis is an acute inflammation of the kidneys. It is not caused by infecting organisms in the kidney. It is caused by an abnormal reaction of the body's immune system. This abnormal reaction is often to a certain type of infection which the patient had about 2–3 weeks before.

Clinical features
A respiratory or skin infection occurs 2–3 weeks before the start of the illness in many, but not all, cases. Then there is suddenly:

- malaise,
- swelling (oedema) of the face and legs,
- only a small volume of urine, which looks like black tea and has positive tests for red blood cells and protein, and
- high blood pressure (developing over a day or two).

See a specialist book for details of diagnosis and management.

Chronic kidney (renal) failure

Chronic kidney failure is present when the kidneys are permanently damaged and cannot excrete (put) all the waste products made by the body into the urine. The amount of waste products in the body increases and damages many functions of the body. There are many causes of chronic kidney failure. You can treat very few of these causes successfully in the health centre. (See Figure 26.10.)

Figure 26.10 A patient with chronic kidney failure. The patient came to the health centre because he had the symptoms of anaemia. Routine treatment of the anaemia did not make him any better. The signs of kidney failure were then looked for and found. The diagnosis was confirmed by a blood urea test.

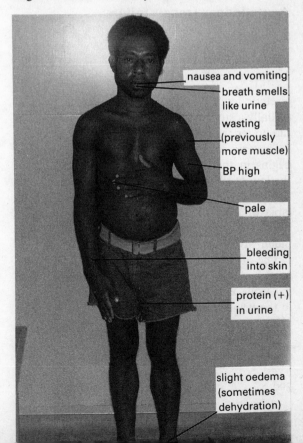

nausea and vomiting

breath smells like urine

wasting (previously more muscle)

BP high

pale

bleeding into skin

protein (+) in urine

slight oedema (sometimes dehydration)

Think of chronic kidney failure in any patient who has:

- anaemia (especially if it does not improve with treatment),
- high blood pressure (higher than 160/100),
- loss of appetite, nausea, and often vomiting (for no obvious reason),
- wasting of muscles (for no obvious reason),
- breath that smells like urine smells,
- deep respirations, even though the patient does not feel short of breath (usually late in the disease), or
- bleeding into the skin (usually only late in the disease)

A history of previous kidney disease makes the diagnosis more likely.

Test the urine for protein. Protein in the urine makes the diagnosis very likely if the other signs are present.

Send blood to the laboratory to confirm the diagnosis; ask for a blood urea test. (See page 281.)

See a specialist reference book for details of diagnosis and treatment.

Do not transfer the patient because no further treatment is possible in the hospital.

Acute kidney (renal) failure

See page 293.

Ureteric (renal) colic

Ureteric colic is a pain caused by something (usually a stone formed in the kidney) going down the ureter from the kidney to the bladder.

Ureteric colic is a very severe pain. It usually begins in the loin (one side of the back, where the lowest ribs join the spine) and then spreads to the iliac fossa (lower outer front of the abdomen), labia or penis or testes or inner leg on the same side. It is a constant pain which may slowly get much worse. It is not a true colic.

The attack may continue for only a few minutes; but sometimes it continues for hours. Passing urine is often painful. Blood is often passed in the urine. Tests show protein and blood in the urine.

Stones never dissolve themselves. But if they are small, they may be passed in the urine. If stones remain in the urinary tract for a long time, infection often occurs.

Treatment includes the following

1. Treat any ureteric colic with IMI pethidine 100 mg (2 ml) and atropine 0.6 mg (1 ml) every 4 hours if necessary.
2. Treat any urinary infection present. Do not use sulphadimidine. Use some other drug.
3. Keep any stone that is passed. Give it to the medical officer for analysis in the laboratory.
4. Give 3–4 litres of fluid daily (to make a large urine volume).

Transfer the patient to a medical officer within two days to check if there is an obstruction of the ureter. This is especially important if there is continuous pain and tenderness over one kidney. The medical officer will do special tests and X-rays.

Some common diagnostic problems and their management

Urinary frequency (Passing urine more often than normal)

Do a full history and examination (see Chapter 6 and page 281).

Do a pelvic examination PR and PV (see Chapter 6 page 284).

Test the urine (See page 284).

Find out if the patient is passing large volumes (amounts) of urine often or if he is passing only small amounts of urine often.

Large amounts of urine passed often
Look for:
1. *Diabetes mellitus*
   - sugar (glucose) in the urine (see Chapter 30 page 295)
   - drinking a lot
   - eating a lot
   - losing weight if young; or overweight if old
   Treat dehydration if present (see Chapter 23 page 224).
   Give the patient has a diet with no sugar in it.
   Refer or transfer to medical officer.
2. *Chronic kidney failure*
   - protein in the urine
   - anaemia which does not get better with rou-

tine treatment
- blood pressure higher than normal
- wasting

See page 289.

3. *Acting out* (drinking more than is necessary)
   - no other abnormalities found on examination
   - urine tests all normal
   - the patient has a mental problem

If you find and solve the problem, and the patient drinks less, the frequency stops.

4. *Rare medical conditions*

If you cannot find the cause, refer or transfer to medical officer.

Do not allow the patient to become dehydrated.

Small amounts of urine passed often

1. *Urinary tract infection*
   - dysuria (pain on passing urine) also
   - urethral discharge if there is urethritis
   - fever if the kidney is infected
   - tenderness over urethra, prostate, bladder or kidney/s if these are infected.

See page 286.

2. *Schistosomiasis*
   - patient in or from an area where schistosomiasis occurs
   - blood in urine, especially at the end of passing urine – worse after exercise
   - eggs or miracidia in urine on examination

See Chapter 18 page 122.

3. *Obstruction of the urethra by an enlarged prostate gland or a urethral stricture*
   - older man if there is an enlarged prostate; or middle-aged man who has a past history of gonorrhoea if there is a stricture
   - for months or years it has been difficult to pass urine – difficult to start, then a thin stream and difficult to pass all the urine
   - sometimes you can feel an enlarged or lumpy prostate on pelvic examination PR
   - no pus or protein in the urine unless there is also a urinary tract infection

If there is pus and protein in the urine, treat for urinary tract infection (see page 287).

If patient is not cured, refer or transfer non urgently to a medical officer (probably for an operation).

4. *Normal pregnancy* pressing on the bladder
   - the patient is well, but is in either early pregnancy (1 or 2 periods missed) or late pregnancy
   - the urine tests are normal

No treatment necessary.

5. *Pelvic disease* such as pelvic inflammatory disease or cancer of the female genital tract pressing on the bladder.
   - vaginal discharge or bleeding
   - abnormal tenderness or enlargement of organs or lumps on pelvic examination PR and PV

Treat pelvic inflammatory disease (see a gynaecology book) and amoebic infections (See Chapter 23 page 231).

Refer or transfer other cases non urgently to a medical officer.

6. *Blood in the urine* when schistosomiasis is not present (no eggs or miracidia in the urine), and you cannot find another disease.

Refer or transfer to a medical officer all patients who have blood in the urine with no obvious cause. It may be disease which can be cured if treated early, but may cause death if not treated until late.

7. *Chronic disease of the bladder* such as a stone or late schistosomiasis or tuberculosis or cancer.
   - long history or urinary symptoms
   - urinary symptoms getting worse
   - blood or protein or pus in the urine

Refer to transfer non urgently to a medical officer.

Dysuria (Pain on passing urine)

Do a full history and examination (See Chapter 6 and page 281).

Test the urine (See page 284).

Do a pelvic examination PR and PV (see Chapter 6 page 19 and page 282).

Pull back the foreskin of the penis and look under it and on the glans of the penis.

Look for:

1. *Sores on, or inflammation of, the penis, vulva or vagina*
   - Urinary frequency may not be present.
   - The urine tests are usually normal.

If sore, see Chapter 19 page 128.
If discharge, see Chapter 19 page 128.

2. *Urethral infection*
   - Urine frequency is present.
   - Ask if there is urethral or vaginal discharge of pus or of white or watery material.
   - Ask about the possibility of a sexually transmitted disease.
   - Still suspect a sexually transmitted disease, even if the patient says it is not possible.
   - Look for urethral discharge.
   - The urine tests may not have much pus or protein in a mid-stream specimen.

   If urethritis is likely, see Chapter 19 page 130.

3. *Prostatitis*
   - Urinary frequency is usually present.
   - Ask about the possibility of a sexually transmitted disease in younger men.
   - Ask about symptoms of an enlarged prostate (increasing difficulty in passing urine, etc.) in older men.
   - Examine for tenderness of the prostate, on pelvic examination PR.
   - The urine test may not have much pus or protein in a mid-stream specimen.

   Treat as for urethritis and urinary tract infection. See page 287.

4. *Cystitis due to bacteria*
   - Urinary frequency is present.
   - Tenderness over the bladder may be present.
   - Symptoms and signs of pyelonephritis may be present.
   - Urine tests show pus and protein.

   Treat for urinary tract infection (see page 287).

5. *Cystitis due to schistosomiasis*
   - patient from or in an area where schistosomiasis occurs
   - blood in the urine, especially at the end of passing urine and after exercise
   - severe pain if clots of blood are passed

   Treatment – see Chapter 18 page 126.

6. *Pelvic disease* irritating the bladder, especially pelvic inflammatory disease.
   - vaginal discharge or bleeding
   - abnormal tenderness, lumps, or enlarged organs on pelvic examination PR or PV

- urine tests normal, unless urine has vaginal secretions in it

Treat for pelvic inflammatory disease (see a gynaecology book) and amoebic infections (see Chapter 23 page 231).

7. *Pyelonephritis*
   - urinary frequency
   - fever, fast pulse, toxaemia
   - tenderness in the loin/s
   - urine tests show pus and protein

   Treatment – see page 287.

8. Note that people often complain of dysuria when they have pains all over or a fever, and pass concentrated urine. The dysuria improves as the person gets better. There is no disease of the urinary tract.

Incontinence of urine (The patient cannot control when urine is passed)

Do a full history and examination (See Chapter 6 page 281).

Examine the urine (see page 284).

Do a pelvic examination PR and PV (see Chapter 6 page 19 and page 282).

Look for:

1. *No proper control of the body and bladder by the brain*
   - children
   - old people with senile dementia – Do not diagnose this until you have done all the examinations below with normal results *and* you find that the patient has a chronic organic psychosis. (See Chapter 35 page 388.)
   - during fitting (convulsions)
   - unconsciousness from any cause
   - some psychoses

   Treat the cause if possible.

2. *Damage to parts of the spinal cord which control the bladder*
   - injury to the back or pain in the back, often with a lump in the spine
   - difficulty in walking or paralysis or the legs
   - loss of sensation in the legs

   Transfer the patient urgently to medical officer care, unless the condition has been present for many months or for years.

3. *Vesico-vaginal fistula or damage to the bladder during labour*
   - present soon after difficult childbirth
   Transfer non-urgently to a medical officer.

4. *Infection in the bladder*
   - dysuria and frequency
   - pus and protein in the urine
   Treatment – see page 287.

5. *Obstruction of the urethra* causing the bladder to be too full. A little urine goes through the narrow urethra constantly
   - Older man if there is an enlarged prostate; or middle aged man who has a past history of gonorrhoea if there is a stricture.
   - For months or years it has been difficult to pass urine – difficult to start, then a thin stream and difficult to pass all the urine.
   - Sometimes you can feel an enlarged or lumpy prostate on pelvic examination PR.
   If there is pus and protein in the urine, treat for urinary tract infection (see page 287).
   If the incontinence is not cured refer or transfer the patient non-urgently to a medical officer (probably for an operation).

Anuria (The patient does not pass urine)

There is usually one of these causes of anuria.
   Look for:
1. *The urine is made by the kidneys but the bladder cannot empty* ('acute retention of urine')
   - You can feel or percuss the bladder in the lower abdomen (See Chapter 36 page 410).
   - The bladder is tender as well as enlarged.
   Find out why the bladder cannot empty.
   - There is a history and signs of an enlarged prostate gland or a urethral stricture (See page 291). *or*
   - There is a history and signs of damage to the spinal cord, usually trauma or tuberculosis. (See Chapter 29 page 324). *or*
   - There are signs of loss of control of the bladder by the brain, such as unconsciousness. (See Chapter 25 page 264).
   Empty the bladder by *gentle*, continuous pressure over the bladder with your hand.
   If this is not possible, insert a urethral catheter with all the special care necessary to avoid infection of the bladder.

2. *The kidneys do not make urine* ('Acute Kidney Failure')
   - You cannot feel or percuss the bladder the bladder because it is not enlarged (it is usually empty).
   - The patient is usually very sick with the condition that caused the acute kidney failure.

Look for the cause of the acute kidney failure
   - Any condition which caused shock which continued for more than a short time before it was cured: external or internal bleeding, and especially antepartum or postpartum haemorrhage; severe dehydration; septicaemia; malaria, etc.
   - Acute haemolysis (See Chapter 21 page 182) especially blood which was wrongly cross-matched or malaria with 'blackwater fever' or some snake bites.
   - Many other causes (see a specialist reference book).
   Immediately treat the condition that caused the acute kidney failure, especially if it is shock (See Chapter 27 page 305).
   Arrange urgent (emergency) transfer to medical officer care.

3. *The patient is not telling the truth*
   - The bladder is not enlarged or tender.
   - The patient has no serious symptoms or signs, and looks well.
   - The patient usually has a big mental problem.
   Admit and observe the patient for 24 hours to see if he is telling the truth or not.

Abnormal colour of the urine

Normally the colour of the urine shows how much waste product is in the urine.

If the person is dehydrated or has no extra water to pass, the concentration of waste product in the urine is high. The urine is 'concentrated'. The colour of the urine is yellow (although the patient may say it is red).

If the person has much water to pass the concentration of waste product in the urine is low. The urine is 'dilute'. The urine colour is clear or like water.

If a person says his urine is an abnormal colour, always look at the urine yourself to see what colour it is and if it is abnormal. Do all the tests for urine. (See page 284.)

Yellow urine
Look for causes of:
1. normally concentrated urine (see above);
2. abnormally concentrated urine, from dehydration (see Chapter 23 page 221);
3. bile in the urine – but this usually makes the urine dark. (See Chapter 24 page 240.)

Clear urine (like water)
Look for causes of:
1. normally dilute urine (see above);
2. dilute urine because the patient has kidney failure and cannot concentrate the urine (see page 289).

Cloudy urine
Look for causes of:
1. pus from a urinary tract infection (see page 295);
2. phosphate crystals – these do not mean any disease at all and they dissolve if acid is added to the urine; the urine then becomes clear.

Red urine
Look for causes of:
1. red blood cells in the urine ('haematuria') (see this page),
2. haemoglobin in the urine (although then the urine is usually brown or black, not red) (no red blood cells are in the urine) – causes for this include malaria with 'blackwater fever', some snake bites, and wrongly-crossmatched blood, the patient is very sick;
3. bile in the urine (the urine is really brown or black, not red) (see Chapter 24 page 240);
4. food, e.g. beetroot, or sweets (lollies) with red colour in them;
5. normally concentrated urine (the urine is really a yellow colour, not red).

Black urine (like tea or coffee without milk)
Look for causes of:
1. bile in the urine (see Chapter 24 page 240), or
2. haemoglobin in the urine (see above).
See page 284 for ways to test urine for pus, blood, bile, haemoglobin, etc. without laboratory help. If a laboratory is available, you can examine the urine for pus cells and red blood cells under the microscope, and for bile, blood, protein, sugar and haemoglobin with test tablets or paper strips.

Blood in the urine (haematuria)

Check that the patient does have blood in the urine and not either:
1. menstrual blood in the urine, *or*
2. red urine not caused by red blood cells (see above).

If there is blood in the urine, look for:
1. *Trauma to the urinary tract*
   • History and signs of trauma are present. Transfer all cases to medical officer care urgently.

2. *Urinary tract infection*
   • dysuria and urinary frequency
   • pus and protein with the blood in the urine
   • treatment removes the blood from the urine and it does not appear in the urine again
   Treatment – see page 287.

3. *Schistosomiasis*
   • patient from or in an area where schistosomiasis occurs and usually a boy;
   • there is more blood at the end when passing urine, and more after exercise;
   • eggs or miracidia are in the urine, on examination see Chapter 18 page 125.
   Management – see Chapter 18 page 126.

4. *Acute glomerulonephritis*
   • throat or skin infection 1–3 weeks before, but not always
   • oedema (puffy face, etc.)
   • blood pressure high
   • urine has protein and blood in it and the volume is small.
   Management – see reference books.

5. *Stone in the urinary tract*
   • ureteric colic (see page 290)
   Management – see page 290.

6. *Causes that you cannot diagnose at the health centre but must be diagnosed* (because some conditions, such as early cancer and tuberculosis, can be cured, but kill if not diagnosed and treated).

Refer or transfer all patients who have blood in the urine for which you cannot find the cause.

Pus in the urine (pyuria)

Look for:
1. urinary tract infection (see page 286); or
2. acute glomerulonephritis (see page 289).

If these conditions are not present, or if treatment is not effective, refer or transfer the patient to medical officer care.

There may be other condition, such as tuberculosis, which must be diagnosed and treated.

Sugar in the urine

You can diagnose sugar in the urine with a positive Benedict's test. There are only two common conditions which cause sugar in the urine:
1. Diabetes mellitus – glucose in the urine
   • Benedict's test and 'Clinitest' tablet test positive
   • 'Clinistix' test also positive
   See Chapter 30 page 333 for management.
2. Pregnancy and lactation – lactose from breast milk in the blood and urine.
   • Benedict's and 'Clinitest' tests positive
   • 'Clinistix' test *negative*
   No treatment necessary.

Protein in the urine (proteinuria or albuminuria)

If you find more than a very little protein in the urine, there is usually a serious disease of the kidneys. Look for the causes:
1. urinary tract infection (see page 286),
2. haematuria (see page 294),
3. pre-eclamptic toxaemia of pregnancy and eclampsia (see an obstetrics book),
4. nephrotic syndrome (see page 287),
5. acute glomerulonephritis (see page 289) or
6. chronic kidney failure (see page 289).

You may find small amounts of protein in the urine of people who have other conditions that do not affect the kidneys directly.
1. heart failure
2. fever of any cause
3. operation

Bile in the urine

See Chapter 24 page 240.

27

Disorders of the Heart and Blood Vessels

Anatomy and physiology

The body is made of many cells. All these cells need food from the intestine and liver and oxygen from the lungs. Waste products and carbon dioxide must also be removed from the cells. The blood takes all things to and from the cells. Many other important things also go from one part of the body to another in the blood (See Chapter 21 page 180). The body, therefore, moves the blood in a big circle through the parts of the body in a special order. The blood moves round this circle in the blood vessels – arteries, capillaries and veins. The heart pumps the blood through the blood vessels. This is called the 'circulation' of the blood (see Figure 27.1). The system of the heart and blood vessels is called the 'cardio-vascular' system. (See Figures 27.2, 27.3, 27.4, 27.5 and 27.6.)

pulmonary artery

pulmonary vein

vena cava

aorta

right auricle

left auricle

right ventricle

left ventricle

portal vein

LUNGS

HEART

hepatic vein

LIVER

INTESTINE

REMAINDER OF BODY

Figure 27.1 (opposite)   Diagram showing circulation of the blood. The blood goes from the lungs to the left side of the heart. This blood contains much oxygen and little carbon dioxide. The left side of the heart pumps the blood through the arteries to the capillaries in the body, and the intestine. Through the walls of these capillaries the blood gives food and oxygen to the cells and removes carbon dioxide and waste products. The blood then goes from the capillaries into veins. The blood in the capillaries of the intestine also takes food from the intestine and it then goes through the portal vein to the liver. In the liver the blood goes into capillaries which put most of the food from the intestine into the liver for storage. The blood from the liver, which contains enough food for the rest of the body, then goes into veins again and travels to the right side of the heart. The blood from the capillaries in the rest of the body travels in veins straight to the right side of the heart. The right side of the heart pumps the blood to the lungs through the pulmonary artery and then into capillaries again. The lungs remove carbon dioxide from the blood and put in oxygen. The capillaries in the lung then join to form the vein which goes to the left side of the heart. The circulation of the blood then starts again.

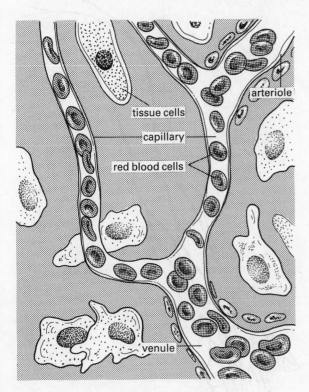

Figure 27.2   Diagram of the smallest arteries (arterioles) and the smallest veins (venules) of the capillaries as seen through the microscope.

Figure 27.3   Diagram showing the main arteries of the body. The names of the arteries are not important.

The heart normally pumps about 70 ml of blood into the blood vessels of the lungs and of the body with every contraction or beat. The heart normally contracts about 70 times every minute.

The blood cannot go back wards into the heart because of the one-way valves (aortic and pulmonary) where the heart is joined to the blood vessels.

The small arteries (arterioles) let the blood go into the capillaries slowly. When the heart beats, the big arteries stretch to let all the blood into them. These stretched big arteries then slowly push the blood through the small arteries and arterioles into the capillaries before the next heart beat. Some blood remains in the arteries before the heart beats again, so there is always pressure in the arteries. When the heart pumps more blood into the arteries the pressure is highest – called the 'systolic blood pressure'. The systolic pressure is

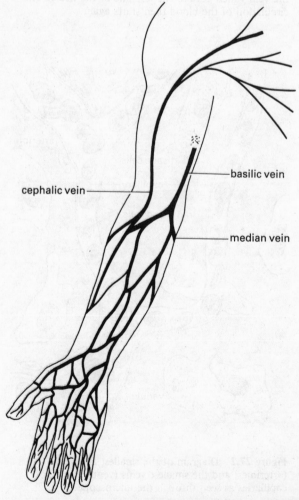

Figure 27.4 Diagram showing the main veins of the body. The names of the veins are not important.

Figure 27.5 Diagram showing the veins of the arm.

aorta

vein bringing blood
from lower body

artery to right lung

veins from right lung

right auricle

right ventricle

vein carrying blood
from upper body

arteries to head and arms

artery to left lung

veins from
left lung

left auricle

left ventricle

Figure 27.6 Diagram showing the internal anatomy of the heart. The arrows show the direction the blood goes. Note the 'one way' valves which make the blood go in one direction only when the heart muscle contracts (gets smaller) and squeezes the blood out of the heart.

normally between 100 and 120 mm mercury when measured with a sphygmomanometer. The pressure in the arteries is lowest just before the heart pumps more blood into the arteries – called the 'diastolic blood pressure'. The diastolic pressure is normally between 70 and 90 mm mercury. The blood pressure (BP) is written with the systolic pressure (e.g. 120) first and the diastolic pressure (e.g. 80) second, like this: BP 120/80.

Pathology

If the blood does not circulate (go round the body), then the body cells cannot work properly. If the circulation of the blood stops, the body cells start to die. If the circulation of the blood to the brain stops for more than 2 or 3 minutes, many of the brain cells die or can never work properly

again – even if the circulation starts again.

The blood does not circulate properly if either of the following things happen.
1. Heart failure. If the heart cannot pump enough blood round the body quickly enough, then heart failure is present.
   For details of heart failure see page 301.
2. Shock. If there is not enough blood in the blood vessels for the heart to pump around the body, then shock is present.
   For details of shock see Chapter 25 page 305.

If the blood pressure remains much higher than the normal blood pressure, this condition is called hypertension (high blood pressure). Hypertension can damage the arteries and the organs they go to. For details about hypertension see Chapter 25 page 300.

Symptoms and signs of cardiovascular disease

Symptoms of cardiovascular disease

Abnormal shortness of breath (dyspnoea)
With mild disease, shortness of breath occurs only after exercise (i.e. walking fast, carrying heavy things, working hard etc.).

With worse disease, shortness of breath also occurs when the patient is sitting or walking slowly.

With severe disease, lying down makes the shortness of breath even worse and sitting up makes it a little better.

There are many causes of shortness of breath other than heart disease. (See Chapter 20 page 177.)

Oedema
Oedema (swelling caused by fluid) of the ankles occurs if the patient usually walks around. Oedema of the back occurs if the patient spends most of the time lying down.

There are many causes of oedema other than heart disease. See Chapter 36 page 398.

Chest pain
Chest pain is not usually caused by heart disease in most developing countries. See Chapter 20 page 179.

Palpitations
Palpitations are present when the patient feels his heart beating faster or harder than normal or irregularly (i.e. out of time). See below.

Signs of cardiovascular disease

Pulse rate (PR) and pulse regularity and pulse volume
The normal PR for adults is 60–80/minute. The normal pulse is regular in time.

The normal pulse has a good volume – you can feel it beat strongly. This means that each contraction of the heart pumps the normal amount of blood into the arteries.

In cardiovascular disease the pulse may be
- fast (more than 100/minutes), or
- slow (less than 60 minutes), or
- small volume (or 'weak') (This means that each contraction of the heart pumps less blood than normal into the arteries.) or
- irregular in time.

If the pulse is irregular or has small volume listen to the heart beat with a stethoscope on the chest to find out the true heart rate. Sometimes the heart beats more quickly than the pulse at the wrist, where you cannot feel some of the small volume beats.

Blood pressure (BP)
The normal BP is

100–140 systolic (*but* it can be lower)

70–90 diastolic (*but* it can be lower)

Many subsistence farmers and rural people have a BP lower than 100/70. If they feel well, the pulse is not fast, and the systolic BP is over 70 and they pass urine, there is no problem.

If the patient has a low BP caused by shock, he will also have the other symptoms and signs of shock – pulse fast (over 100) and weak; breathlessness; pallor; skin usually cold and moist; etc.

If the BP is higher than 160 systolic (or 120 if pregnant) or 100 diastolic (or 90 if pregnant), the patient has high blood pressure or hypertension.

Signs of heart failure (see page 301)
1. Raised jugular venous pressure ⎫
2. enlarged liver ⎬ (almost always)
3. oedema ⎭
4. fast pulse (usually)
5. cyanosis (often)
6. crackles in the lungs (sometimes)

Signs of shock (see page 306)
1. The patient is dizzy, faint, restless or even unconscious.
2. The pulse is fast (over 100) and small volume (sometimes you cannot feel it at all).
3. The blood pressure is low (less than 100 and often less than 70 systolic) (sometimes you cannot record it at all).
4. Shortness of breath (usually deep breaths)
5. Pallor or paleness
6. Skin cold and moist (occasionally warm and dry; but only in *some* severe infections)
7. The patient makes little or no urine.

Heart failure

Definitions and diagnosis

Heart failure is present if the heart cannot pump enough blood around the body quickly enough. Heart failure may be acute or chronic, severe or mild.

You can check the amount of blood the heart is pumping round the body by examining these things.

1. *The pulse* – in heart failure it is usually fast (more than 100/minute) and has a small volume (it feels weak). But a very slow pulse less than 40/minute or an irregular pulse can also occur in heart failure.
2. *The blood pressure* – in heart failure it is usually normal or low. But high BP for a long time may cause heart failure.
3. *The colour and temperature of the body tissues, especially the skin* – in heart failure the skin is often cool and cyanosed (blue).

Acute severe heart failure can cause shock if the heart can only pump a very little blood round the body (see Chapter 25 page 305).

Also blood can return to the heart from the body more quickly than the heart can pump it out again. This causes the veins behind the heart to become overfilled and they distend (or stretch). Some fluid from the blood leaks (goes out) of the distended veins and causes oedema (swelling) of the organs nearby. You can check for overfilling of the veins by looking for these things:

1. oedema of legs and sacral area (lower part of back),
2. enlargement of the liver,
3. distension of the veins in the neck (raised jugular venous pressure) (see Figure 27.7), and
4. oedema of the lungs causing crackles in the lower parts of the lungs.

Figure 27.7 Diagrams showing jugular venous pressure. (1) Note that in all positions in all persons (as in this patient), the vertical height of the sternal angle remains 5 cm above the level of the middle of the right atrium. (2) Note that the jugular venous pressure is normally not higher than the level of the sternal angle. (3) Therefore, in a normal person, the jugular veins are full when he is lying flat. You can see the top of the pulsation of the jugular veins of a normal person best when the patient is lying at 45° (i.e. half way up). If he is lying lower the veins are normally full. If he is lying higher the top of the pulsation is behind the clavicle, and too deep in the neck to see. (4) So, as the jugular venous pressure rises, the patient must sit further upright for you to see the *upper level* of the pulsation (otherwise the upper level is in the head). But you can see the venous pulsations of the neck at a higher level that normal (the sternal angle level).

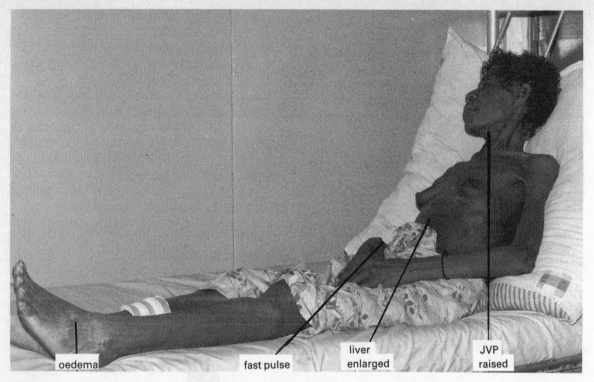

Figure 27.8 A patient with heart failure. Note the usual feature of heart failure.

It is also possible to examine the heart for signs of heart failure. But this is difficult and you should not try do it.

Diagnose heart failure by
almost always (1) raised jugular venous
    pressure (2) enlarged liver (3) oedema
and usually (4) fast pulse
and often (5) cyanosis
and sometimes (6) crepitations in the chest

When you diagnose heart failure, always look for the cause.

Unfortunately it is not possible to treat many of the causes of heart failure. But you can cure or help some of the causes of heart failure. It is important that you quickly diagnose and treat causes that will result in death unless treated. If you cannot diagnose the cause or if you cannot treat the cause in the health centre, then refer or transfer the patient for the Medical Officer to diagnose and treat. However, if you can diagnose the cause

and there is no treatment possible for the cause, then do not transfer the patient.

Common causes of heart failure which you can treat include:
1. *Severe acute pneumonia*. The toxins from the organisms damage the heart muscles. Also the heart does not get enough oxygen from the blood which has gone through the diseased lung. But the heart must pump faster and do more work because of the infection. These things can cause heart failure.
2. *Chronic lung disease* usually caused by chronic obstructive lung disease (COLD) (but in some countries caused by schistosomiasis). Chronic lung disease destroys many blood vessels in the lungs. The remaining blood vessels contract and become narrow. The heart tries to pump the normal amount of blood through these few narrow vessels. So the pressure rises and makes the heart work harder. Finally the heart cannot do all this work, and it fails. Little blood then goes through the lungs. Much blood distends the veins behind the heart. This causes congestion (overfilling of the veins) and oedema of the organs behind the heart.

If acute lung infection (acute bronchitis or pneumonia) then occurs, the toxins damage the heart, less oxygen goes to the heart and the heart failure gets worse. The heart failure may start or get worse during an acute chest infection (acute bronchitis or pneumonia) in a patient with COLD (chronic obstructive lung disease).

The most common cause of heart failure is an acute chest infection in a person with chronic lung disease.

---

3. *Other infections* which affect the heart, including:
   Typhus fever
   Trypanosomiasis both acute and chronic (Chagas Disease in South America and East African Trypanosomiasis in Africa)
   Typhoid fever
   Relapsing fever
   Septicaemia.
4. *Severe anaemia*
   The blood contains a small amount of haemoglobin, so the heart must pump it around the body more quickly to take enough oxygen to the body. But while it does this extra work, the heart gets less oxygen. This can cause heart failure.
5. If you give a *large volume of intravenous fluid* (or a smaller volume too quickly) to someone who already has a condition (such as anaemia) which can cause heart failure, the extra work of pumping this extra fluid can make the heart fail.
6. *Beriberi*. If the diet is poor and there is not enough vitamin B_1 (also called aneurine or thiamine) in it, the heart muscle cannot pump properly. The lack of vitamin B_1 also makes the blood vessels dilate (get bigger) and so the heart must pump more blood to fill the blood vessels. These things cause heart failure. Sometimes the lack of vitamin B_1 also stops the nerves in the legs working properly, and this causes pain and weakness in the legs. Beriberi occurs most often in poor people, in people during a famine or in alcoholics.
7. *Acute rheumatic fever*.
8. *A patient with heart failure stops his treatment*.

9. *'Epidemic dropsy'*
   If a group of people eat food which contains mustard oil and then develop heart failure and other symptoms and signs, notify the Medical Officer immediately (and tell the people not to eat mustard oil until the Medical Officer has it tested for a poison).

You can diagnose all, and treat most, of the above conditions at the health centre.

There are some other conditions which a medical officer can diagnose and treat but you cannot. There are other conditions which the medical officer can diagnose but cannot treat. These diseases include:
congenital heart disease,
thyrotoxic heart disease,
hypertension,
pericarditis (especially tuberculous pericarditis),
chronic rheumatic valvular disease,
infective endocarditis,
syphilitic heart disease,
coronary artery disease
endomyocardial fibrosis, and
cardiomyopathies of various sorts.

Differential diagnosis

Check that the patient does not have another cause for the symptoms or signs of heart failure:
- *oedema* – toxaemia of pregnancy, nephrotic syndrome, chronic liver disease or filariasis, etc. See Chapter 36 page 398.
- *enlarged tender liver* – especially amoebic abscess. See Chapter 24 page 247.
- *shortness of breath* – especially pneumonia, acute bronchitis, asthma or tuberculosis. See Chapter 20 page 177.

If you think the patient could have heart failure always look for raised jugular venous pressure (almost always raised if there is heart failure).

Treatment

1. Treat the heart failure itself.
2. Look for and treat the cause of the heart failure.

Treat the heart failure itself

> 1. Rest
> 2. Oxygen if acute and severe
> 3. Diuretics
> 4. No salt in food
> 5. Potassium chloride if necessary
> 6. Aminophylline if necessary
> 7. Digoxin, only in special cases

1. Rest
Sit the patient up in bed if he is in an acute stage and short of breath. The patient must rest for some weeks if he is in a chronic stage; but do not stop him walking around.

2. Oxygen if acute and severe
Give intranasal oxygen 1–2 litres/minute. Give only in acute heart failure. *Do not* give more than 2 litres/minute if he has COLD. There is not usually enough oxygen available for treatment of chronic heart failure from COLD.

3. Diuretics
Give frusemide 40 mg (4 ml) IVI immediately for acute heart failure. You can repeat this in ½–1 hour if necessary and increase the dose to 60–80 mg (6–8 ml) if necessary.

Give hydrochlorothiazide 50–100 mg (1–2 tabs) every morning in the acute and the chronic stage.

Give frusemide 40–160 mg (1–4 tabs) also every morning if the hydrochlorothiazide tabs are not effective.

> Diuretics are the most effective and important treatment in most cases

However, do not give a diuretic if the patient has shock. If the patient has shock, give digoxin.

4. No salt in food
Tell the patient not to put salt in his food.

5. Potassium chloride if necessary
Give potassium chloride 1200 mg (2 tabs) three times a day if on diuretics *and if*
(a) the patient is taking frusemide *and* hydrochlorothiazide; *or*
(b) he is *not* on a tuber diet (e.g. sweet potato, yam, taro, etc.); *or*
(c) he *is* taking digoxin.

6. Aminophylline or theophylline if necessary
Give aminophylline by *slow* IVI –
For a large adult (> 50 kg), give 375 mg (15 ml)
For a small adult (< 50 kg), give 250 mg (10 ml)
Give it by *slow* IVI (take 10 minutes by the clock).

Give aminophylline for acute severe heart failure after the frusemide and for acute heart failure that is not responding to all the other treatment.

Also give for chronic heart failure that is not responding to all other treatment.

After this large starting dose, give only a small dose, 100 mg (1 tab) twice daily for a small adult or 100 mg (1 tab) three times a day for a large adult (i.e. about half (½) of the dose for asthma).

Stop if there is nausea or vomiting not caused by digoxin. Increase the dose every 2–3 days until the heart failure is controlled or nausea or vomiting occurs. Do not give more than 400 mg daily if heart failure.

7. Digoxin, only in special cases
Give digoxin *only if*
(a) there is heart failure from acute severe pneumonia in a previously healthy person (with no COLD) *or*
(b) the patient has shock (Do not give diuretics if the patient has shock. Use digoxin instead.) *or*
(c) all the other treatment for heart failure (above) and treatment of the cause (below) does not control the heart failure.

Digoxin is not given often in health centres.
The signs of too much digoxin are:
(a) loss of appetite or vomiting or
(b) pulse slow (< 60) or irregular (if the pulse was not slow or irregular before starting digoxin).

If the signs of too much digoxin develop *then*:
(a) *stop the digoxin* for 48 hours,
(b) *after* 48 *hours* start the digoxin again at *only half of the previous dose.*

Digoxin dose
– 0.5 mg (½ mg) or 500 mcg (2 ml or 2 tabs) every 6 hours for 2 doses *for large, young adult* IMI or orally
– 0.5 mg (½ mg) or 500 mcg (2 ml or 2 tabs) once

only *for small or old adult* by IMI or orally *then*

– 0.25 mg (¼ mg) (1 tab) daily *for* large young adult orally
– 0.125 mg (1/8 mg) (½ tab) daily *for small or old adult* orally

> You must always give potassium chloride (2 tablets three times a day) if you are giving diuretics with the digoxin.

> If a patient on digoxin loses his appetite or vomits or his pulse is slow or irregular, **stop the digoxin** for 48 hours and **then** give it at only **half of the previous daily dose**.

Look for and treat the underlying cause

1. Chest infections – give antibiotics, etc. See pneumonia (Chapter 20 page 164).

> Antibiotics are an essential part of the treatment in most cases of heart failure as chest infection is a common cause.

2. Chronic obstructive lung disease. See Chapter 20 page 171.
3. Other infections and septicaemia. See Chapter 12.
4. Anaemia. See Chapter 21 page 182.
5. Beriberi – aneurine (thiamine or vitamin B_1) 50 mg (1 ml) IMI immediately, then aneurine 50 mg (1 tab) orally daily for 2 weeks.
   Give a good mixed diet.
   Give aneurine to all patients who have no obvious underlying cause for heart failure; especially if the patient is on a poor diet (famine, old, drinks a lot of alcohol or has bad dietary habits), or is anaemic, or has weak or painful legs.
6. IV saline or blood given too fast – stop or slow down the drip.
7. A patient on treatment who has stopped his drugs – start treatment again.

Refer or transfer to medical officer

1. All cases of heart failure who do *not* have COLD or anaemia or another treatable cause (for diagnosis – because they may have a curable cause) (non urgent).

2. All cases of heart failure with an irregular pulse (urgent if acute heart failure).

Shock

The medical term shock means collapse because not enough blood is circulating through the body. Shock is always acute and very serious. (Shock, in the medical sense, has nothing to do with the 'shock' people are said to have when they get a big surprise or very bad news and are mentally upset.)

There are two causes of shock:

1. There is not enough volume of blood. This can be caused by loss of blood itself through broken blood vessels, or loss of just the water and salt from the blood through blood vessel walls (as in dehydration, burns, septicaemia, etc.) or not enough water and salt absorbed into the blood vessels (as in late stages of dehydration especially from gastro-enteritis).
2. There is widening of some of the venous and capillary blood vessels. Blood collects in these blood vessels and does not return to the heart.

In either case, there is not enough blood for the heart to pump around the body and fill the arteries, and so the blood pressure falls.

The body then tries to keep the blood going to the most important parts of the body (brain, heart and liver) by closing down the blood vessels to the less important parts (skin, muscles, gastro-intestinal tract and later kidneys). These parts then become pale and do not work properly. Also the heart pumps all the blood there is fast round the body, i.e. the pulse rate is fast.

If, after this, there is still not enough blood for the heart to pump round to the brain, liver and heart, these organs also do not work properly. If the blood volume is not quickly increased the patient soon dies.

Shock can sometimes occur when the heart cannot pump the blood around the body even when there is enough blood (acute severe heart failure). See page 301.

Diagnosis

The diagnosis of shock is usually obvious from the symptoms and signs (see Figure 27.9).

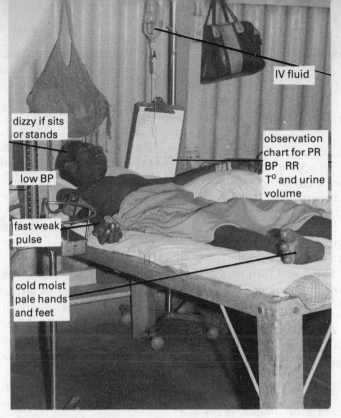

dizzy if sits or stands

low BP

fast weak pulse

cold moist pale hands and feet

IV fluid

observation chart for PR BP RR T° and urine volume

Figure 27.9 A patient who has shock. Note the usual features of shock. Note two essential things in treatment.

1. The patient feels weak, faint and dizzy (especially when he stands up, but often also when sitting). In severe cases, he is restless or unconscious. This is because not enough blood is going to the brain.
2. The pulse is fast (over 100/minute) and has a small volume.
3. The blood pressure is low (less than 100 and usually less than 70 systolic).
4. There is shortness of breath (deep breaths).
5. There is pallor or paleness.
6. The skin is cold and moist (sometimes in some infections the skin may be warm and dry).
7. Little or no urine is made.

Cause

The cause of shock is usually obvious. If it is not, find out from the history and examination of the patient (see Chapter 6). *Do this while you are starting treatment* for the shock. The cause is usually one of these things:

1. Loss of blood or fluid from the blood vessels.
   - external bleeding

   - internal bleeding (e.g. from ruptured spleen or ectopic pregnancy)
   - burns
   - gastro-enteritis
   - malaria
   - severe infections (peritonitis, septicaemia, typhus fever, relapsing fever, etc.)
   - allergic reactions.
2. Dilation of blood vessels.
   - infections
   - allergic reaction
   - severe pain
   - fright or fear   'fainting' – usually a
   - standing still for a   *slow* pulse
   long time
3. The heart not pumping properly.
   - severe infections with toxaemia and low oxygen e.g. severe pneumonia malaria, acute tryponosamiasis, typhus fever, relapsing fever, 'heart attack'
   - chronic trypanosomiasis (Chagas Disease).

306

Management of a patient with shock

Immediately put up an intravenous drip of 0.9% sodium chloride (even before you diagnose the cause).

Diagnose the cause. The cause is usually obvious. If it is not, diagnose it from the history and examination of the patient (or from a history given by the patients relatives or friends). *Do this while you are putting up the drip.*

Shock is usually caused by:
1. loss of fluid ⎫
2. loss of blood ⎭ (common)
3. septicaemia or infection ⎫
4. allergy ⎬ (uncommon)
5. heart not pumping properly (very uncommon).

If no cause is obvious, look carefully for internal bleeding (especially ruptured spleen or ectopic pregnancy). If you cannot find the cause, treat for shock from septicaemia.

Management
1. Keep the airway clear. Give artificial ventilation if necessary.
2. Give oxygen.
3. Give analgesics, if severe pain.
4. Keep the patient lying down and warm.
5. Diagnose and treat the cause.
   (a) If loss of fluids – give IV fluids
   (b) If loss of blood – stop bleeding
   Give IV fluids and/or plasma volume expander and/or blood.
   (c) If septicaemia – Give IV chloramphenicol, quinine, fluids, digoxin.
   (d) If acute allergic reaction –
   Give IM or IV adrenaline
   Give IV antihistamine
   Give IV fluids
6. Look for signs of heart failure. Treat heart failure if it occurs.
7. Transfer patient if necessary.

Treatment depends on the cause (see below). But do the following in all cases,
1. Make sure the airway is clear. If the patient unconscious, give routine care of the airway for an unconscious patient (see Chapter 25 page 264). If he is not breathing enough, give artificial ventilation (see Chapter 37 page 416).

2. Give intranasal oxygen, 4 litres/minute.
3. If there is severe pain give pethidine (75 mg (1½ ml) for small adult or 100 mg (2 ml) for large adult *slowly* over 5 minutes by IVI.
4. Keep the patient lying down flat with the legs raised. Keep the patient warm but not hot.
5. *Treat the cause* (see below).

When loss of fluid (dehydration) is the cause (usually from gastro-enteritis) treat as described below.

IV 0.9% *sodium chloride* as fast as possible until signs of shock go. Check the patient after each litre. Give up to 4 litres. If the patient is still shocked after 3–4 litres, he needs IV plasma volume expander.

IV *plasma volume expander* (e.g. 'Haemaccel' or SPPS) as fast as possible until the signs of shock disappear. Give 0.5–1.5 litres (1–3 bottles).

When the signs of shock go, finish that bottle of plasma volume expander, then change back to 0.9% sodium chloride.

IV 0.9% *sodium chloride* 1 litre every hour until the signs of dehydration go.

See gastro-enteritis (Chapter 23 page 224) for details of replacement of continuing fluid losses and maintenance fluids.

If the 3–4 litres of 0.9% sodium chloride and the 1.5 litres of plasma volume expander do not cure the patient's shock, there is probably also another cause of the shock, e.g. septicaemia *or* hidden blood loss. See below for treatment.

When loss of blood is the cause (e.g. bleeding peptic ulcer, obstetric bleeding, trauma, etc.) treat as described below.

Stop the bleeding if possible. If you cannot certainly stop the bleeding arrange an urgent blood transfusion and emergency transfer.

Give IV 0.9% *sodium chloride* as fast as possible. Give up to 1500 ml. If the signs of shock go, finish off that bag of saline and then change to maintenance fluids (0.18% sodium chloride in 4.3% dextrose, 1 litre every 8 hours – see Chapter 23 page 224).

If the signs of shock are still present after

1500 ml 0.9% sodium chloride, give: IV *plasma volume expander* (e.g. 'Haemaccel' or SPPS) as fast as possible. If the signs of shock go, finish that bottle of plasma volume expander and change to maintenance fluids (See above or Chapter 23).

If the signs of shock have not gone when you are giving the third bottle i.e. 1000–1500 ml, the patient needs *blood*.

If possible transfer the patient to a medical officer before blood is necessary. If you cannot transfer the patient quickly, see a reference book for details of how to crossmatch and give blood.

> When septicaemia or other acute severe infection is the cause treat as described below.

Treat for septicaemia if:
(a) the history, symptoms or signs suggest septicaemia; *or*
(b) there is no obvious cause for shock.

Give IV *chloramphenicol* 2 g immediately then 1 g every 6 hours.

Give 2 g (2 bottles) by IVI immediately. If *immediate* IVI is not possible, give 1 g (1 bottle) by IMI. Then give an IV 1 g dose also as soon as an IVI possible.

If an IV dose is still not possible 1 hour after the first IM dose, then give another 1 g (1 bottle) by IMI.

Give 1 g by IVI or by IMI every 6 hours after the first dose.

Give by IVI if – shock is still present or
– a drip is necessary.

For details about antibiotics, see acute severe bacterial infections (Chapter 11 and Chapter 12).

Give IVI *quinine* 10 mg/kg (if unable to weigh patient, 10 ml if large adult and 7½ ml if small adult) in 500 ml 0.18% sodium chloride slowly over the first 4 hours in another (a second) drip. Give by IMI if another IV drip is not possible. Complete the treatment course. (See malaria Chapter 13 page 55.)

Give IV *fluids* as in 'Loss of fluids' (above). But do not give more than the least fluid necessary to correct the shock. Look carefully for heart failure; treat it, if it occurs (stop IV fluids and see page 301).

> When acute allergic reaction is the cause (anaphylactic reaction) treat as described below.

Give IMI *adrenaline* tart. 1–1000 solution 0.5 ml (½ ml) immediately. (If the patient is about to die, you can give the adrenaline intravenously slowly at 0.1 ml (or 1/10 ml) every minute i.e. 0.5 ml (or ½ ml) in 5 minutes).

Give IVI *promethazine* 50 mg (2 ml) immediately.

Give IV *fluids* as in 'Loss of fluids' (above). Watch carefully for heart failure; treat it if it occurs (page 301).

Repeat the antihistamine and adrenaline after 10 minutes if necessary.

6. When you give intravenous fluids, look carefully for signs of heart failure.

Signs of heart failure are high jugular venous pressure or shortness of breath and crackles in the lungs that were not present before the IV fluids started. Later the liver enlarges and becomes tender and oedema develops.

Heart failure is not probable in shock from dehydration or blood loss until the fluid or blood loss is cured.

When mild heart failure occurs –
• Change to 0.18% sodium chloride in 4.3% dextrose and slow the drip to 1 litre every 12 hours.
• Give digoxin 0.5 mg or 500 mg (2 ml) IV slowly over 2 minutes immediately *or* 0.5 mg (2 tabs) immediately. See page 304 before you give further doses.

When severe heart failure occurs (patient becomes very breathless or has a lot of crackles in his chest)
• Stop the IV fluids.
• Give frusemide 40 mg (4 ml) IVI immediately once and repeat in ½ to 1 hour if necessary.
• Give aminophylline once. Give 375 mg (15 ml) for a large adult (> 50 kg) or 250 mg (10 ml) for a small adult (< 50 kg) slowly – take 10 minutes by the clock. See Chapter 20

page 171 before you give more doses. See heart failure page 301.

- Give digoxin (see above).

Transfer to medical officer care

1. Any case which needs blood transfusion (urgent – emergency).
2. Any case which does not greatly improve with treatment in 3 hours (urgent – emergency).
3. Any case for which you cannot find or treat the underlying cause successfully in a health centre (urgent – emergency).

Prevention

Prevention is by carefully observing and giving proper treatment early to all patients who have a condition which can cause shock.

Ischaemic heart disease or coronary artery disease

Definition

Ischaemic heart disease is a condition caused by narrowing of the coronary arteries which take blood to the heart muscle. Not enough blood can go to the heart muscle and this damages the heart muscle.

Frequency and cause

This disease is uncommon in village people in non-industrialised countries who still live in their traditional ways. But, it occurs in middle-aged town people who have western ways of living, eating, smoking, working and not exercising. It is more common in people with high blood pressure or diabetes mellitus, especially if they are not treated properly. It is very common in middle-aged and old people in industrialised countries.

Pathology, symptoms and signs, complications

The blood vessels that take blood from the aorta to the heart muscle are narrowed or completely blocked. So the heart muscle does not get enough blood.

Narrowing of the arteries can cause central chest pain or discomfort (like a tight band around the chest or the feeling of a heavy weight in the centre of the chest). The pain is sometimes also in the jaw or the arms but it is almost always in the centre of the chest. This pain or discomfort comes when the patient exercises but goes quickly when he stops the exercise. This is called 'angina pectoris' or just 'angina'. The narrowing of the arteries can also make the heart beat irregularly. It can also make the heart weak and cause heart failure.

Sometimes a coronary artery becomes completely blocked. Then a part of the heart muscle will die. This causes a constant severe central chest pain which often also goes to the jaw and to the arms. The heart beat and the pulse may be irregular. There may be shock or cardiac failure. This is called a 'myocardial infarct' or a 'heart attack'.

Differential diagnosis

Check that it is not another cause of chest pain (see Chapter 20 page 179) or heart failure (see page 301) or shock (see page 305).

Treatment

Treatment of a 'heart attack'

1. Make the patient rest and sit or lie down.
2. If pain is present give morphine 10–15 mg (1–1.5 ml) or pethidine 100–150 mg (2–3 ml) IMI and repeat the dose when necessary.
3. Treat any heart failure present in the usual way including diuretics, oxygen and digoxin (see page 304).
4. If the pulse is irregular give an injection of lignocaine 100 mg IMI immediately (10 ml of a 1% solution or 5 ml of a 2% solution), and repeat 50 mg (5 ml of a 1% solution or 2.5 ml or a 2% solution) every hour if the pulse remains irregular.

Treatment of other conditions

1. Carefully look for and treat any anaemia present.
2. Glyceryl trinitrate 600 mcg (0.6 mg) tablets are used for treatment of angina. The patient must dissolve one tablet under the tongue when angina occurs or before exercise which causes angina in that patient. He must repeat the dose as often as necessary but not as often as causes

side effects such as headache, feeling hot or fainting.
3. Treat heart failure in the usual way.
4. Consult with a medical officer about the treatment of these and other conditions which may present.

Consultation – transfer – referral

Arrange immediate emergency transfer to medical officer care for any 'heart attack' patient.

Arrange non-urgent transfer or consultation with the next visiting medical officer for any patient you think has one of the other conditions caused by this disease.

Prevention

People should not eat too much animal fat or refined carbohydrates (such as white sugar); not get fat; not smoke; exercise regularly; and get proper treatment for hypertension or diabetes mellitus, etc.

28

Disorders of the Bones and Muscles

Anatomy

See Figure 28.1.

Osteomyelitis

Osteomyelitis is an infection of the bone.

Acute osteomyelitis is caused by bacteria, usually staphylococci (which may be resistant to penicillin), and, in some parts of the world, salmonellae (which are usually resistant to penicillin).

Chronic osteomyelitis can develop from acute osteomyelitis that is not treated properly. Chronic osteomyelitis can also be a chronic infection from the start and is then often caused by tuberculosis bacteria, usually in the spine. Chronic osteomyel-

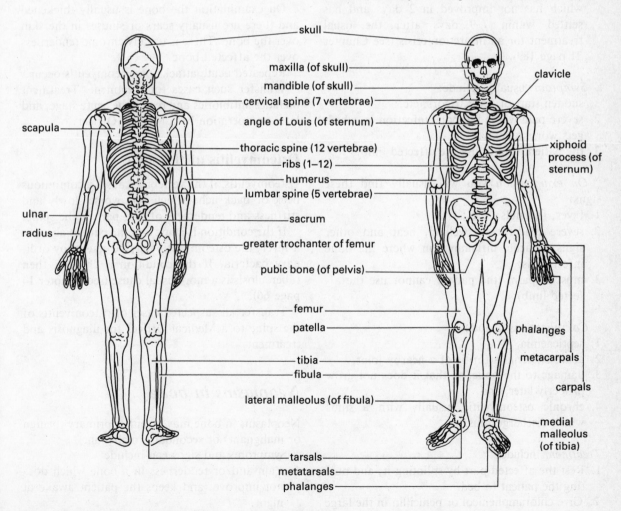

Figure 28.1 Diagram showing the skeleton (or bones of the body).

- skull
- maxilla (of skull)
- mandible (of skull)
- cervical spine (7 vertebrae)
- angle of Louis (of sternum)
- thoracic spine (12 vertebrae)
- ribs (1–12)
- humerus
- lumbar spine (5 vertebrae)
- sacrum
- greater trochanter of femur
- pubic bone (of pelvis)
- femur
- patella
- tibia
- fibula
- lateral malleolus (of fibula)
- tarsals
- metatarsals
- phalanges
- scapula
- ulnar
- radius
- clavicle
- xiphoid process (of sternum)
- phalanges
- metacarpals
- carpals
- medial malleolus (of tibia)

itis in the other bones is usually caused by ordinary bacteria.

Acute osteomyelitis

The organism carrying the bone infection usually goes to the bone through the blood.

The *history* from the patient usually includes:
1. A recent skin infection that may be still present (often).
2. A recent injury to the bone (often).
3. The sudden start of symptoms and signs.

Another history suggestive of acute osteomyelitis is
1. A patient with sickle cell disease.
2. The sudden onset of symptoms and signs in a bone (often the fingers or toes, but any bone) which has not improved in 2 days and has settled within 7–9 days after the usual treatment for an infarction crisis (see Chapter 21 page 189).

Symptoms usually include:
1. sudden start of fever, rigors, etc.;
2. severe pain where the bone infection is, which gets worse quickly;
3. the patient cannot use the affected limb.

On examination you will usually find these signs:
1. fever, fast pulse, etc.;
2. severe tenderness, swelling, heat and other signs of acute inflammation where the bone infection is;
3. muscle spasm (the patient cannot use the affected limb).

Complications include:
1. septicaemia,
2. acute bacterial arthritis of a nearby joint,
3. damage to the bone, so that it does not grow properly later, and
4. chronic osteomyelitis, usually with a sinus which discharges pus.

Treatment includes
1. Rest the affected part by splinting it, and putting the patient to bed.
2. Give chloramphenicol or penicillin in the large doses as for any acute severe bacterial infec-

tion. (See Chapter 11 page 42.) But you must continue the antibiotic for at least 4 weeks. You can reduce the dose when the patient appears to be cured; but you must still continue the antibiotic until at least 4 weeks.
3. Analgesics (See Chapter 7 page 28).

Transfer the patient for operation if:
1. the affected area is not much improved in 2 days, or
2. it does not appear to be completely cured in 2 weeks.

Chronic osteomyelitis

Symptoms may include continuous or repeated discharge of pus from a sinus over the affected bone.

On examination the bone is usually thickened and there are usually scars or sinuses in the skin over the bone. There is usually chronic tenderness over the affected bone.

Repeated acute attacks of osteomyelitis occur.

Transfer such cases for treatment. Treatment includes antibiotics and rest in the acute stage, and later an operation by a Medical Officer.

Osteomyelitis of the spine

Osteomyelitis of the vertebrae causes a continuous neck or back ache which gets worse slowly and stiffness and tenderness of that part of the spine.

If the condition is acute and the patient also has a fever, the osteomyelitis may be caused by ordinary bacteria. If the condition is chronic, then tuberculosis is a more usual cause (see Chapter 14 page 66).

Transfer all suspected cases of osteomyelitis of the spine to a Medical Officer for diagnosis and treatment.

Neoplasms in bone

Neoplasms in bone may be either primary (benign or malignant) or secondary (malignant).

Symptoms and signs can include:
1. Pain and/or tenderness in a bone which does not improve, and keeps the patient awake at night.
2. A deformity of a bone – most often a lump.

3. A pathological fracture (a fracture after only a small injury or no injury, because the bone was weak because it had been partly replaced by a cancer).
4. Compression of the spinal cord, if vertebrae affected by the cancer collapse.
5. Anaemia.

See a reference book for diagnosis and management.

Pyomyositis or tropical myositis

Pyomyositis is an acute bacterial infection of one or more of the large skeletal muscles. An abscess usually forms in the muscle and general symptoms and signs of infection develop. If you do not give treatment the condition can become chronic.

Pyomyositis is common only in developing and tropical countries.

Symptoms and signs include:
1. General symptoms and signs of infection – malaise, fever, fast pulse etc. If a large abscess or septicaemia develop, these become severe.
2. Pain in the affected muscle, which is present at rest and much worse when the patient moves the muscle. The affected muscle is firm and tender and painful if stretched during examination.
3. The general and local symptoms and signs of infection get much worse in the next few days. The muscle may become fluctuant; but only if it is just under the skin.
4. If it is not treated, the affected muscle becomes a bag of pus, and the patient becomes wasted, with anaemia etc. Septicaemia and death can occur.

Differential diagnosis of painful muscles:
1. generalised illness, e.g. malaria, influenza
2. unusual exercise
3. trauma to muscles
4. parasitic diseases of the muscle (e.g. trichinosis)
5. pain in nearby structures
   – joints,
   – bones (osteomyelitis or fracture),
   – tendons
6. referred pain
7. others – see a medical reference book.

If the diagnosis is not certain, put a needle into the affected muscle. You can usually aspirate pus if the condition is pyomyositis.

Treatment is simple, if you make the diagnosis.
1. Antibiotics.
   If possible use tetracycline, as it needs no injections and the organisms are usually sensitive to it. Penicillin is often also effective. Chloramphenicol may be needed. (See Chapter 11 page 42.)
2. Incision and drainage, if pus has formed.
   This is best done under general anaesthetic. Bleeding is sometimes severe and may need packing of the abscess cavity and local pressure to stop it.

29

Disorders of Joints (Arthritis)

B Fibrous joint -
no movement possible

Example: skull joints

Anatomy

There are three types of joints in the body (see Figure 29.1).

A freely moveable joint.

Example: elbow joint

C Cartilaginous joint -
some movement possible

Example: spine

Figure 29.1 Diagram to show three types of joint. Note that in the freely moveable type joint the articular cartilage is often not present. (For details of the anatomy of the spine see Chapter 25 page 271.)

Pathology, symptoms and signs

Arthritis is inflammation of a joint. Arthritis may be acute or chronic.

Symptoms and signs in the affected joint itself

The joint can have any of the usual symptoms and signs of inflammation.
1. Pain – acute and chronic cases
2. Tenderness – acute cases only
3. Swelling – acute and chronic cases
4. Heat – acute cases only
5. Redness and shinyness – acute cases only
6. Loss of function – i.e. not able to move properly (active and passive) and not able to work properly or bear weight – acute and chronic cases
7. Abnormal fluid in the joint itself (called 'effusion') – acute and chronic cases

The patient complains of
- pain,
- swelling, and
- loss of function (cannot move or use the joint).

On examination (depending on the type of arthritis):
Inspection
- swelling
- redness
- deformity
Palpation
- swelling
– fluid
– bone overgrowth at edges of joint
– soft tissue swelling
- tenderness
- heat
- movement
– passive (patient rests and you move the joint), less than mormal, painful, sometimes with crepitus (a grating feeling or noise)
– active (patient moves the joint), less than normal, painful, sometimes with crepitus
Work or weight bearing
- less than normal or not possible

Symptoms and signs in the muscles which move the affected joint

In acute arthritis the muscles go into spasm so that the joint cannot be moved normally (movement causes pain). Later, and in chronic arthritis, the muscles waste and become thin and weak.

Even later, if the patient does not have physiotherapy, the muscles and tendons become shortened and changed into bands of fibrous tissues and cannot be stretched. These hold the joint in abnormal positions. These muscle and tendon changes are called contractures.

General symptoms and signs

These can include fever, fast pulse, malaise, wasting, etc.
1. Some may be the result of the cause of arthritis e.g. rheumatic fever.
2. Some may be caused by the effect of the arthritis e.g. toxins from the bacteria causing acute bacterial arthritis.

Disease in other parts of the body may be present and cause symptoms and signs

An example is tuberculosis of the lungs in a patient with tuberculous arthritis.

Note on examination of the spine

Check for:
1. deformity (lump or twisting) of the spine,
2. tender areas on palpation or percussion of the spine,
3. movement of the spine in all directions,
4. legs – movement and sensation,
5. abdomen – bladder enlargement or incontinence of urine

Tests

The only important test you must do at a health centre is *the aspiration of a joint if the joint may be infected with bacteria (septic arthritis).* (Put a needle into the joint and suck out any fluid with a syringe.) If pus is present, you must give antibiotics in high dosage.

Always use careful aseptic procedure when you aspirate a joint. Do not introduce bacteria into the joint and cause acute bacterial (septic) arthritis. Scrub up. Use mask gown and gloves. Prepare the skin carefully with iodine in spirit or another suitable antiseptic. Use sterile needles and syringes. Always give a local anaesthetic before putting the large needle into the joint. Suck out all of the fluid which is in the joint. Put a sterile dressing over the needle hole.

Method of aspirating joints

These diagrams show where you can put a needle into the various joints (see Figures 29.2, 29.3, 29.4, 29.5, 29.6 and 29.7). But do *not* try to aspirate a hip joint unless you have had special training. Transfer a patient who needs aspiration of the hip joint to a Medical Officer.

Figure 29.2 Methods of aspirating the knee joint. The top diagrams show an anterior method you can use when the knee is flexed (bent). The lower diagram shows a lateral method you can use when the knee is extended (straight). Usually you will use the lower method as a patient with acute arthritis usually cannot flex (bend) the knee.

316

Figure 29.3 Method of aspirating the ankle joint.

Figure 29.4 Method of aspirating the hip joint. Do not try to aspirate the hip joint unless you have had proper training.

Figure 29.5 Method of aspirating the wrist (radio-carpal) joint.

Figure 29.6 (left) Method of aspirating the shoulder (scapulo-humeral joint).

Figure 29.7 (below) Method of aspirating the elbow (radio-humeral) joint.

Details of joint conditions

Table 29.1 The common causes of acute and chronic arthritis

Acute		Chronic
1. Traumatic	The most common	1. Osteo-
2. Acute bacterial (septic)	The most important as (1) treatment cures (2) joint destroyed if not treated	2. Chronic bacterial (septic) 3. Tuberculous
3. Rheumatic fever		
4. Tropical arthritis	Acute, recurrent or chronic	4. Tropical artritis
5. Rheumatoid	Usually chronic	5. Rheumatoid
6. Others See page 326	Usually acute See page 326 and Medical Reference Book	6. Others See page 326

Traumatic arthritis

Traumatic arthritis is an acute arthritis caused by an injury to the joint. There is usually *a history* of an injury.

On examination you will find:
1. acute arthritis with tenderness over the damaged area of the joint or of the ligaments around the joint; and usually and effusion;
2. no general symptoms and signs of infection.

Aspiration shows clear yellow fluid or blood.
Treatment includes:
1. aspiration of the joint;
2. splint until the acute stage is finished;
3. exercise muscles in the splint – 10 contractions of the muscles which move the joint in the splint, 4 times a day (but without letting the joint bend);
4. aspirin if necessary.

Transfer to Medical Officer if:
1. there are signs which may be caused by a fracture, or
2. the joint is unstable (ligaments are torn and it bends more than normal in any direction).

Acute bacterial (septic) arthritis

Acute bacterial arthritis is not common; but it is very important. Treatment will cure it. If it is not treated, it will destroy the joint.

Symptoms, signs and tests
Symptoms and signs of infection in another part of the body (especially skin infection but also urethral or lung or other infection, etc.) were often present *before* the arthritis. The infection was carried to the joint by the blood. Sometimes there was a wound which entered the joint. Sometimes there was a soft tissue or bone infection which got bigger and went into the joint. Sometimes there was an aspiration of the joint with an unsterile needle.

Symptoms in the joint are usually extreme pain and swelling of the affected joint, which the patient cannot move.

Signs in the joint (see Figure 29.8) are usually:
• swelling, caused by an 'effusion' made of pus,
• tenderness,
• heat,
• redness or shininess, and
• severe pain on moving the joint with guarding of the muscles which move that joint. This is usually so severe that the patient will not allow any movement of the joint.

Figure 29.8 Acute bacterial ('septic') arthritis of the right knee. Note the large amount of swelling. Note that because of severe pain the patient is lying with the knee slightly bent over a pillow and would not allow the examiner to bend it during examination. This joint needs *immediate* aspiration. The patient needs *immediate* large doses of antibiotics.

General symptoms and signs of infection caused by the toxins from the arthritis are usually severe – fever, rigors, fast pulse etc.

Aspiration of the joint shows pus.

Treatment

1. Aspirate all the pus from the joint. Use strict aseptic precautions. Send pus for Gram stain, culture and sensitivity if possible. Repeat the aspiration when more pus forms (daily or more often if necessary).
2. Give antibiotics as for any acute severe bacterial infection. (See Chapter 12.) Give chloramphenicol 1 g (4 caps) orally immediately and repeat every 6 hours. Give 1 g (1

bottle) by IMI or IVI if necessary. Continue the antibiotic for at least 2 weeks. Reduce dose when the patient improves.
3. Splint the joint (usually with a well padded plaster-of-Paris (POP) back-slab). Elevate (raise up) the affected limb.
4. Give aspirin 600–1200 mg (2–4 tabs) or codeine compound tablets 2 tabs every 6 hours if needed for pain.
5. Give antimalarial drugs as indicated; usually chloroquine 450–600 mg (3–4 tabs) daily for 3 days, if there is fever.
6. When the acute inflammation starts to improve, begin physiotherapy. Supervise the patient doing active exercises three times a day in the splint (the patient should contract all the muscles which normally move the joint 20–30 times; but without bending the joint). Move the joint through all its movements out of the splint, once daily. Remove the splint and start active exercises of the joint when all the signs of acute inflammation have gone.

Transfer to Medical Officer care:
1. all severe cases (urgent – but not emergency);
2. all cases of acute arthritis of the hip joint (urgent – but not emergency);
3. any case not much improved in 2 days (urgent – but not emergency);
4. any case where you have not aspirated all the pus for 2 days running (urgent – but not emergency); and
5. any case not cured in 2 weeks (non-urgent).

Rheumatic fever

Rheumatic fever is an acute non-infectious inflammatory disease of the joints and heart, and other parts of the body.

It is caused by an abnormal reaction of the immune system of the body to an infection (usually a throat infection) the patient had about 2 weeks before.

It usually affects children and young adults.

Symptoms and signs
1. Usually fever is present, with two or more of the other signs and symptoms.
2. Acute arthritis. The arthritis usually
   • starts quickly
   • affects a large joint

- affects only 1 or 2 joints at a time
- is a typical acute arthritis.
- gets completely better in the affected joint after a few days,
- then affects another joint or joints
- lasts for 1–5 weeks moving from joint to joint.

3. Carditis (inflammation of the heart). This causes:
   - fast pulse and at times heart failure (this can get better),
   - damage to the heart valves, (this does not cause immediate trouble, but it does not get better, and can slowly get worse and cause heart failure many years later).
4. Chorea or abnormal twisting movements of the body which the patient cannot stop.
5. Skin rash
6 . Nodules under the skin.

Treatment
1. Rest if there is acute arthritis or heart failure.
2. Aspirin in large doses regularly (see Chapter 7 page 29)
3. Usual treatment of heart failure if this develops (see Chapter 27 page 301)
4. Procaine penicillin 900,000 units (3 ml) IMI for 10 days to kill any of the bacteria left from the infection which caused the abnormal reaction.
5. Routine antimalarial treatment, if in a malarious area.

The arthritis usually gets better very quickly with treatment.

Prevention of further attacks is necessary so that the heart is not damaged again. Give long acting penicillin injections, e.g. benzathine penicillin, 1.2 million units, every month for 10 years, or until the age of 20 years.

If bacteria get into the blood (during operations or dental extractions etc.), they can start to grow on the damaged valves before the body can destroy them. To stop this give all patients with damaged heart valves benzyl (crystalline) penicillin 2,000,000 units (4 ml) and streptomycin 1 g (2 ml) and procaine benzyl penicillin 900,000 units (3 ml) 1 hour before the operation or dental extraction; and after the operation, procaine benzyl penicillin 900,000 units (3 ml) daily for 3 more days.

'Tropical arthritis'

Tropical arthritis is an unusual type of chronic (but sometimes acute) arthritis that occurs in some tropical countries.
The cause is sometimes infection with filaria. Most times the cause is not known.

Clinical features
Young adults are usually affected; but patients can be any age.

It affects one or two (only sometimes more) joints, usually the knees or ankles.

Symptoms include swelling or pain of the joint.

Signs include marked swelling (caused by effusion) and painful movement of the joint (see Figure 29.9). Tenderness and heat may occur in acute cases. Limited movement and deformity may occur in late severe cases. Usually no general signs are present.

Figure 29.9 Tropical arthritis affecting the left knee. The patient was treated first with chloramphemicol in large doses for 2 weeks (but joint fluid aspirated and examined in the laboratory did not confirm the diagnosis of bacterial infection). He was then treated with diethylcarbamazine for 3 weeks. He had large doses of aspirin during this time, and a splint and physiotherapy. At 6 weeks he still has arthritis with a lot of swelling but not much pain. This is common in 'tropical arthritis'.

Aspiration gives fluid which is green or yellow and clear or cloudy; but the fluid is usually different from pus.

Send thick smears for microfilaria to laboratory. (See Chapter 22 page 202.)

Sometimes the arthritis goes away without treatment. Sometimes it returns later. Sometimes chronic pain and swelling continue for months or years. In severe or prolonged cases, the joint is destroyed.

Management of a case of tropical arthritis
Always check that it is not:
1. acute infective arthritis, by aspirating the joint;
2. traumatic arthritis and rheumatic fever and rheumatoid arthritis, by history and examination;
3. tuberculous arthritis, if possible, by history and examination (if this is not possible, transfer the patient for investigation).

Admit all suspected cases.

Send thick blood smears (taken at midnight on 3 nights) for examination for microfilaria.

Treatment
1. Aspirate all the fluid from the joint. Use strict aseptic precautions. Send the fluid for Gram stain, culture and sensitivity (if possible). If you think the fluid may be pus, treat as for acute bacterial (septic) arthritis. (See page 319.)
2. Splint the joint (usually in a well padded POP back-slab) until the acute stage finishes. When you are certain that no further improvement will occur (e.g. after 6 weeks), remove the splint
3. Physiotherapy
   Make the patient do active exercises three times a day in the splint. Show the patient how to contract all the muscles which normally move the joint but without moving the joint itself. Tell the patient to do this 20–40 times three times every day.
   Move the joint through all its movements out of the splint once daily; but only after the acute inflammation has started to improve (if it was present).
   Make the patient do active exercises with movement of the joint after all the signs of acute inflammation have gone.
4. Aspirin 900–1200 (3–4 tabs) four times a day.

5. Antimalarial drug as indicated usually chloroquine 450–600 mg (3–4 tabs) daily for 3 days, if there is any fever.
6. Diethylcarbamazine 100 mg (2 tabs) three times a day for 3 weeks if the patient is in (or has been in) an area where filariasis occurs. See Chapter 22 page 203 about reactions to diethyl-carbamazine.

Transfer to medical officer care if:
1. the arthritis may be acute bacterial (septic) arthritis which is not improving with antibiotics (urgent); or
2. the arthritis may be tuberculous arthritis (non-urgent).

Rheumatoid disease

Rheumatoid disease is a chronic disease that affects the whole body but especially the joints. The cause is not known. Often patients are middle-aged adults; but it can affect people of any age.

First general symptoms and signs of ill health are present for some weeks – malaise, fever, aches and pains, etc. Then there can be severe anaemia, weight loss, etc.

The arthritis usually:
1. is chronic, but it can start with an acute attack and become acute from time to time;
2. is roughly symmetrical (i.e. same joints on both sides of body);
3. starts in the small joints of hands and feet (especially the first joints of the fingers) see Figure 29.10;
4. then spreads to larger joints (wrists, ankles, knees etc. and sometimes the spine)
5. has symptoms of pain and stiffness, worse in the morning or after rest and a little improved by use or exercise.
6. has, at first, signs of
   (a) swelling of soft tissues around the joint
   (b) effusion and
   (c) inflammation.
7. has, later, severe joint destruction with deformity, stiffness and loss of use of the joint, especially if not treated properly.

Aspiration is usually not necessary for diagnosis (as many joints are involved and the arthrits is not very acute); but aspirated fluid is yellow and cloudy if you do this.

Figure 29.10 Late severe rheumatoid disease affecting hands. Note the swelling of the first joints of the fingers, which suggests rheumatoid disease.

Figure 29.11 Tuberculous arthritis of the left hip. Note that any patient with chronic arthritis of one joint must be transferred for test. Note the typical severe wasting of the muscles of the left thigh.

Sometimes acute bacterial arthritis can develop in a joint affected by rheumatoid arthritis.

Treatment includes aspirin in large doses e.g. 900–1200 mg (3–4 tablets) four times a day regularly for months or years; the patient should wear splints made to hold the joints in their proper positions at night if deformity is developing and he should also have physiotherapy.

Tuberculous arthritis

Tuberculous arthritis is a chronic inflammatory arthritis caused by infection of the joint with tuberculosis bacteria.

Tuberculous arthritis is not common; but it is important. Treatment will cure it. If it is not treated, it will destroy the joint.

Most often if affects the hip or knee (see Figure 29.11); but it can affect any joint.

Most often the patient is a child or young adult; but it can affect people of any age

Symptoms include pain and stiffness of the joint, or a limp.

Signs include:

1. *chronic arthritis which slowly gets worse* (swelling, tenderness, warmth, pain on moving joint, limited movement of joint, the patient cannot use joint properly, etc.);

2. *severe wasting of the muscles* which move the joint;
3. nearby lymph glands usually enlarged;
4. a sinus discharging pus near the joint late in the disease;
5. symptoms and signs of tuberculosis in other parts of the body (e.g. chronic cough or enlarged lymph glands);
6. the tuberculin test is usually positive.

> You should suspect tuberculous arthritis in any chronic arthritis which gets progressively worse over months and refer or transfer the patient for tests. This is especially important if only one joint is affected and if the tuberculin test is positive.

Do not diagnose a case of arthritis as osteoarthrosis if there are signs of *inflammation* which *get slowly worse*. Osteoarthrosis does not usually have inflammation of the joint and it has times when it gets better and times when it gets worse. Think instead of tuberculous arthritis and transfer the patient for tests and treatment.

Vertebral tuberculosis

Vertebral tuberculosis is a special type of tuberculous arthritis. It starts in the joints between the vertebrae and then spreads to the bones of the vertebrae.

Symptoms include:
1. back pain and stiffness which lasts for weeks or months and does not get better but gets increasingly worse;
   and later
2. a lump or deformity in the spine (if some infected bones collapse);
   and sometimes
3. weakness or paralysis and loss of sensation in the legs and the patient cannot pass urine properly (if there is spinal cord pressure).

Signs include:
1. tenderness and stiffness of part of the spine; and later
2. a lump or deformity of the spine; and sometimes
3. weakness or paralysis and loss of sensation in the legs and an enlarged bladder or urinary

Figure 29.12   Tuberculosis of the spine. Note the deformity of the spine (often called a 'gibbus'). Tuberculosis of the spine is often called Pott's disease. This patient needs urgent transfer before she becomes paraplegic.

incontinence (if there is spinal cord pressure).

4. There may be symptoms or signs of tuberculosis in other parts of the body e.g. chronic cough or enlarged lymph glands.
5. The tuberculin test is usually positive.

Transfer the patient for diagnosis by X-ray, if you suspect vertebral tuberculosis. Transfer for treatment, if cord pressure occurs.

Suspect vertebral tuberculosis at the stage of chronic, constant, increasing backache with stiffness and tendernss of the spine, before a lump forms or the spinal cord is damaged. (See Figure 29.12.)

Osteoarthrosis (osteoarthritis)

Osteoarthrosis is a degeneration or 'wearing out' of joints.

It occurs in older adults in the joints they use most – hips, knees, spine, etc. *or* in younger persons in a joint which has previously been seriously injured.

Osteoarthrosis is not an *arthritis*. There is no inflammation of the joint (unless it has been injured again or used a lot, just before examination). There are no general symptoms or signs of inflammation or infection.

Clinical features

Symptoms are usually of pain in a joint during and after use. The pain is improved by rest.
Signs include:

1. swelling caused by overgrowth of the ends of the bone at the 'worn out' joint;
2. crepitus (a 'crackling' you can feel or hear) when the joint is moved:
3. full movement of the joint is not possible;
4. some wasting of muscles which move the joint is present;
5. *if recent injury or hard work* by the joint, there may be some tenderness and sometimes an effusion.

If you aspirate any effusion present the fluid will be clear yellow. It is not pus.

Usually there is a slow start of the symptoms and signs. Very slowly the condition gets worse. Usually there are times when there is little or no pain and times when the symptoms are much worse.

Always check that the conditon is not tuberculous arthritis. If there is inflammation of the joint, and if the arthritis gets worse and worse over weeks or months, and if there is severe muscle wasting, and especially if only one joint is affected, then suspect tuberculous arthritis.

Other diseases you should check for include chronic infective (bacterial) arthritis, 'tropical' arthritis and rheumatoid arthritis.

Outpatient or inpatient treatment is possible.

Treatment

1. Rest.
   The patient should use the affected joint as little as possible. Tell the patient how to lose weight if the patient is fat.
2. The patient should do exercises to strengthen the muscles which move the joint without putting weight on the joint during the exercises. *Show* the patient how to contract the muscles which move the joint without letting the joint move, or how to move the joint without putting weight on it. *Tell* the patient to do 20–40 of these exercises three times every day.
3. Give aspirin 900–1200 mg (3–4 tabs) four times a day, when pain is present.

Transfer to Medical Officer care is not necessary unless tuberculous arthritis is a possibility (see page 323)

Osteoarthrosis of spine

Osteoarthrosis of the spine is the same as osteoarthrosis of other joints, except that if affects the spinal joints. The nerves that go from the spinal cord to the body may *sometimes* be pressed on. This can *sometimes* give pain radiating to the arms, truck or legs and/or weakness of the muscles of the arms or legs.

Symptoms include:

1. pain and stiffness in the neck or back, often worse after exercise and improved by rest;
2. pain radiating to the trunk or the limbs (sometimes);
3. weakness of some muscles (sometimes).
Signs include:
1. stiffness of the neck or back (which will not bend properly in all directions); pain on some movements of the spine; and sometimes tenderness on percussion of the spine;

2. loss of sensation of part of a limb (sometimes);
3. muscle weakness of part of a limb (sometimes).

The symptoms and signs may be severe, then greatly improve only to return again (i.e. there are good and bad times).

Treatment is as for osteoarthrosis of other joints, and especially 'extension exercises' to strengthen muscles along spine.

Check that the patient has no weakness of the legs, loss of control of the bladder, signs of inflammation of the spine, increasing worsening of the disease, or symptoms and signs of tuberculosis in other parts of the body. If the patient has any of these things, transfer the patient for the Medical Officer to check that it is not tuberculosis of the spine.

Deformity of spine

Causes include:
1. fracture
2. tuberculosis
3. others – see a specialist reference book.

Acute arthritis of many joints from other causes

The causes of 'tropical arthritis' (see page 321) and rheumatoid disease with arthritis (see page 322) are not known in most cases. But both of these diseases have characteristic clinical features. Even if you are not certain that the patient has one of these when you first see him, the characteristic clinical course usually makes you certain after some weeks.

Sometimes also you will suspect rheumatoid disease or tropical arthritis; but the arthritis gets better quickly or has a course not typical of these diseases.

There are a large number of other conditions which can cause arthritis similar to rheumatoid disease or tropical arthritis; and these are often hard to diagnose in a health centre.

Whenever you see a case of arthritis first *check that it is not acute bacterial arthritis* or *tuberculous arthritis*; although these usually affect only one joint. Other conditons which the patient may have are:
1. *Reiter's syndrome* is a condition which causes arthritis, conjunctivitis, urethitis and other skin and mucous membrane lesions. It often follows a sexually transmitted disease or gastro-enteritis. Tetracycline treatment and aspirin sometimes helps.
2. *Virus infections such as hepatitis and rubella* can cause an arthritis that affects several joints. The arthritis is usually not severe. Other signs of the virus infection are present.
3. *Virus infection carried by mosquitoes and other insects* (arbor viruses) can cause both single cases and epidemics of arthritis of several joints. Fever and rashes of various types are often present at first; but the disease gets better after some weeks or months.
4. *Allergic reactions of various types* (see Chapter 10 page 37), especially the 'serum sickness' type and those caused by drugs (including intravenous iron infusions) can cause acute and chronic arthritis of many joints which finally gets better. Reactions in leprosy (Chapter 15 page 86) can also cause arthritis.
5. There are also a large number of *other causes*.

If the patient has arthritis which you cannot diagnose and which continues to get worse, refer or transfer to a Medical Officer for diagnosis.

Diagnosis and management of joint problems

Acute arthritis of one or a few joints

Admit all cases for inpatient treatment.

Find cause by history and examination (see Chapter 6 page 16 and page 315 of this chapter and Table 29.1):
acute bacterial infection
trauma
'tropical'
rheumatic fever
rheumatoid disease (usually chronic and many joints affected)

Do a diagnostic joint aspiration on all cases of acute arthritis unless you are certain that the diagnosis is *not* bacterial infection.

Treatment
1. Aspirate any joint which has fluid in it. Use proper aseptic precautions (see page 315).

Aspirate (suck out) any fluid in the joint until no more fluid remains. If you find pus, repeat the aspiration whenever more pus is formed (daily or more often if necessary).

2. If aspiration shows pus, or if aspiration does not get any fluid out, give chloramphenicol 1 g (4 caps) orally immediately and repeat every 6 hours. Continue chloramphenicol for at least 2 weeks. (See Chapter 12 page 46)
3. Splint the joint (usually with a well padded POP back-slab). Elevate (raise up) the affected limb.
4. Aspirin 900–1200 mg (3–4 tabs) every 6 hours.
5. Antimalarial drugs as indicated (see Chapter 13 page 55) usually chloroquine 450–600 mg (3–4 tabs) daily for 3 days if there is fever.
6. Give diethylcarbamazine 100 mg (2 tabs) three times a day if the patient is in (or has been in) an area where filarasis occurs and the aspirated fluid is yellow or green but does not look like pus. See Chapter 22 page 203 first.
7. When the acute inflammation improves, start physiotherapy. Make the patient do active exercises three times a day in the splint. Show the patient how to contract all the muscles which normally move the joint without moving the joint itself. Tell the patient to do this 20–40 times three times each day. Move the joint through all its movements out of the splint once daily. Remove the splint and start active exercises (with the patient moving the joint) when all the signs of acute inflammation have gone.

Transfer to a Medical Officer if:
1. It is a severe case (urgent – but not emergency).
2. The hip joint is affected (urgent – but not emergency).
3. The patient is not greatly improved in 2 days (urgent – but not emergency).
4. Pus is present but you cannot aspirate it for 2 days (urgent – but not emergency).
5. The patient is not cured in 2 weeks (non-urgent).

Chronic arthritis of one or a few joints

Do a history and examination. See Chapter 6 page 16 and page 315 of this chapter to find the cause.
Outpatient or inpatient treatment is possible.

Treatment
1. Rest. (The patient should do things which put weight on the joint, or make it work, as little as possible.) The patient should use the affected joint as little as possible. Tell the patient how to lose weight if he is fat.
2. The patient should do exercises to strengthen the muscles which move the joint without putting weight on the joint. *Show* the patient how to contract the muscles which move the joint without moving the joint, or how to move the joint without putting weight on it. *Tell* the patient to do 20–40 of these exercises three times a day.
3. Aspirin 900–1200 mg (3–4 tabs) four times a day when pain is present.

If the joint improves with this treatment and there are no important signs of inflammation of the joint (not warm, red or shiny, tender, etc.), then the condition is probably osteoarthrosis. Repeat the treatment whenever it is necessary.

If
• there are signs of inflammation of the joint (warm, shiny, tender, etc.) *or*
• there is a sinus near the joint *or*
• the joint does not improve much with treatment, or later the joint gets slowly worse *or*
• muscle wasting becomes severe –
then the arthritis may be caused by tuberculosis or chronic bacterial infection.
Transfer these patients to Medical Officer care.

Arthritis of many joints

Do a history and examination (see Chapter 6 page 16 and page 315 of this chapter) to find the cause:
rheumatoid disease
viral infection
serum or drug or allergic reaction
rheumatic fever
leprosy reaction
Give treatment for any cause.
Give aspirin 900–1200 mg (3–4 tabs) four times a day.
Look carefully for signs and symptoms of acute bacterial arthritis – aspirate any joint which may have bacterial infection (see page 319).
If the patient is not cured in one month transfer to a Medical Officer non-urgently for diagnosis and treatment.

Backache

Look for disease in the organs listed below.

Do a full history and examination (see Chapter 6 page 16). Test the urine for pus, protein and blood.

> Examine the spine for tenderness and movement. Do a pelvic examination PV if necessary.

1. Spine
Direct traumatic injury
Acute back strain (muscle or joint damage from lifting something heavy)
- sudden start during lifting
- pain, tenderness and stiffness of part of the spine

Chronic back strain
- The patient is often a student or a clerical worker or a woman.
- chronic ache
- usually lower back or neck
- often worse after the back is used
- no abnormalities on examination of spine
- often improves if patient improves posture and strengthens muscles by 'extension exercises'

Osteoarthrosis of spine (see page 325)
- pain, stiffness and tenderness varies from time to time

Tuberculosis of spine (see page 324)
- slow start; but constant and increasing pain and tenderness and stiffness of part of the spine

2. Kidney
Ureteric colic (see Chapter 26 page 290)
- pain from where lowest rib joins spine to genitalia
- kidney often tender
- blood in urine often

Pyelonephritis (urinary tract infection) (see Chapter 26 page 286)
- fever
- urinary pain and frequency
- kidney tender
- urine shows pus and protein

3. Reproductive system
Pregnancy
Labour of miscarriage
Painful menstrual period (dysmenorrhoea)
- on examination, no abnormalities found

Pelvic inflammatory disease
- pelvic examination PV shows pus in vagina, tenderness on moving cervix and tenderness or masses in pelvis.

4. General diseases
Malaria (see Chapter 13)
Viral diseases, especially influenza.

Deformity of the spine

See page 326.

30

Disorders of the Endocrine Glands

Anatomy and physiology of the endocrine glands

Glands which make secretions which flow into the blood (and not outside the body or into one of the mucous membrane lined tubes, such as the gastrointestinal tract) are called endocrine glands.

The secretions of the endocrine glands are called 'hormones.'

Hormone means messenger. Hormones have effects on the other parts of the body they travel to in the blood. See Figure 30.1

Pathology of the endocrine glands

Diseases of endocrine glands cause symptoms and signs in three ways.

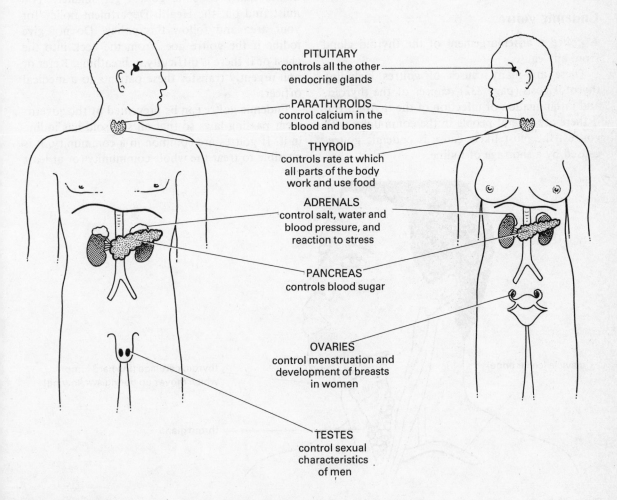

PITUITARY
controls all the other
endocrine glands

PARATHYROIDS
control calcium in the
blood and bones

THYROID
controls rate at which
all parts of the body
work and use food

ADRENALS
control salt, water and
blood pressure, and
reaction to stress

PANCREAS
controls blood sugar

OVARIES
control menstruation and
development of breasts
in women

TESTES
control sexual
characteristics
of men

Figure 30.1   Diagram to show the location and function of the endocrine glands.

1. More hormone is secreted than is needed.
2. Less hormone is secreted than is needed.
3. Effects of the disease in the gland – the most common effects are (a) swelling of the gland and (b) spread of any malignant cancer cells from the gland to another part of the body.

Diseases of the thyroid gland

The thyroid gland normally makes the right amount of thyroid hormone to allow all the cells of the body to work normally. (See Figure 30.2.)

Diseases of the thyroid gland which you may see in a health centre include:
1. endemic goitre,
2. endemic cretinism, and
3. hyperthyroidism or thyrotoxicosis.

Endemic goitre

A goitre is an enlargement of the thyroid gland from any cause.

There are many causes of goitres including thyrotoxicosis (page 332), cancer of the thyroid, and inflammation or infection of the thyroid. But if there are several people in the community with goitres, the most likely cause is endemic goitre, caused by a shortage of iodine.

Endemic goitre occurs when there is not enough iodine in the food and so there is also not enough iodine in the blood. The thyroid gland grows bigger (i.e. a goitre forms) to try to take more iodine from the blood. This shortage of iodine usually occurs only in mountainous areas.

Usually it affects girls at puberty and women during pregnancy.

Symptoms and signs include
1. swelling in the neck caused by a goitre (see Figure 30.3) (This is usually the only symptom and sign.);
2. difficulty in breathing; but not usually;
3. difficulty in swallowing; but not usually.

Many textbooks and many medical officers say you should not treat patients with endemic goitre with iodine. But in some parts of the world, iodine makes many endemic goitres get smaller. You must find out the Health Department policy for your area and follow this policy. Do not give iodine if the goitre goes from the neck into the chest or if there is difficulty in breathing. Refer or non-urgently transfer these patients to a medical officer.

Endemic goitre can be prevented by the government passing laws so that all salt sold has iodine in it. If goitres are common in a community, it is possible to treat the whole community (or at least

clavicle (collar bone)

thyroid cartilage (the hard lump which moves up during swallowing)

throid gland

Figure 30.2 Diagram to show the position of the thyroid gland in the neck.

Figure 30.3 An enlarged thyroid gland. This is called a 'goitre'. See Figure 30.2 for normal position and size of the thyroid gland. A normal gland is not usually visible except in some females at puberty and in the child-bearing years; but even then it should not be very large.

the women and girls) with prophylactic iodised oil fluid injection. The main reason for giving iodine is to stop endemic cretinism occuring in the children of affected women (see below).

If you find a few people with endemic goitre, or if you find only one patient with endemic cretinism (see below) in the community, then notify the medical officer so that he can arrange a survey and iodine prophylaxis.

Endemic cretinism

A patient has endemic cretinism if he has:
1. deafness from birth and cannot speak;
2. spastic legs and was slower than normal children in learning to sit, walk etc.;
3. mental subnormality;
4. squint.

Not all patients with endemic cretinism have all these symptoms and signs – deafness and lack of speech are the most common. (See Figure 30.4.)

Figure 30.4 Endemic cretinism. Note that the child cannot walk (he has 'spastic' legs). He is deaf, cannot talk and is mentally dull. He has a large abdomen and an umbilical hernia, which are also common in cretinism.

Endemic cretinism is caused by a shortage of iodine in the mother's blood before the child was born. So endemic cretins are born only in areas where adults have goitres.

Notify the medical officer if you find any case of endemic cretinism of if you find several adults with a goitre in an area. The medical officer will arrange a survey and, if necessary, mass treatment with iodine, to prevent more endemic cretinism.

No treatment is possible for cases of cretinism.

Prevention is by everyone eating salt with iodine in it; or, if this is not possible, by giving all girls and women prophylactic iodised oil fluid injections.

Thyrotoxicosis or hyperthyroidism

Thyrotoxicosis or hyperthyroidism is present when too much thyroid hormone is made by the thyroid gland. The most common cause of this is a reaction of the immune cells of the body which affects the thyroid gland and the eyes and is called 'Graves' Disease'.

Thyrotoxicosis is not common, but it is important. It usually affects adults.

Thyrotoxicosis may cause any of these 3 groups of conditions (all of them need not be present).
1. All parts of the body work faster than normal but not as well as normal. (This is caused by too much thyroid hormone.) Look for:
   (a) weight loss and weakness of the muscles, although the patient eats well;
   (b) pulse fast; even while the patient is at rest or asleep; pulse irregular (sometimes with some weak beats so that the heart rate counted with the stethoscope on the chest is more than the pulse rate felt at the wrist):
   (c) heart failure for no other obvious cause;

Always think of thyrotoxicosis in anyone (especially older adults) who have heart failure and you cannot find the cause, especially if pulse irregular.

   (d) shaking of the hands. (Look for this when the patient holds his hands out straight ahead of him);
   (e) nervousness or mental illness;
   (f) feels hot and sweaty all the time (more than before).

Figure 30.5 The eyes in thyrotoxicosis. Note the whites of the eyes above the corneas. The patient appears to be staring and does not blink often (lid retraction). When you look from the side, you can see that the eyes are pushed out (exopthalmos).

2. The eyes may seem to be staring (i.e. the patient does not blink often; and when he looks up and then down, the whites of the eyes show above the brown). (See Figure 30.5.) The eye or eyes may be pushed out (exopthalmos).
3. A goitre (swelling of the thyroid gland) is present or comes. (But only if there are also some of the other signs.) (See Figure 30.3.)

It is possible to cure thyrotoxicosis. But if it is not treated, it can cause death from heart failure or blindness from exopthalmos.

If you suspect a patient has thyrotoxicosis because of any the above features refer or non-urgently transfer the patient to a Medical Officer for diagnosis and treatment.

Diabetes

Diabetes mellitus is a condition where the pancreas does not make enough insulin to keep the blood sugar (glucose) normal. The blood sugar becomes very high and causes these symptoms and signs and complications.

Think of diabetes in anyone who
1. had weight loss, even though
2. he is eating well (often more than normal), and
3. is passing much urine, and
4. is thirsty and drinking much fluid.

Also think of diabetes if you see patients with complications which can be caused by diabetes, including
1. repeated infections (especially skin, urinary or vaginal infections, and all cases of tuberculosis),
2. blindness,
3. nephrotic syndrome,
4. coma (unconsciousness), and
5. gangrene of the toes or feet.

In all the cases, test for sugar in the urine (with e.g. Benedict's solution). If the patient is pregnant or breastfeeding a baby, the sugar from the breast milk can get into the blood and urine (and give a positive test for sugar with Benedict's solution), even when the patient has no glucose in the urine and does not have diabetes. Test patients who are pregnant or breastfeeding a baby with 'Clinistix' or another test which is positive for glucose only.

If there is glucose in the urine, transfer the patient ot medical officer care for confirmation of the diagnosis and treatment.

The treatment for diabetes includes:
1. The patient should have a diet containing as little sugar as possible. Most traditional village diets, except for sugar cane and sweet fruits, are usually all right. The patient should eat enough food to be at the normal weight for his height and age. Then the patient should eat only enough to remain at this normal weight.
2. The patient should have daily physical exercise.
3. Some patients need insulin injections every day. (Some patients can take tablets of a drug such as insulin instead.) Do not stop the insulin if the patient gets sick or has gastro-enteritis. if vomiting, continue the insulin and give IV 4.3% dextrose in 0.18% sodium chloride.
4. Treat any complications quickly and properly.

If a patient is on treatment for diabetes with insulin and develops any of these – weakness, sweating, shaking, mental abnormality or unconciousness – then immediately give two large spoonfuls of sugar in water by mouth or by intra-gastric tube (or, if available, 50 ml of 25% or 50% dextrose solution for injection by IVI if the patient is unconscious). Then urgently consult a medical officer. It is most likely that the symptoms and signs were caused by too much of the insulin.

Prevention of diabetes is by not eating too much (especially refined carbohydrate foods) and not getting fat.

Acute adrenal insufficiency

The adrenal gland of the body normally makes a small amount of cortisone each day and a large amount of cortisone at a time of stress (e.g. acute infection or accident or operation).

Medical officers give cortisone or cortisone-like drugs including hydrocortisone, prednisone, prednisolone and dexamethasone for some conditions.

After some weeks of taking cortisone-like drugs, the adrenal glands of the body stop making cortisone, and cannot make it again even at times of stress. If the patient suddenly stops taking his drug he will have no cortisone in his body and may die. Also, if the patient does not take an extra dose of the cortisone-like drug at a time of stress, he may die.

Also the high dose of cortisone makes the patient more likely to get infections, especially malaria and tuberculosis.

If you have a patient who is taking a corisone-like drug, see a specialist reference book for details. Remember these rules:
1. The patient must take the drug as indicated and not stop it (unless the Medical Officer stops it).
2. If there is a time of stress the patient must take 3–4 times the normal dose of the drug immediately, and then daily. You must consult the medical officer urgently.
3. The patient must take prophylactic anti-malarials and prophylactic INAH, if he is in an area where malaria occurs or if tuberculosis is common.
4. Treat any infection quickly and well with antibiotics and antimalarials.

31

Disorders of the Eye

Figure 31.1 Diagrams to show the structure of the eye and the tear gland and ducts.

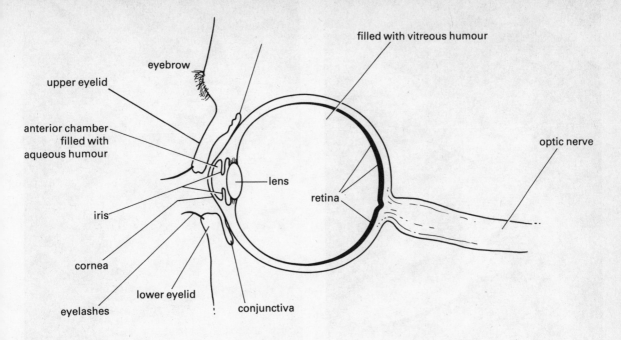

Figure 31.2 Diagram of the eye in section from front to back, to show the structure of the eye in more detail.

History and examination

Symptoms of eye diseases

1. loss of vision
2. pain in the eye
3. eye red; watering; or sticky (from pus)

Signs of eye diseases

Examine structures of the eye from the outside ones to the inside ones to find any signs present

1. *Look at the site, shape and size etc. of the eyes*
   - exopthalmos?
   - orbital cellulitis?

2. *Look at the eyelids*
   - 'stye'?
   - entropion?
   - infection?
   - oedema?
   - haematoma?

   Ask the patient to open and close his eyes.
   - ptosis?
   - lagopthalmos?

Figure 31.3 Examination of the conjunctiva of the lower lid.

335

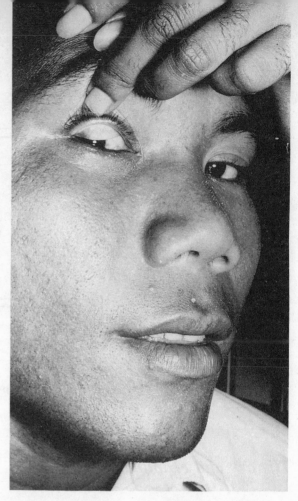

Figure 31.4 Examining the conjunctiva of the upper eye lid. Left photograph, first step. Right photograph, second step. See text for details. The conjunctivae may be red and inflamed all over with or without the formation of pus (conjuntivitis). They may be inflamed just around the cornea (acute iritis). A vascular fleshy growth may be growing across it to the cornea (pterygium). A foreign body may be present.

3. *Look at the conjunctiva*
   (a) over the sclera,
   (b) inside the lower lids (see Figure 31.3),
   (c) inside upper lids (turn upper lid inside out)
   (see Figure 31.4).
   • foreign body?
   • inflammation of all conjunctiva or just around cornea?
   • pus?
   • nodules?
   • pterygium?

4. *Look at the cornea*
Anaesthetise with 2% amethocaine sterile eye drops, 2 drops into the outer side of the eye every minute for 2–3 minutes, as necessary (see Figure 31.5) Note that anaesthetic is only needed if the patient has pain.

Stain with fluorescein. Put one drop of sterile solution, or lay the end of a sterile ophthalmic strip, on the conjuctiva of the sclera (white part of the eye) on the lateral (outer) side of the eye for a few seconds. Then get the patient to blink. Corneal ulcers will show as green areas.

Shine a light in from side and ask the patient to look up, down, right and left.

Use a torch and a loupe if available. Otherwise use an auriscope without a speculum (see Figure 31.6)
   • foreign body?
   • ulcer?
   • clear or cloudy?
   • scar?

Figure 31.5 Putting local anaesthetic and fluorescein drops into the eye. Local anaesthetic is only necessary if the patient has pain. Fluorescein is necessary in all patients. Note that the drops are put in the outer side of the eye while the patient looks towards the other side.

5. *Look at the anterior chamber by shining a light into it*
   - clear?
   - cloudy?
   - pus or blood at the lower part?

6. *Look at the iris and the pupil*
   - pupil shape round or irregular?
   - pupil size normal, large or small?
   Shine a light into the pupil
   - pupil constricts (gets smaller) when light goes in and dilates (gets bigger) when light goes away, or not?

7. *Look at the lens*
   - cataract?

8. *Test eye movements*
   Ask the patient to follow with his eyes one of your fingers which you move up then down then to the right and then to the left
   - double vision?
   - squint?

9. *Visual acuity*
   Check vision with an eye chart at 6 metres (6/6 or less) *or*
   - count fingers *or*
   - see light
   - read small print

Figure 31.6 If you use an auriscope with a magnifying lens you can examine the eye more closely and accurately.

Table 31.1 Clinical findings of the common eye disorders

History and examination	Acute conjunctivis	Foreign body in cornea	Corneal ulcer	Acute iritis (infection from outside)	Acute iritis (from other diseases)	Acute glaucoma	Cataract
History of injury	no	often	at times	corneal ulcer or penetrating injury	no	no, sometimes yes	sometimes
Red discharging eye	yes, pus	yes, watery	yes, watery	yes varies	yes, watery	yes, watery	no
Pain in eye	no	yes	yes	yes	yes	yes	no
Loss of vision	no	often	often	yes	yes	yes	yes
Conjunctiva	all inflamed, pus	inflamed	inflamed	inflamed – only around cornea or all	inflamed only around cornea	inflamed around cornea only	normal
Cornea	normal	foreign body	ulcer	ulcer or injury often	normal	cloudy	normal
Anterior chamber	normal	normal	normal	cloudy or hypopyon	cloudy or hypopyon	not easily seen	normal
Pupil	normal	normal	normal	small irregular, will not dilate	small irregular, will not dilate	large, oval, will not constrict	normal
Lens	normal	normal	normal	normal	normal	normal	white
Other disease present	at times	no	no	no	often yes	no	not usually

Check for symptoms and signs of disease in the rest of the body, if the eye condition is not just an eye injury.

Using these symptoms and signs, you can easily diagnose the most important eye diseases. See Table 31.1.

Treatment of eye diseases

Most of the important eye diseases are infective or traumatic (and traumatic injuries often get infected), so it is important always to do certain things if a patient has an eye condition.

1. Always look for foreign bodies in the eye. (This is especially important if the eye is red and painful.) Carefully look all over all surfaces of the conjunctiva. Carefully look all over the cornea.
2. Always look for corneal ulcers. Always stain the eye with fluorescein. Then shine a light into the eye from each side, and above and below.
3. If an infection or injury is present, use any antibiotic ointment in the eye. Remember that sulphacetamide is not very strong in killing organisms; but is usually soothing.
4. If any eye infection is serious, chloramphenicol is the most powerful antibiotic usually available. It should be put into the eye at least every 3 hours. If the infection is inside the eye, give chloramphenicol capsules (or injections, if vomiting is present). (Penicillin alone is not very effective for most infections inside the eye.)
5. If there is any injury or infection inside the eye or a severe injury or infection on the cornea, always dilate the pupil with atropine eye ointment or drops. Use atropine 3–4 times daily until the pupil dilates. The pupil will stay dilated for a week, sometimes more. If necessary, continue the atropine once daily. Injuries or infections in the eye may fix the iris, so that the pupil cannot get bigger or smaller. It is better for sight and for other reasons if the iris is fixed with the pupil big rather than small. This is the reason for using atropine.
6. Always put a pad on an eye with a serious injury or infection in it or on the cornea. But pad is not good treatment for conjunctivitis. Hold the pad on the eye with strip of adhesive cellulose tape or sticking plaster. Put the strips diagonally across the corners of the eye (and

not across the centre of the eye).
7. If a patient has only one eye, the patient and you must take great care of this good eye. If the patient develops injury or disease in his one good eye, transfer him quickly, if you are not certain of the diagnosis and treatment.
8. Before transferring any eye case, first check that the Medical Officer at the hospital will take the case. He may prefer a non-urgent case to wait until the opthalmologist (eye specialist) is visiting the hospital.

Some common eye diseases

The common stye

The common stye is an abscess or pimple in the gland of an eyelash.

Symptoms
Pain and swelling of the eyelid.

Signs
A swollen tender red hot area in the eyelid (see Figure 31.7).

After a few days it points to the edge of the eyelid, then discharges pus, and gets better without treatment.

Treatment
Hot bathing three or four times a day.

Figure 31.7 A common stye affecting the medial (centre) part of the lower lid.

Antibiotic compound eye ointment three or four times a day. This does not cure the disease, but often stops the pus starting new styes.

Conjunctival foreign bodies

Conjunctival foreign bodies cause pain, redness and watering of the eye.

Remove foreign bodies from under the lower eyelid with the patient looking up. See Figure 31.3,

Remove them from under the upper lid with the patient looking down. Turn the upper lid inside out over swab stick or a finger. See Figure 31.4,

Chemicals in the eye

Lime is the most common and dangerous chemical that gets into the eye. Chemicals can quickly cause damage to the eye. Give immediate proper first aid.

Hold the affected eye open and pour large amounts of water across it for 10–15 minutes, even though this causes pain.

Then anaesthetise the eye with a local anaesthetic, see page 336.

Stain the cornea with fluorescein, see page 336

Remove any foreign bodies very carefully.

Wash the eye with water again if necessary.

If the cornea is clear, treat with antibiotic compound eye ointment 3 or 4 times a day.

If the cornea is not clear, treat as for iritis, (see page 343) but the oral chloramphenicol is not necessary.

Transfer the patient to Medical Officer's care if he is not much better in 1–2 days.

Acute conjunctivitis

Conjunctivitis is inflammation of the conjunctiva of the eye with or without the formation of pus.
   Causes include:
1. gonorrhoea organism in infants at birth (from the mother's cervix or vagina),
2. infection with other kinds of bacteria,
3. viral infections,
4. allergic reactions, and
5. acute stage of a chronic conjuntivitis.

Spread of most infectious types of conjunctivtis is by direct contact, or by a vehicle (e.g. towel), or by vectors (especially flies).

Symptoms include:
1. red watering eyes,
2. eyelids stuck together with pus in the morning, and
3. some discomfort (but no pain).

If there is pain, another serious disease is present as well as conjunctivitis

---

Signs include:
1. inflammation of the conjunctivae, over the sclera and under the eyelids of both eyes; and
3. discharge, which may be watery, or pus

You must always stain the cornea with fluorescein and examine it for any corneal foreign body or corneal ulcer. Examine the anterior chamber and pupil for iritis.

(These things are especially important if the conjunctivitis is only on one side because conjunctivitis almost always spreads to both eyes. If conjunctivitis is only in one eye there is usually a local cause in that eye, such as forgein body, entropion (rolling in of the eyelid) or blocked tear duct, etc.)

These things are especially important if the inflammation is only around the cornea, because conjunctivitis causes inflammation of all of the conjunctivae. If the inflammation is only around the cornea, then a corneal ulcer or foreign body or iritis is probably present.

A mild chronic conjunctivitis with swelling of the conjunctivae which does not respond to the usual treatment for conjunctivitis can occur from onchocerciasis.

Vitamin A deficiency, especially in children, can cause dry conjunctivae with dry corneas and this can result in painful conjunctivitis. (See page 345.)

Treatment
1. *Show* the patient how to put antibiotic eye ointment under the lower eyelids. *Tell* the patient to do this four times daily to both eyes. *Give* the patient a tube of antibiotic compound eye ointment to take home. Treat for 5 days. Do not pad the eye.
2. If possible, admit the patient for hourly treatment for the first 8–12 hours by member

of your staff. This is usually much more effective than the patient giving himself the treatment. The patient can then continue the treatment at home.

3. See a specialist reference book for treatment of gonococcal, allergic, and other acute types of conjunctivitis.

Explain how the infection spreads, and how to stop this spread.

If the patient is not cured, look carefully for foreign bodies, iritis, Vitamin A deficiency, onchocerciasis and trachoma.

Trachoma

Trachoma is a chronic inflammation of the conjunctivae and cornea caused by trachoma bacteria.

Trachoma is common all over the world. But it is much more common, and causes much more severe disease, in areas which are hot, dry and dusty, and where there is not enough water for people to wash regularly.

Spread of the trachoma bacteria is by direct contact with the eye discharge from infected people. Infected people are much more infectious early in the infection. Flies may also spread the disease. It is usually children who have active infection. Older children and adults usually have the results of the infection, which is often blindness.

There are four stages in the development of trachoma.

1. *Early trachoma*

First the eyes are uncomfortable and watery, and the conjunctivae inflamed, like any other conjunctivitis. However the condition is chronic. After about a month, small pink-grey lumps, called 'follicles', develop under the upper eyelid (see Figure 31.8). There is little pus is the eye, unless there is secondary infection by other bacteria.

2. *Pannus formation*

Small blood vessels start to grow into the top of the cornea. This is called 'pannus'. Use a loupe or magnifying glass to look for the grey colour of *early* pannus at the top of the cornea.

3. *After some years the lesions heal without treatment.*

Figure 31.8 Trachoma. Note the follicles on the conjunctiva of the upper eyelid.

The follicles leave white scars on the inside of the upper eyelid. The pannus (which may spread over much of the cornea) leaves a whitish colour on the cornea (the cornea is normally clear).

4. *Entropion and trichiasis occurs*

The scarred tissue inside the eyelid, like any scar tissue, becomes smaller over the years. This turns the edge of the eyelid in, and this is called 'entropion'. This makes the eyelashes scrape over the cornea every time the patient blinks. This is called 'trichiasis'. The entropion and trichiasis causes more corneal damage, and finally blindness.

At any stage the patient may get an acute bacterial infection in the eye which can cause a lot more damage to the cornea.

Treatment

In the early stages, before entropion and trichiasis
Treat the patient with tetracycline or sulphonamide or both.

The usual method is:

1. Tetracycline 3% eye ointment (not the usual 1% which does not sting) at least once every day (better if more often) *and*

2. Sulphadimidine (or other sulphonamide) orally for 2 weeks, the dose depending on the weight

341

of the child (for adult dose see Chapter 11 page 42).

In the late stages of entropion and trichiasis

1. Remove any eyelashes which are scraping over the cornea. Pull them out with a pair of forceps.
2. Transfer the patient to a Medical Officer for an operation for the entropion, and other operations if necessary.

If there is acute bacterial infection at any stage treat quickly, as for corneal ulcer (see this page).

Control and prevention

1. Kill the organism in the reservoir.

   Treat all infected cases early, when they are most infectious. School surveys may be necessary every 6 months, to find cases early. If trachoma is very common, give the teacher enough 3% tetracycline eye ointment to treat all the children once daily for 5 days, every month for 6 months.
2. Stop the means of spread.

   It is very important that there is enough water for regular washing of the hands and face.
   Give education about personal hygiene.
   Control of flies may help.
3. Immunisation is not possible.
4. Prophlactic treatment (see 1 above).

Corneal or scleral foreign bodies

Usually there is a *history* of something going into the eye.

Symptoms include:
1. pain in the eye,
2. the patient cannot open the eye properly, and
3. red, watering eye.

Examination shows:
1. inflammation of the conjunctiva, and
2. foreign body on the cornea if you anaesthetise the cornea and stain it with flourescein and examine with a light and loupe or an auriscope.

Treatment

1. Anaesthetise the eye with amethocaine 2% sterile eye drops (see page 336).
2. Stain the cornea with fluorescein (see page 336).

3. If the foreign body does not penetrate (go right through) the cornea into the eye, remove it. Remove the foreign body with the point of a large hypodermic needle. Hold the needle parallel to the surface of the eye with your hand resting on the patient's face. If the foreign body is iron, also remove any rust stain surrounding it.
4. Then treat as for corneal ulcer (see below).
5. Look for signs of infection inside the eye (pus in the anterior chamber, or the pupil small or irregular). If either of these are present, also treat for acute iritis (see page 343).

Transfer to Medical Officer care

1. if the foreign body penetrates through into the eye (Do not try to remove it. (Urgent – emergency.) Meanwhile treat for acute iritis – see page 343 and give tetanus prophylaxis – see Chapter 25 page 264.);
2. if you cannot remove the foreign body (urgent); or
3. if you cannot see a foreign body but it may have gone right into the eye and still be there. This is especially important if the foreign body is made of iron.

> Always look for a foreign body in anyone who has a painful or red eye.

Corneal ulcer

A corneal ulcer is present when there is loss of part of the outside surface of the cornea (see Figure 31.9).

Corneal ulcers are caused by foreign bodies, abrasions, drying (when the eyelids will not close on e.g. leprosy), other injuries, bacterial infections, herpes virus infections, onchocerciasis, Vitamin A deficiency, chemicals especially lime, etc.

Symptoms include:
1. pain in the eye,
2. red watery eye, and
3. some loss of vision.

Signs:
1. The conjunctiva are inflamed.
2. You can see the ulcer on the cornea but often only if you give a local anaesthetic and stain with fluorescein and use a torch and loupe or

Figure 31.9 Corneal ulcer.

an auriscope. In areas where onchocerciasis occurs you may find white areas deep in the cornea (but no surface ulcer); these slowly become bigger.

3. There is some loss of vision, if the ulcer is central.
4. Iritis (small pupil and pus in the anterior chamber) may be present if the ulcer penetrates (goes through) the cornea.
5. You may see a foreign body if it caused the ulcer.

Treatment
Admit for inpatient treatment, unless the ulcer is very small.

1. Give antibiotic compound eye ointment four times a day. (Do not use any ointment or drops which contain hydrocortisone or predniso-lone or cortisone-like drug.)
2. Keep a firm pad on the eye all the time. But do not pad the eye if there is a discharge from the eye.
3. Examine the eye (after staining with fluor-escein) every day.
4. If the ulcer gets worse or iritis develops, treat for iritis – see this page.
5. If there is any possibility of Vitamin A deficiency, give Vitamin A 100,000 IU immedi-atly and daily.

Transfer to Medical Officer care
1. if the ulcer gets worse (urgent);

2. if the ulcer does not improve within 2 days of the start of treatment (urgent);
3. if the ulcer has not almost healed after 5 days of treatment (non-urgent).

Note – There may be a scar for which no treatment is possible. Do not transfer if there is only a scar.

> Always look for a corneal ulcer in anyone with a red painful eye.

Acute iritis

Acute iritis is an acute inflammation of the eye, including the anterior chamber and iris.

Causes include:
1. infection from outside the eye (e.g. after in-juries or corneal ulcer);
2. infection which started inside the eye i.e. taken there by the blood (e.g. leprosy, onchocerciasis);
3. non-infective causes (e.g. rheumatoid disease, leprosy reaction, etc.); and
4. no cause diagnosed (most cases if it is not infection).

Symptoms include:
1. severe pain in the eye, made worse by light, and
2. loss of some vision.

Signs include:
1. inflammation of the conjunctiva around the edge of the cornea only (not under the eyelids);
2. pus in the anterior chamber (cloudy anterior chamber or hypopyon);
3. pupil irregular and small and does not contract and dilate normally;
4. eye tender when touched;
5. loss of some vision;
6. you may find the cause of the iritis (see above).

See Figures 31.10 and 31.11

Treatment
Try to find the cause. Always stain the cornea with fluorescein, and look for foreign body and ulcer – see page 336 and page 342.

If the cause is obvious, e.g. corneal injury or ulcer, treat as below.

If the cause is not obvious, always look for leprosy, and especially a leprosy reaction, (see

343

Figure 31.10 Acute iritis. Note that: (1) There are dilated blood vessels in the conjunctiva around the cornea (not present all over the conjunctiva). (2) The anterior chamber is not clear. (3) The pupil is small and irregular – it does not dilate in a dark place.

Figure 31.11 Acute iritis with hypopyon. Note that: (1) The circum-corneal conjunctival vessels are enlarged. (2) A corneal ulcer is present (the cause of the iritis). (3) The pus has settled to the bottom of the anterior chamber (called hypopyon). (4) The anterior chamber is all cloudy, so that you cannot see the small irregular pupil clearly.

Chapter 15 page 86); also look for onchocerciasis (see Chapter 32 page 365).

If the cause is leprosy or you cannot find the cause, treat as below, *and* transfer to Medical Officer care (urgent).

1. Antibiotic eye ointment – use chloramphenicol or antibiotic compound ointment, put under the lower lid every 3 hours.
2. Atropine sulphate 1% eye ointment – put under the lower lid four times a day, until the pupil is widely dilated, and then once daily.
3. Keep a firm pad on the eye all the time. But do not pad the eye if it is discharging.
4. Chloramphenicol 1 g (4 caps) every 6 hours – Give by IMI if necessary. Reduce the dose to 750 mg (3 caps) four times a day when the patient improves.
5. Aspirin 600–1200 mg (2–4 tabs) or codeine compound tablets (2 tabs) should be given every 6 hours for pain, if necessary.

Continue the treatment for 10 days, or until all the redness goes and the eye is completely better (up to 3 weeks), whichever is the longer.

Transfer to Medical Officer's care if

1. It is caused by leprosy (urgent) or onchocerciasis (urgent if acute).

2. You cannot find then cause (urgent).
3. The patient is not improving after 2 days of treatment (urgent).
4. The patient is not completely cured after 2–3 weeks of treatment (non-urgent).

> Always look for acute iritis in anyone with a painful red eye.

Cataract

A cataract has formed if the clear lens of the eye becomes cloudly.

Causes include:
1. old age,
2. injury, and
3. others.

Symptoms:
Slow loss of vision which continues to get worse, is usually the only symptom.

Signs include:
1. The pupil seems white not black when you shine a light into it.

2. There is some loss of vision or total loss of vision.

Treatment
Transfer the patient to the eye specialist when there are cataracts in *both* eyes and he cannot see enough for normal living. (The eye specialist will operate on the worst eye, and give him special glasses.)

No other treatment is possible.

Onchocerciasis (river blindness)

See Chapter 32 page 365 for description and treatment.

See also Conjunctivitis (page 340), Corneal Ulcer (page 342) and Acute Iritis (page 343).

Vitamin A Deficiency

Vitamin A deficiency, affecting the eyes, is common between the ages of 6 months and 6 years. It is uncommon in adults but can occur in pregnant or breastfeeding women or in both sexes in times of famine or war.

The earliest symptom or sign is often not being able to see properly at night – night blindness.

Dryness of the conjunctiva and cornea (called 'xerophthalmia') is an important sign. The conjuntiva look dry, roughened and wrinkled. The eyelids can be red and swollen. The eye can become painful and there is pain on looking into the light. The cornea is then not clear and colourless as normal, but looks dry and a little dull and hazy.

In severe disease, a spreading white spot appears on the cornea and the cornea my break open.

Prevention is by eating a diet with enough Vitamin A. If this is not possible, a single oral dose of 200,000 IU Vitamin A each six months will prevent the condition.

Treatment is by synthetic Vitamin A 5000–10,000 IU daily for several day; but if the cornea is involved, larger doses of up to 100,000 IU daily are recommended.

Long sight and short sight

The patient slowly loses his vision of things close to the eyes if he has long sight; or of things far away if he has short sight.

Examination shows that the patient cannot see the small part of the eye chart if he has short sight, or small printing if he has long sight. There is no other abnormality. But if you give the patient with short sight a card with a small hole (pin hole) in it to look through, he can see things much better.

If the patient cannot see enough for normal living, refer or transfer him non-urgently to the eye specialist, who will give him glasses to wear.

Strabismus (squint)

The two eyes do not look in the same direction at the same time.
Causes include:
1. abnormal development in a child,
2. trauma, and
3. disease of brain or the nerves to the eye.

Treatment
If a child has a squint, refer or non-urgently transfer the patient to the eye specialist. It is essential that this is done before he is seven years old.

If an adult has a squint which started recently, refer or transfer the patient to the Medical Officer for investigation.

If an adult has a squint which has been present for many years, do not transfer the patient as no treatment is possible.

Eye injuries

Bruising of eye lids
No treatment is necessary.

Sub-conjunctival haemorrhage
No treatment is necessary, but check that there is no facture of the skull. If there is a skull fracture transfer the patient to Medical Officer care.

Corneal abrasions
Treat as for a corneal ulcer.

Hyphaema (blood in the anaerior chamber)

Order complete rest in bed and an eye pad until all the blood goes.

Transfer urgently to Medical Officer care if most of the anterior chamber is filled with blood (for urgent surgery).

Iris damage

Treatment does not help. Treat other conditions present.

Cataract after injury

No treatment is possible. If there is severe pain, transfer urgently for surgery.

Wounds of the eyelids

Carefully suture to make the edges of the eyelids level.

All penetrating wounds of cornea and sclera

Urgent transfer to Medical Officer's care is necessary. Meanwhile, treat as acute iritis and give tetanus prophylaxis

Problems of diagnosis and management

Painful or red eye

Take a history of the present illness and also about the loss of sight, pain, redness and discharge.

Do a full examination of the eye, see page 345.

1. Find out where the redness is

If it is all over the conjunctiva (on the undersurface of the eyelids as well as around the cornea) then diagnose:

- conjunctivitis (see page 340) or
- foreign body or chemical in eye (see page 340).

If it is mainly around the cornea, then diagnose

- corneal ulcer, or
- corneal foreign body, or ⎱ (see 2
- iritis, or ⎰ below)
- acute glaucoma.

2. Put fluorescein into the eye (see page 336)

If the cornea stains green in some parts, then diagnose:

- corneal ulcer (see page 342) or
- corneal foreign body (see page 342).

If the cornea is normal, then diagnose

- iritis, or ⎱ (see 3 below)
- glaucoma. ⎰

3. Find out the size of the pupil.

If the pupil is small, then diagnose iritis. See page 343.

If the pupil is large then diagnose glaucoma. Transfer to Medical Officer (urgent if there is still some sight in the eye).

32

Disorders of the Skin

The skin has a number of functions:
1. protection of the body from things outside the body – mechanical injury, heat, cold, light, chemicals, organisms etc;
2. keeping salt and water and other things inside the body;
3. keeping the temperature of the body normal, e.g. by sweating when the body is too hot; and
4. taking sensations into the body, e.g. touch, pain, heat, cold etc.

Pathology

There are many different types of lesion of the skin. See Figure 32.2, for illustrations of them.
1. *Macule* (or macular lesion)

   A macule is an area of skin which is different from the surrounding skin. It is not raised above the level of the skin surface. You can see (e.g. different colour) and/or feel it in the skin.

Anatomy and physiology

horny layer of keratin

prickle cell layer of cells which make the keratin

sweat gland duct

hair

sebaceous gland

sweat gland
blood vessels and nerves etc. running to and from the skin in fatty tissue

epidermis

dermis

sub cutaneous tissue

Figure 32.1 Diagram to show the structure of the skin under the microscope. In certain parts of the body certain parts of the structure of the skin are more marked than usual (e.g. thick horny layer on the soles of the feet).

Figure 32.2 Diagrams showing some of the different types of skin lesion.

2. *Papule* (or papular lesion)
   A papule is like a macule, but it is raised above the level of the skin surface.
3. *Vesicle* (or vesicular lesion)
   A vesicle is like a papule, but there is clear fluid under the surface of the lesion.
4. *Pustule* (or pustular lesion)
   A pustule is like a vesicle, but the fluid contains pus.
5. *Crust*
   A crust is dried exudate (fluid which comes from the lesion) and may consist of:
   • serum (yellow),
   • blood (red or brown),
   • pus (grey green), or
   • mixtures of these.
6. *Scales* are built up surface layers of the skin. They may be:
   • yellow and greasy (e.g. seborrhoeic dermatitis),
   • silvery (e.g. psoriasis), or
   • grey (e.g. eczema)
7. *Ulcers* are areas where the skin has been destroyed.
8. *Dermatitis* is any inflammation of the skin. There are many different types of dermatitis.
9. *Eczema* (or eczematous reaction or eczematous dermatitis)
   Eczema is the most common type of dermatitis (see Figures 32.3 and 32.4). In the acute stage the affected area gets red, shiny and warm because the blood vessels widen. Then small vesicles appear on the surface of the skin. These vesicles soon burst. The exudate dries and forms a crust. Secondary bacterial infection may occur. After some time chronic eczema develops. The affected area may be thick, dry, scaly and the normal lines in the skin become very deep. Cracks can develop deep into the flesh underneath.

Diagnosis and treatment of skin conditions

Sometimes you can easily recognise the symptoms and signs of a certain disease. If you cannot, then do a full history and examination and test the urine (see Chapter 6). Look at the skin all over the body. Decide which of the two main groups of skin conditions your patient is in:

Figure 32.3   Acute eczematous dermatitis.

Figure 32.4   Chronic eczematous dermatitis. The area has become 'lichenificated' – the skin is thick and dry and the normal creases are deep.

1. Generalised illnesses with a skin condition, e.g. chickenpox, measles, syphilis, yaws, leprosy or other infections; malnutrition; allergic reaction to a drug; etc.
2. *Localised skin conditions*, i.e. conditions affecting only the skin.

Important causes include:

(a) external parasites, e.g. scabies, lice;

(b) fungal infections, e.g. tinea;

(c) bacterial infections, e.g. impetigo;

(d) eczematous dermatitis which has many causes;

(e) itching which causes scratching which causes damage to the skin (i.e. dermatitis) which causes more itching ...

Localised skin conditions are very common and important, and so you should know about

1. the preparations that are available to treat localised skin conditions; and

2. how to use these skin preparations.

Preparations often available for treatment of skin conditions

You do not need all of these preparations.

1. *Antibacterial preparations*
   - Eusol[1] solution
     – use for dressings if there is much pus or dead tissue;
     – stop when the lesion is clean
   - Antiseptics
     (a) hexachlorophene 3% emulsion (e.g. 'Phisohex') – use with water to clean the skin or a lesion
     (b) chlorhexidine compound solution (e.g. 'Savlon') in either water or spirit (alcoholic) solution – use to clean the skin or a lesion
   - Antibiotics
     (a) antibiotic compound ointment
     (b) antibiotic compound powder
     (c) powder from inside a tetracycline capsule
   - Crystal (gentian) violet 1% solution in either water or spirit (alcoholic) solution; but better further diluted to 0.25% (¼%) solution
   - Iodine 2.5% solution in spirit (alcohol) – use to clean a lesion or the skin
   - Acriflavine emulsion (use only with strong 3% saline[1] dressing); stop when infection goes or it will stop healing.
   - Potassium permanganate (Condy's crystals) 1–10,000 solution[1] in water

Give also an oral or injected antibiotic (see Chapter 11 page 42) if there is a severe infection.

2. *Antifungal preparations*
   - Benzoic acid compound ointment (Whitfields ointment)
   - Salicylic acid 10% paint
   - Gentian violet 1% solution in either water or spirit (alcohol) it is best diluted to ¼%)(for Candida 'thrush' only)
   - Potassium permanganate (Condy's crystals) 1–10,000 solution[2] in water
   - Iodine 2.5% solution in spirit (alcohol)

3. *Anti-inflammatory preparations*
   These are used for eczema and other dermatitis and to help healing.
   - Potassium permanganate (Condy's crystals) 1–10,000 solution[2] in water
   - Aluminium acetate 10% solution (Burrows solution) in water
   - Weak 1% saline[2] solution
   - Calamine lotion
   - Zinc cream
   - Glycerine and ichthamol
   - Cod liver oil ointment
   - Wool fat anhydrous (lanoline)
   - Ammoniated mercury ointment 2.5% (Ung HAD)

4. *Anti-itch preparations*
   - Weak 1% saline[2] solution
   - Potassium permanganate (Condy's crystals) 1–10,000 solution[2] in water
   - Give also an antihistamine orally or by injection if required

5. *Anti-external parasite preparations*
   - Gamma benzene hexachloride 1% solution
   - Benzyl benzoate 25% solution
   - Iodine solution 2.5%. *Dilute immediately before use* with an equal volume of water
   - DDT 2% emulsion
   - DDT 10% powder

A number of preparations have more than one function and can be very useful if the diagnosis is not certain, or if two or more conditions are present e.g.:

Potassium permanganate solution

– anti inflammatory

---

1 For details of how to make this, see page 351.

2 For details of how to make these, see page 351

– anti itch
– anti fungal
– anti bacterial
Crystal violet
– anti bacterial
– anti fungal (for Candida ('thrush') only)
Iodine solution
– anti bacterial
– anti fungal
– anti scabies
– (but this can itself cause a rash)

How to make simple useful skin preparations

1. Eusol solution

Mix chlorinated lime 12.5 g (20 ml) with enough water to make a paste. Add a little more water and shake. Add boric acid 12.5 g (20 ml) and shake. Add enough water to make 1 litre. Shake well. Leave overnight. Filter. Store in a dark coloured bottle. Note that Eusol is a clear solution with the smell of chlorine. It does not store well and you should use it within a week. If the solution is more than a week old, or does not smell of chlorine, throw it away.

2. Potassium permanganate 1–10,000 solution.

Dissolve 1¼ ml or ¼ of a teaspoonful (not heaped) of potassium permanganate (Condy's

crystals) in 10 litres (½ bucketful) of clean water. It is a dark pink colour.

3. Strong (3%) saline.

Dissolve 7½ ml (1½ teaspoonsful, not heaped) of salt in 200 ml (1 cup) of clean water.

4. Weak (1%) saline.

Dissolve 2½ ml (½ teaspoonsful, not heaped) of salt in 200 ml (1 cup) of clean water.

Dressings

Use a *wet gauze bandage* for all painful conditions on legs, arms, feet, hands, and head, especially if you think it will heal slowly.

Use *adhesive plaster* for all small painless conditions on rounded parts of the body, joints, etc.

Use *crepe bandages* for all painful conditions on joints and thighs, and for large deep ulcers, wounds, etc. anywhere.

Use *elastic plaster bandage* on soles, palms and early boils.

Use dry *gauze bandages* only for tinea of the feet.

Note these things about treatment

1. Do not make a dermatitis worse by treatment which irritates the already damaged skin. (e.g. do not immediately use Whitfields ointment on

Table 32.1. Dressings for skin conditions

		Cost	Pain relief?	Helps healing?	Stays on?	Pain when removed?
Gauze bandage (WOW)	Wet	Cheap	Good	Good	Good	No pain
	Dry	Cheap	Some	Some	Poor	No pain
Adhesive plaster		Very cheap	None	None	Good in dry weather	A little painful
Elastic plaster bandage		Expensive	Some	Some	Good	Very painful
Crepe bandage		Expensive	Very good	Very good	Good	No pain

an acutely inflamed fungal infection. It is better to use postassium permanganate solution wet dressings to start with until the condition is not acute. Then you can use the Whitfield ointment (see Figure 32.8).

2. You must treat any bacterial infection.
3. Always look for signs of scabies and lice if there is (a) an itch or (b) if there is skin infection, especially if more than one area is affected and especially if it returns after treatment.
4. Always treat an itch which causes scratching. If you do not treat the itch, the scratching causes dermatitis and the dermatitis causes more itch and more scratching . . . . .
5. Always think of the possibility that drugs or skin treatment have caused the skin problem. Treatment for a condition which has gone, may have caused a new skin condition.

The common skin conditions

Tinea

Tinea is a fungal infection of the skin. *Complaints* include itching and worry about the appearance of the skin.

Examination usually shows affected areas that are roughly circular. The edges are often a little raised and a little inflamed. Sometimes there are small papules, vesicles or pustules at the edge. The skin in the rest of the lesion is often peeling. The centre of the lesion may appear to be healing.

There are many types of tinea – see Figures 32.5, 32.6, 32.7 and 32.8.

Make sure the lesion is not caused by leprosy. Do tests for loss of sensation, etc. If you have real doubt, do a biopsy (but not on face).

Routine treatment
(but *not* for an acutely inflamed area)
Treat as an outpatient.
1. Remove any hair from the affected area.
2. Wash the affected area with soap and water every day. Rub off any scales. Dry the skin well after washing. Keep the skin as dry as possible.
3. Put either salicylic acid paint *or* benzoic acid compound ointment (Whitfields ointment) on the affected area twice daily. Also put it on the normal skin for 2 cm round the edge of the affected area. Do not cover more than one-quarter of the body every day.
4. Change and wash the clothes every day.
5. Continue the treatment every day until all the tinea goes and then for 2–4 weeks after this.

Figure 32.5 Tinea of the body.

Figure 32.6 Tinea imbricata. There is an abnormality in the immunity of many of these patients. This is probably inherited, because the disease is common in certain families. The disease usually returns, even after successful treatment.

Figure 32.7 Tinea of the body, with secondary bacterial infection. You must treat the bacterial infection and the skin inflamation before you treat the tinea infection.

Figure 32.8 Tinea of the nails.

Treatment of an acutely inflamed area of tinea

1. Do not treat with Whitfields ointment or salicylic acid paint at first.
2. Bathe the area with potassium permanganate 1–10,000 solution and then put on a *little* acriflavine emulsion on a dressing soaked in strong 3% saline.
3. Also give procaine penicillin 900,000 units (3 ml) IMI daily or tetracycline 250 mg (1 cap) four times a day for at least 5 days for infection if necessary.
4. Give routine treatment (as above) only when the acute inflammation improves.

The above treatment by itself will not cure –
  tinea of the nails
  most cases of tinea of the scalp
  many cases of tinea of the skin
See a reference book about griseofulvin tablets.

Tinea versicolor (white spot)

Tinea versicolor is a fungus infection which causes many small lesions which are pale and covered with powdery skin (see Figure 32.9). The patient may complain of the appearance or of the itch.

Treat with 10% or 20% sodium thiosulphate solution ('hypo' or X-ray fixer) on the whole body twice daily or Whitfields ointment daily on the affected areas (but not more than ¼ of the body daily).

If this is not successful, see a reference book about the use of selenium sulphide.

Griseofulvin does not help.

Mycetoma ('Madura foot')

Mycetoma is a fungus infection which spreads to deep structures (such as the bones). It is common in dry areas of Africa, the Middle East and parts of Asia. It is common in people who do not wear shoes, especially farmers. Most often it affects the patient's foot.

Figure 32.9   Tinea versicolor.

354

Figure 32.10 Foot affected by mycetoma.

First there is a painless swelling of the area. The area affected slowly becomes larger. Lumps may appear in the swollen area. The lumps may burst and sinuses may form. Pus, with little lumps of coloured material (e.g. black, red, yellow), comes out of the sinuses. There is still no pain or fever, and the patient can still use the affected area. But over months or years the affected area becomes larger. The infection does not often spread to the lymph glands or to other parts of the body.

After many years the infected area (usually the foot) is so badly affected that the patient cannot use it. (See Figure 32.10.)

Treatment of some of these infections with drugs is possible. However surgery is usually necessary. Refer or non-urgently transfer affected patients to a medical officer.

Prevention may be possible if you tell people in the areas where the disease is common to wear shoes.

Impetigo

Impetigo is a bacterial infection of the skin. It is very infectious and spreads to others by direct contact or by vehicles, such as towels.

First a blister forms. This bursts and leaves a red wet surface. A thick yellow crust forms. Then new blisters form. There are other types of impetigo. (See Figure 32.11.)

Management
1. Gently rub off the scabs and crusts with antisceptic solution (see 2 below.).
2. Wash the whole area with antiseptic solution twice a day, and then daily, when it improves. Suitable antiseptics include chlorhexidine comp. antiseptic in water (e.g. 'Savlon') or hexachlorophene emulsion (e.g. 'Phisohex').
3. Put a dressing over the affected area especially if it is large or has pus coming from it.
4. Put antibiotic compound ointment *or* a *little* acriflavine emulsion on a dressing wet with strong 3% saline on to the affected area. Do this three times a day at first; and then daily, when it improves.
5. Change and wash the clothes daily.
6. Give antibiotics for 5–10 days *if*
   - the patient develops general symptoms and signs of infection *or*
   - the skin lesions are very large or inflamed *or*
   - the condition does not respond to the above treatment *or*
   - the condition continually returns *or*
   - you are not certain that the patient will do the treatment properly.

Figure 32.11 Impetigo with vesicles. Sometimes the vesicles develop into large bulbous lesions.

Give procaine penicillin 900,000 units (3 ml) daily or tetracycline 250 mg (1 cap) four times a day.

7. Look very carefully for scabies and lice, especially if there is an itch. (The lesions of scabies and lice are not always typical.) Treat if present (see pages 361–3).

8. If the condition appears in new areas, or returns after it was cured and treatment was stopped, then wash the *whole body* (including the perineum and inside the nose) with the antiseptic solution daily. Then give all the above treatment, especially 6 and 7.

9. Tell the patient that the infection spreads by pus from the infected areas taking germs to new areas. He should not touch the infected areas. He should wash his hands often. He should not allow others to touch his towel and clothes until he is cured.

Furuncle or boil

A boil is an infection by bacteria of the skin in the place where a hair grows. A boil starts as a small tender lump in the skin. It becomes bigger over

Figure 32.12 Furuncle or boil.

some days, and has all the signs of acute inflammation. It then 'points' – softens in the centre as pus forms. The skin bursts and the pus comes out. A day or two later the 'core' comes out – the dead part of the skin which made the hair. (See Figure 32.12)

In an area where myiasis occurs, check that any slowly developing 'boil' is not caused by the myiasis (see page 363)

Treatment

At early stage – only inflamed swelling:
1. Paint the lesion (and several cm all round it) with iodine solution 2.5%
2. Cover the area with a large square of elastic plaster bandage (e.g. 'Elastoplast'). Stretch the elastic plaster as you stick it on to the skin. (This will 'splint' the area.)
3. Give aspirin 300–900 mg (1–3 tabs) four times a day for pain, if necessary.
4. Test the lesion under the elastic plaster for fluctuation every day.
5. If the lesion goes, remove the plaster; but only when it has *completely* gone.
6. If *definite* fluctuation develops, remove the elastic plaster with one quick pull. This will probably also pull off the thin skin over the surface of the boil and allow it to drain – incision will then not be necessary.

At other stages
See Chapter 11 about antibiotics and a surgery book about incision and drainage.
If repeated boils
Treat as for repeated impetigo (see 8, page 356).

Tropical ulcer

Tropical ulcer is a skin infection with special types of bacteria, which cause an acute severe infective ulcer, which may become a chronic ulcer.

The special bacteria which cause tropical ulcer spread by direct contact and by flies.

A tropical ulcer usually comes on exposed areas, usually the legs. First a vesicle forms. This bursts and leaves an ulcerating, dirty surface. The ulcer spreads very quickly. It is painful and itchy. The edge is slightly raised. The surface is covered with a smelly grey-green or bloody membrane. (See Figure 32.13.)

Figure 32.13 Tropical ulcer. You can diagnose the ulcer by its very quick growth, its typical appearance (raised edge, a grey bloody membrane on the surface). There are very few general symptoms and signs.

The patient has no general symptoms and signs of infection. The ulcer may remain for months or years. When it heals, if forms very thin skin, which often breaks down and forms an ulcer again.

Treatment
If the ulcer is severe or large, admit for inpatient treatment. If it is small, treat as an outpatient.
1. Give procaine penicillin 900,00 units (3 ml) IMI daily until the ulcer is healing well or at least 7 days (this is very important if it is a true Tropical Ulcer).
2. If possible, rest the affected area. Keep the leg with the ulcer on it higher than the rest of the body. If this is not possible, firmly bandage a cotton wool pad over the dressing (see 3 and 4), using a crepe bandage if possible.
3. Dress the ulcer twice daily (or more often if necessary) with Eusol, or strong (3%) saline solution, until the ulcer is clean.
4. When the ulcer is clean, dress with any non-irritating dressing, e.g. cod liver oil ointment, or antibiotic compound ointment on gauze, or vaseline gauze. Change the dressing only when it is really necessary (so that you do not damage new skin growing).

5. Skin graft the ulcer if it is larger than 3 cm in diameter.

Transfer to Medical Officer's care non-urgently if:
1. The ulcer does not improve with treatment.
2. You cannot do the skin graft.
3. The ulcer is very large, or there is bone at the base (bottom) of the ulcer.

Yaws

Yaws is a bacterial infection spread by direct contact or by flies.

It affects children much more often than adults.

The first (or primary) lesion is a sore, usually on the leg (see Figure 32.14). It is itchy, becomes 1–2 cm wide, and is raised. It has an irregular white-yellow crust with a bleeding surface with yellow spots, if you remove the crust. After 1–2 months it goes. The nearby lymph nodes are enlarged but not tender.

Figure 32.14 An early yaws skin lesion.

Figure 32.15 Secondary yaws lesions affecting the soles of the feet.

358

Figure 32.16 Late yaws affecting the face.

Figure 32.17 Late yaws affecting the bones.

Secondary skin lesions are similar to the primary lesions (see Figure 32.15). There are many of them all over the body and they appear when the primary lesion is getting better or has gone. If a lesion appears on the sole of the foot, it is painful and the patient limps. Bones and joints may become painful, tender and thickened at this stage. The long bones may become curved, or the fingers swollen. After some weeks or months, all these things may go. But they may often return.

Late yaws develops in some patients. This can cause skin ulcers, thickening and cracking of the skin of the feet, and destruction of the bones of the nose and face. (See Figures 32.16 and 32.17.)

The VDRL test becomes positive in yaws.

Penicillin cures yaws. But, if you find a case arrange for a survey to find out if control measures are necessary. if a survey shows only a low frequency (less than 5% of the population) you only need to treat the family and obvious contacts of a case. If there is medium frequency (5–9%) treat all children in the community. If there is high frequency (more than 10%), treat everyone in the community. For prophylactic treatment one dose of procaine penicillin of 1,200,000 units for adults and 600,000 units for children is very effective (especially procaine penicillin with aluminium monostearate (PAM)).

Bejel (endemic syphilis) and pinta

Endemic syphilis (called Bejel or other local names) occurs in the Middle East and Africa and is caused by non-sexually transmitted syphilis in childhood. Spread is by close personal contact, and by cups etc. Children can develop all the lesions of secondary syphilis (see Chapter 19 page 134) and sometimes skin lesions which are the same as yaws (see above). After some years these conditions go; but after some more years, severe destruction of the skin and the bones of the face can occur (as in late yaws). The VDRL test is positive. (See Figure 32.18)

Treatment is with penicillin, as for syphilis (see Chapter 19 page 134)

Pinta (which has other local names) occurs in Central and South America and the Middle East. It is caused by an organism related to the syphilis and yaws bacteria. Spread is by non-sexual transmission, like yaws. First there is an itchy scaly

Figure 32.18 Secondary rash caused by Bejel (endemic syphilis).
(Source: W. Peters and H. M. Gilles. *A colour atlas of tropical medicine and parasitology*. London, Wolfe Medical Publications, 1981) (Dr A. Buck)

papule. This slowly enlarges and joins with new papules which continue to appear around its edge. The papule becomes up to 10 cm in diameter. Nearby lymph nodes are enlarged. This lesion often remains, but later many other lesions appear on the exposed parts of the skin. These lesions are most often dark. After many years, the lesions on the limbs become symetrical (i.e. the same on both sides) depigmented (pale) and thin. The VDRL is positive. (See Figures 32.19.)

Treatment is with penicillin, as for syphilis (see Chapter 19 page 134)

Anthrax

Anthrax is normally a bacterial infection of cattle and sheep etc. It can infect people on exposed parts of their skin, most often on the face. A papule forms quickly. This soon becomes a vesicle filled with blood-stained fluid. Small vesicles appear around the original vesicle. The area

around the lesion becomes very swollen, and looks inflamed; but it does not pit on pressure, and it is not very tender. After some days the vesicle dries, becomes black, and starts to heal.

Usually there is some enlargement of the nearby lymph glands, but few general symptoms and signs of infection. But the infection can spread and cause septicaemia and death. Other more severe forms of the disease can occur.

If you suspect a patient has anthrax, immediately start treatment with penicillin, and check with your Medical Officer for methods of control and prevention.

Mycobacterium ulcerans ulcer

Mycobacterium ulcerans is a bacterium which can cause a chronic skin ulcer. The reservoir and means of spread is not certain.

The lesion usually starts as a papule which bursts to form an ulcer. The ulcer grows slowly

Figure 32.19 Depigmented lesions caused by pinta. (Source: W. Peters and H. M. Gilles, *A colour atlas of tropical medicine and parasitology*, London, Wolfe Medical Publications, 1981)

Figure 32.20 A *Mycobacterium ulcerans* infection. A probe can go several centimetres under the apparently normal skin at the edge of the ulcer.

over weeks or months. It goes down to the muscle, and sideways underneath the skin. This causes a very typical appearance, where the skin overhangs the edge of the ulcer, some times by several centimetres. (See Figure 32.20.)

Diagnosis is by the typical appearance and by a biopsy sent for examination in the laboratory.

If you diagnose this condition, non-urgently transfer the patient for excision or curettage of the ulcer and skin grafting. Special drugs may sometimes help.

Cellulitis

Cellulitis is an inflammation of the cellular and other tissues underneath the skin. These tissues normally join the structures under the skin. The inflammation in cellulitis usually spreads along the divisions between the organs under the skin. If cellulitis is not cured quickly, pus can form. Abscesses can then form and even gangrene of the skin can occur.

There is usually pain in the area, but not at one definite place. There is swelling, redness and tenderness of the affected part of the body, but again it is not usually in one particular place. Blisters can form on the skin. There is usually malaise, fever, fast pulse, etc.

Treatment is by rest and antibiotics. Benzyl (crystaline) penicillin 1,000,000 units by IMI every 6 hours until the condition improves and then procaine benzyl penicillin 900,000 units daily by IMI is usually enough. If the condition gets worse, the antibiotic should be changed to chloramphenicol 1 g (4 caps) orally every 6 hours and if pus has collected in any area, and it can be drained easily without risk of damaging any important structure, incision should be made over the area. Should pus be deep, however, or should the inflammation be in an area where there are many important structures, such as the neck or hand, transfer the patient urgently to a medical officer.

Cutaneous Leishmaniasis ('Oriental Sore' and 'Espundia')

See Chapter 18 page 166.

Scabies

Scabies is an infestation of the surface layer of the skin by an insect, the scabies mite. The scabies

Figure 32.21 Scabies

mite spreads from one person to another during close personal contact. It usually infests all people who live in the same house as a person with scabies.

The patient usually complains of an itch in part of the body or of repeated sores in part of the body.

The usual lesion of scabies is a dark papule, several mm in diameter. You can sometimes see the path the mite made through the skin. The patient scratches the lesions and often causes an eczematous reaction or a bacterial infection (such as impetigo) in the area.

Most often it affects the areas between the fingers, the front of the wrists, the elbows, the breast, the penis, the pubic region and, in babies, the sides of the feet.

Treat as an outpatient.

1. Apply gamma benzene hexachloride (BHC) 1% lotion or cream like this:

    (a) Wash all the body with soap, using a cloth. Rinse and dry the skin.

    (b) Shake the bottle very well, and put the BHC lotion on all the body below the neck especially in the folds of the skin. The medicine must remain on the skin for 24 hours.

Figure 32.22 Diagram to show the usual distribution of scabies lesions.

362

(c) After 24 hours, wash the BHC lotion off and put on clean clothes.

(d) Four days later, repeat the treatment as in (a), (b) and (c).

Give the patient a private room where he can completely undress. The patient can wash himself. **But a health worker must apply the lotion** to all the skin of the patient (except the face). The patient cannot do it well enough.

If the patient is a mother, wash the breasts before breastfeeding. After breastfeeding, put the application on again.

2. If the lesions are infected, give antibiotics: procaine penicillin 900,000 units (3 ml) IMI daily, or tetracycline 250 mg (1 cap) four times each day starting on the day of the first gamma benzene hexachloride treatment until the infection goes. If impetigo is present, treat this first (see page 355) before giving the gamma benzene hexachloride treatment.

3. Treat (or show the patient how to treat) all members of the patient's family, and anyone else who lives with him.

4. Change and wash the clothes and bedclothes, and put them in the sun, at the end of every 24 hour treatment.

5. Educate the patient about the cause and prevention of the disease. Encourge the patient and his family to wash regularly with soap. Encourage the patient to keep clean and regularly wash his clothes, bedclothes, and house.

Tell the patient to come for treatment when any new lesions appear (before they are bad or there are many).

Lice (Pediculosis)

Lice are insects which can infect people. They can carry dangerous disease (e.g. typhus). But usually they only caɪse itching and skin rash. There are 3 types of lice.

The head louse lives on the scalp and puts its eggs on the hair ('nits'). It causes severe itching of the scalp. Scratching often causes eczema or results in bacterial infection of the scalp. The glands in the neck are aften enlarged. You can diagnose lice by finding them or their eggs on the scalp or hair.

Body lice cause itching, scratching and eczema or bacterial infections of the body; especially around the waist. You will find the lice and eggs in the clothes (especially under the edges).

Pubic lice affect the pubic area, and also the eyelashes.

Treatment is with gamma benzene hexacloride (BHC) 1% cream or lotion or benzyl benzoate 25% solution or DDT 2% emulsion or 10% powder.

Put one of these insecticides on the hair and scalp. Cover the hair with a cloth for some hours. The next day wash and carefully comb the hair to remove all the eggs. Repeat the treatment a week later.

For body lice boil or iron the clothes and bedclothes during each treatment. Treat the patient and his clothes with insecticide. See Chapter 17 page 107 for methods of mass treatment in epidemics.

For pubic lice, it may be necessary to shave off the pubic hair. But do *not* shave or cut the eyelashes.

Control and prevention is by treatment of cases, good personal hygiene, and using repellents in epidemics of typhus.

Tungiasis

Tungiasis occurs mostly in South America and Africa. It is an infestation with the chigoe or jigger flea, which affects man and pigs.

Most often it affects the feet. The flea goes into the skin, and grows to the size of a small pea. It then pushes eggs through the skin lesion. First there is itching. Later there can be secondary bacterial infection. Tetanus can occur.

In treatment you must remove the whole flea in one piece with a sterile needle and prevent and treat secondary bacterial infection and tetanus. If there are very many lesions, soak the affected area in a 5% solution of benzene hexachloride.

Myiasis

Myiasis is an infestation with the larvae (maggots) of flies. The larvae can go into the skin and make a lesion like a furuncle or boil. In areas where myiasis occurs, always think of this condition

Figure 32.23 The distribution of onchocerciasis. (Based on: WHO Technical Report Series No. 597, 1976 (Report of a WHO Expert Committee on the Epidemiology of Onchocerciasis))

Endemic onchocerciasis

Onchoceciasis known to occur but distribution and prevalence uncertain when a patient has an inflamed swelling of the skin.

In treatment put oil (such as liquid parafin) on the lesion so that the larvae cannot breath and so start to come out of the skin to get air. If you put more oil on and press the sides of the lesion this will usually remove the larvae. Sometimes surgery is necessary. Treat any secondary infection with antibiotics.

Onchoceriasis

Onchocerciasis is a chronic disease of the skin and eye. It is caused by an infestation with a filarial worm. The adult worm causes nodules in the skin. The larvae (microfilaria) cause dermatitis and blindness.

Onchocerciasis is common only in parts of Africa, the Middle East and in Central and South America. (See Figure 32.23.)

The bite of an infected *Simulium* (a small black fly) injects infective larvae of the worm. These flies breed only in fast flowing rivers; but they can fly many kilometres from the rivers.

The larvae develop into adult worms in the skin of the infected person. The adults cause painless nodules under the skin. These may become large lumps and are most common where bones are just under the skin (e.g. around joints, hips, ribs, back of head). The adults make many larvae (called microfilaria) which travel around the body in the tissues of the skin and eye (but not in the blood).

The microfilaria cause dermatitis with itching and form macules and papules. The skin can become lichenified (or thickened) and wrinkled. This is sometimes called 'lizard' or 'elephant' skin. After some years of severe itching and scratching, the skin can become thin and loose (called 'tissue paper' skin) and patches of the skin become pale (called 'leopard' skin). Folds of skin can form in the groin ('hanging groin). (See Figures 32.24, 32.25 and 32.26.)

The microfilaria can cause many sorts of damage to the eyes, which can lead to blindness (River Blindness). They can causes conjunctivitis or a chronic oedema of the conjunctivae and eyelids. They can also cause whitish spots on the cornea and later a thickening and loss of clearness of the cornea, often with blood vessels growing in the affected area. This change starts at the bottom of the cornea and grows up over the cornea so that the patient cannot see through it. Microfilaria can also cause iritis and later glaucoma and cataract. The retina of the eye may be damaged. From any one or more of these things the patient often becomes blind.

You can diagnose onchocerciasis like this:

1. remove a nodule, cut it across and see an adult worm in it; *or*
2. take a 'skin snip', put it into saline on a slide under the microscope and see microfilaria.

Treatment is not necessary in patients who do not have symptoms or signs other than lumps.

Treat if there are eye lesions, or severe dermatitis, or many nodules.

Treatment needs:

1. diethylcarbamazine and antihistamine to kill the microfilaria (see Chapter 22 page 203 for dose of diethylcarbamazine, you need to use an anthistamine e.g. promethazine with it), and
2. surgical removal of all the nodules which contain adult worms, or the killing of the adults

Figure 32.24 Nodules of onchocerciasis. If you remove and cut a nodule you can see the adult worms lying inside.

Figure 32.25 (above) Skin changes and itching caused by onchocerciasis.

Figure 32.26 Characteristic pale patches on the skin caused by itching.

with suramin (which is a toxic drug – give it only if you have had specially training about it).

Control and prevention is by stopping the spread of the worm by the insects. Use insecticides to kill the larvae and adult fly at its breeding places in rivers. Use clothing and repellents to stop the fly biting. There are no other useful methods.

Loiasis

Loiasis is an infestation of the subcutaneous tissue with a filarial worm *Loa loa*. It occurs in Africa.

The adult worms are up to 7 cm long. They can cause areas of oedema, and often pain, in the skin ('Calabar swellings'). The swellings are often many centimetres in diameter and may last for a number of days. Sometimes you can see the adult worms wriggling under the skin or crossing the conjunctiva of the eye.

The adult produces microfilaria which circulate in the blood. These infect *Chrysops* ('mango' or 'softly-softly' flies) which then give the infection back to man.

Treat people who have repeated swellings as for onchocerciasis (see above).

Prevention is by control of the *Chrysops* fly.

Guinea worm

Guinea worm infestation occurs in parts of Africa, the Middle East, India and South America.

The Guinea worm is a long (e.g. 1 metre) worm which lives under the skin of people and dogs and cats. Adult worms cause irritation of the skin in one area, usually a leg. A blister forms. The blister bursts and a very itchy ulcer forms see Figure 32.27. The itch is helped by putting the leg in water. When the patient puts the leg in water, the end of the worm comes out through the ulcer and

Figure 32.27 A Guinea worm emerging from an ulcer in the patient's leg.

passes its larvae into the water. The worm larvae go into little animals in the water, and develop into larvae which are then infective for people. If people drink water with these infective larvae in it, the larvae develop into new worms under their skin; and the cycle starts again.

Symptoms and signs include:
1. There are allergic reactions, fever or vomiting as the worm starts to go through the skin.
2. A blister forms where the worm goes through the skin. This is usually on the foot or leg or part of the body that is cool and often wet. The blister bursts and an itchy ulcer forms. You can see the end of the worm passing white larvae when the ulcer is in water.
3. After 3–4 weeks the worm leaves the body.
4. If the worm goes into another part of the body, or if it dies, or if other infections go into the ulcer, the patient may develop
   (a) abscess,
   (b) arthritis, or
   (c) tetanus.

Treatment includes:
1. Treat any bacterial infection with antibiotics (see Chapter 11 page 42).
2. Prevent tetanus (see Chapter 25 page 263).
3. Put the affected part into cold clean water so that the worm will pass all its larvae. Tie the end of the worm to a sterile stick with sterile cotton. Slowly wind the worm out of the ulcer round the stick. Do only a little each day, and take care not to break the worm. Cover with antiseptic and a sterile dressing.
4. If available give thiabendazole or niridazole to kill the worm.

Control and prevention is by supplying safe drinking water; or if this is not possible, by boiling or filtering drinking water.

Warts (Verrucae)

Warts are caused by a virus infection of the skin.

The virus makes the cells which make the surface layer of the skin grow too much. They make too much skin in that place and cause a lump. The surface is often rough, or even like cauliflower (see Figure 32.28). If warts develop under the feet, they are pressed flat and make a hole in other tissues of the foot. This can be

Figure 32.28 Warts on the hand.

painful. In other areas they do not usually cause symptoms.

Most warts eventually go away without treatment. If you cover warts with sticking plaster they often go away more quickly. If you decide that the warts need treatment, apply salicylic acid (e.g. 12% in collodion) to the wart once a day until the wart falls off. It is important that you do not put this treatment on nearby normal skin because it will cause severe damage.

Molluscum contagiosum

Molluscum contagiosum is an infectious disease caused by a virus.

It is passed from a patient to another person by close contact or sexual intercourse. It is common in children.

The lesions may occur anywhere on the body. There are almost always many of them. They may vary in size from 2 mm up to 2 cm although large ones are uncommon. They are small white tumours of the skin tissue, but the centre is sunk in and is darker. If you press the larger lesions, a white discharge comes out of the centre.

Treatment is not usually necessary as the lesions

Figure 32.29 Molluscum contagiosum. (The dark centre is often more obvious than in the photograph.)

368

go away in time. If treatment is necessary make a small incision in the centre of the nodule. Then squeeze out the white contents. Then put on tincture of iodine 2.5% solution.

Prevention is by avoiding contact with infected persons.

Pellagra

Pellagra is a condition caused if there is not enough group B vitamin in the food. It is only common in places where maize (corn) is the main food, and little else is eaten (e.g. some parts of Africa).

Pellagra causes 3 conditions:

1. dermatitis – the most common condition;
2. diarrhoea – often with a sore tongue and other gastro-intestinal symptoms; and
3. dementia – more often only anxiety and depression; though dementia and even coma can occur.

Figure 32.30 A severe case of acute pellagra.

The dermatitis of pellagra occurs in areas exposed to sunlight – usually the face and arms. At first there is redness, swelling and discomfort (like sunburn). In acute cases the skin cracks, crusts and ulcerates, and may become infected. In chronic cases the skin becomes dark, thick, dry, rough and scaling. By this stage dermatitis of the vulva, perineum and perianal area is usually also present. (See Figure 32.30.)

In treatment, give vitamin B compound tablets (containing nicotinamide) three or four times a day until the patient improves; but more importantly, improve the diet by including as much animal products and legumes (peas etc.) as the patient can afford.

Eczema or eczematous dermatitis

The patient usually complains of an itch or rash. Examination shows an acute or chronic eczematous reaction (see page 349).

You must then find the *cause* of the eczematous reaction. *Always* think of these four things:

1. contact, especially with chemicals, drugs, cosmetics and clothing,
2. infections or infestations, specially with scabies and lice,
3. drugs, and
4. scratching.

There are two special types of dermatitis for which the cause is not known:

1. *Atopic dermatitis* occurs in allergic patients. Usually it affects areas behind the knees and in front of the elbows in adults.
2. *Seborrheic dermatitis* affects the scalp, eyebrows and eyelids, the sides of the nose and the front of the chest. There are usually thick greasy scales on the affected area.

Treatment – see page 349.

Psoriasis

In psoriasis patches of redness and inflammation of the skin covered by silvery scales appear. The lesions do not itch or cause pain. The edges of the patches, where they join the normal skin, are very definite (see Figure 32.31). The finger nails are often pitted.

Treatment – see a specialist reference book.

Figure 32.31 Typical skin lesions of psoriasis. Note the definite edge. These patches are covered by scales.

Figure 32.33 Photograph showing a close up view of skin affected by acne. You can usually see 'blackheads' on the patient more easily than in this photograph.

Acne vulgaris

In acne, blackheads and pimples form in the skin. Some may become infected and cause boils. Scars and keloids may occur. (See Figures 32.32 and 32.33.)

Treatment – see a specialist reference book.

Vitiligo or leucoderma

In vitiligo patches of normal skin lose their pigment and become white (see Figure 32.34). The skin is otherwise perfectly normal. There is no loss of sensation over the patches.

Do not mistake leprosy, late yaws, late onochoceriasis, etc. for vitiligo.

No treatment for vitiligo is necessary or possible at the health centre, except to protect the skin from sun burn. Vitiligo is not dangerous and is not infectious.

Albinism

Albinism is a hereditary condition in which there is not enough pigment formation in the body.

The irises of the eyes are pink or red, and the hair and the skin are white. The skin does not become darker in the sun.

Figure 32.32 Diagram to show the parts of the body where lesions of acne vulgaris most commonly occur.

Figure 32.34   Vitiligo affecting the skin of the legs. The skin is normal except that it is milky white.

Figure 32.35   The child on the right side of the photograph is an albino. Note the sun-damaged white skin.

The main complication is skin cancer caused by the sun continually burning the skin which is not protected by pigment.

This is no cure for this condition.

Treatment includes wearing clothes to keep the sun off the skin – hat, long sleeved shirt and long trousers or dress, etc. all the time during the day. The person should keep away from the sun as much as possible. He should put a sunscreen on (e.g. 5% para aminobenzoic acid in ethanol or 'UV Cream') twice daily or more often, before going in the sun.

If the patient develops any sores which do not heal, refer or transfer him non-urgently for biopsy and probable excision of lesion, in case it is a skin cancer.

Common skin symptoms and signs

Itch (with or without rash)

Do a full history and examination (see Chapter 6 page 16)
Test the urine for protein, sugar and bile.
Note especially
1. where the itch is, and

2. the details of any skin lesions (rash) present. Diagnosis depends on where the itch and rash is. Treat as in this book (see Index) or see a specialist medical reference book.

Rash between fingers or on wrists or on elbows or on genitalia; but not on face, then
- scabies – see page 361.

Rash in hair or around waist or in eyelashes or in public area, then
- lice – see page 363.

Rash only on uncovered areas (arms, legs, face), then
- insect bites, or
- contact with irritants (contact dermatitis), or
- sunshine and a drug taken or put on skin (photo-sensitive dermatitis).

Itch around anus, then
- tinea – see page 352, or
- enterobius (threadworm) – see Chapter 23 page 219, or
- haemorrhoids or anal fissure, or
- diabetes mellitus (sugar in urine) – see Chapter 30 page 333.

*Itch of vulva,*then
- all conditions as for anus, or
- Candida (thrush) or trichomonas infection, or
- after menopause.

Itch all over, then
- onchocerciasis if there are skin nodules over bony areas and especially if there is trouble with the eyes – see page 365, or
- drugs and other causes of allergy – see Chapter 10 page 37, or
- jaundice – see Chapter 24 page 248, or
- chronic kidney failure – see Chapter 26 page 289

Itch where there is a rash of round patches which are worse at the edges, anywhere on the body, then
- tinea – see page 352.

Itch where there is a rash on face or behind knees and in front of elbows and is either
1. lesions which are thick and very dry or
2. small blisters which burst leaving moist red areas, then
- eczematous dermatitis – see page 369.

Rash (For rash and itch – see also itch)

Do a full history and examination (see Chapter 6 page 16).
Note:
1. where the lesions are, and
2. the type of the lesions they are.
Test the urine for protein, bile and sugar.
Diagnosis depends on the features below.
Treat as in this book (see Index) or see a specialist reference book.

Acute start; fever; general rash (face, trunk and limbs) then
- chickenpox – see Chapter 16 page 98, or
- measles – see Chapter 16 page 97, or
- other viral diseases – see Chapter 16 page 99.

Vesicules, pustules, yellow crusts, then
- impetigo – see page 355.

Dry skin patches –
1. *no loss of sensation; itching, healing in centre,* then
- tinea – see page 352.
2. *loss of sensation and thick nerves,* then
- leprosy – see Chapter 15 page 77.

Nodules
1. *severe itchy dermatitis and eye trouble,* then
- onchocerciasis – see page 365
2. *other signs of leprosy,* then
- leprosy – see Chapter 15 page 77
3. *drugs given recently or other causes of allergy,* then
- allergic reaction – see Chapter 10 page 37
4. *other signs of leprosy and patient is sick or has tender nerves or iritis,* then
- leprosy reaction – see Chapter 15 page 86.

Eczematous reaction (small blisters which burst leaving moist red areas with itch or thick dry areas). Then
- eczematous dermatitis – see page 369.

Skin ulcer

Do a full history and examination (see Chapter 6 page 16).
Test the urine for protein, sugar and bile.
Note especially where the ulcer is – there are 3 common places:
1. genitalia, 2. breast, and 3. leg.
But ulcers can occur anywhere.

Diagnosis depends on the features of the ulcer (see below).

Ulcer on genitalia
Then most likely syphilis or – see Chapter 19.

Ulcer on breast
Acute start in young woman. Then
- most likely breast abscess see Chapter 36 page 401 and a surgery book.

Chronic start in old woman. Then
- most likely cancer. See a surgery or gynaecology book.

Ulcer on leg or foot
Ulcer started acutely and spread very quickly and was itchy and painful and smelly. Ulcer becomes chronic, if untreated. Then
- tropical ulcer – see page 357

Ulcer started after injury or infection.
Ulcer is like an ulcer anywhere but is slow to heal. Then
- bacterial infection. (Treat as for tropical ulcer)

Ulcer started as a blister with general allergic reaction, fever and often vomiting. Blister burst and itchy ulcer developed, relieved by cold water. Outline of worm under skin or end of worm seen in ulcer. Then

- guinea worm – page 367.

Ulcer after chronic anaemia, often jaundice, no bile in urine, infarction crises and especially attacks of bone pain. Then
- sickle-cell anaemia ulcer (Treat as for Tropical Ulcer; but eusol and antibiotics are not necessary if there is no infection.)

Ulcer most often under foot
Loss of sensation under foot
Enlarged nerves or patches with loss of sensation. Then
- leprosy – See Chapter 15 page 77.

Ulcer most often under foot
Loss of sensation under foot
No enlarged nerves or patches with loss of sensation
Sugar in urine, Then
- diabetes mellitus – Chapter 30 page 333;

Ulcer anywhere
Ulcer anywhere, you can see pus and bone. Then
- chronic osteomyelitis – see Chapter 28 page 311.

Ulcer anywhere, in an area where dermal leishmaniasis occurs. Then
- dermal leishmaniasis (oriental sore) – see Chapter 18 page 114.

33

Bites and Stings

Snakebite

If a snake injects venom when it bites, the effects of the injected venom may include any or all of the following three groups of conditions.

1. Paralysis of the motor part of the nervous system so that muscles become weak or paralysed.
   - If the throat muscles become paralysed, the patient's airway may become blocked. The patient cannot breathe and dies.
   - If the swallowing muscles become paralysed, the patient aspirates (breathes in) saliva into his lungs and gets severe pneumonia or even 'drowns in his own saliva'.
   - If the breathing muscles become paralysed, the patient cannot breathe and suffocates.
2. The blood will not clot.
   - The patient can bleed to death.
3. The venom may poison certain body cells.
   - There may be pain where the bite occurred and in the nearby lymph glands.
   - There may be abdominal pain.
   - Inflammation and even necrosis of the area where the bite occurred with swelling, blisters, cellulitis and even large ulcers, may develop.
   - Shock may develop.
   - Haemolysis (break-down of red blood cells with dark urine) may occur.
   - Damage to the muscles themselves with (a) aching, stiffness, and weakness of the muscles

and (b) dark urine (caused by the insides of damaged muscle cells going into the blood and urine) may develop.

If early signs of any of these conditions develop (called 'envenomation'), then *give antivenom*. Antivenom is a serum which contains antibodies which destroy the venom, and stop more signs and death occurring.

If signs of envenomation do not occur, *do not give antivenom*. Often when snakes bite people, they do not inject enough venom to cause envenomation, and the patient does not need antivenom.

The type of antivenom you give depends on which type of snake bit the patient.

You must find out for your area:
1. What types of snake are present.
2. What the effects of their bites are.
3. What antivenoms are available.
4. When you should give these antivenoms.
5. What does of these antivenoms you should give.

In Papua New Guinea, for instance, on the Papua side of the country, all of the venomous snakes which occur in PNG are found. Usually therefore, in Papua, CSL polyvalent venom is given. On the New Guinea side however, almost all serious bites are due to the Death Adder. Occasionally a significant bite may be from a small-eyed snake. In New Guinea therefore CSL Death Adder antivenom is used. If this antivenom is not effective, or if it is known that the snake was a large one (Death Adders do not grow to more than one metre), CSL polyvalent antivenom is given.

First aid

1. The patient should not move. Tell the patient to lie down, keep still and rest. The patient must not walk. Take transport to the patient, or carry the patient to transport or the health centre.
2. Wash the wound; but only if there is water available immediately. Gently wipe away venom on the skin.
3. Do *not* cut the wound.
4. If the patient comes to you with something tied round the limb just above the bite, do not

remove it, as long as you can feel a pulse below it.

5. Bandage and splint the limb.

Bandage the bite area and then the all the limb firmly (as tightly as for a sprained ankle). Use a bandage or torn up clothing. Then put all the limb in a splint. If you are in an area where snake bites cause swelling of the bite area, check the colour and temperature and pulse of the limb, below the bandage, every half hour. If the limb becomes cold or white or blue, or if the pulse becomes weak or is not present, or if there is a lot of swelling of the bitten area, then remove the bandages.

> The patient must not move the bitten limb or walk. Bandage the bite area and then all the limb firmly. Then put all the limb in a splint.

Management

> Management includes:
> Admit all patients who say they have been bitten.
> 1. Comfort the patient.
> 2. Make the patient rest.
> 3. Set up an IV drip.
> 4. Take blood. Test it for the time it takes to clot.
> 5. Examine to see if there are signs of envenomation. Repeat the examination every hour. Look for:
>   (a) paralysis,
>   (b) abnormal bleeding, and
>   (c) poisoning of other body cells.
> 6. Give antimalarial drug if you are in a malarious area.
> 7. Give antivenom carefully, but ONLY if signs of envenomation are present or develop. Look carefully for reactions. Treat any reactions quickly.
> 8. Treat any complications in the usual way.
> 9. Do not give morphine or pethidine.
> 10. Give tetanus prophylaxis.
>
> Transfer to medical officer, if envenomation is probable or present and if there is no antivenom available; or you cannot give antivenom because a reaction occurred; or if another complication occurs.

Admit all patients who say they have been bitten by a snake (for observation and treatment if treatment becomes necessary).

You cannot always tell if envenomation is probable by looking at the bite area.

1. Comfort the patient.
2. Make the patient rest in bed.
3. Set up an intravenous drip of 0.9% sodium chloride (1 litre every 12 hours).
4. Put 5 ml of venous blood in a test tube; note the time; tilt the tube every minute (do *not* shake it); note the time the blood takes to clot.
5. Examine for any clinical signs of envenomation (see below). Repeat and write down these observations:
   • hourly for 12 hours if suspected snakebite,
   • hourly for 24 hours if a definite snakebite,
   • 1/4-hourly if signs of envenomation are present or develop.

> Write the headings on the observation chart so that your staff know what observations to take.

Observations include:

(a) Symptoms and signs of paralysis, which are –
• ptosis (drooping of eyelids),
• double vision or paralysis of movements of the eyes,
• speech 'thick', or like a drunken man,
• jaw hanging open, by more than one inch,
• cannot swallow properly, or saliva collects in the throat, and
• cannot take a deep breath and cough.

(b) Symptoms and signs of abnormal bleeding, which are –
• venous blood put in a test tube does not clot in 15 minutes (do this once only on admission; but repeat it later if you suspect abnormal bleeding),
• bleeding from the place of the snakebite,
• blood in the sputum, vomit, urine, stool, nose, etc., and
• bleeding into the skin.

(c) Symptoms and signs of poisoning of other body cells, which are –
• pulse fast,
• BP low,

- respiratory rate fast,
- level of consciousness below normal,
- swelling and tenderness of lymph glands,
- abdominal pain and vomiting,
- swelling and blisters at the place of the bite, and up to the knee or elbow (if the bite was on the foot or hand), and
- urine is pink or brown or black from haemolysis (examine urine every time it is passed).

6. Give an antimalarial drug as indicated (usually chloroquine) if you are in a malarious area (see Chapter 13 page 55). If a rigor occurs later, then it will probably not be caused by malaria.

7. Antivenom

Give antivenom only if

(a) any signs of envenomation are already present when you first see the patient – give 2 full dose ampoules of the type indicated;

(b) signs of envenomation develop while you are observing – give 1 full dose ampoule of the type indicated;

(c) signs of envenomation are the same or are getting worse 4 hours after you gave antivenom – give 2 full dose ampoules of polyvalent antivenom.

You must find out the *type of antivenom* indicated for your area.

Dose of antivenom

You must find this out for your area. The dose of antivenom in one CSL ampoule neutralises the amount of venom injected by one usual snakebite. The size of the dose in ampoules in your area may be different.

(a) one usual bite – give one full dose ampoule.

(b) if more than the usual amount of venom was injected and there was more than one bite – give more than one full dose ampoule (usually two; but more than two may be necessary)

(c) children – dose as for adults

How to give antivenom

(a) Make sure the antivenom is clear.

If it is cloudy it is probably not active, and may be dangerous.

(b) Give antivenom by IVI.

(c) Put the antivenom into a drip which is running.

(d) First inject promethazine 25 mg (1 ml) IV.

Keep the syringe at the bedside with another ampoule of promethazine.

(e) Then inject adrenaline tartrate 1–1000 solution one half (1/2) of the usual dose given for asthma (i.e. 0.25 ml (1/4 ml) for an adult) subcutaneously. Draw up into the syringe 0.5 ml (1/2 ml) of adrenaline tartrate 1–1000 solution and keep this syringe at the bedside with another ampoule of adrenaline.

(f) Draw up the antivenom, and inject a few drops.

(g) Wait 5 minutes. Take PR and BP, look for skin rash or itch, look for swelling of the face or neck and listen for cough and rhonchi.

(h) If there is no reaction after 5 minutes, inject the rest of the antivenom, slowly over 30 minutes (never in less than 10 minutes).

(i) Observe as in (g) every 15 minutes for 1 hour.

(j) Remove the bandage and splint from the bite area when you have given the antivenom.

If a reaction to the antivenom occurs –

(a) stop giving the antivenom,

(b) give the adrenaline tart. 1–1000 solution 0.5 ml (1/2 ml) IMI immediately, and

(c) give the promethazine 25 mg (1 ml) IVI and 25 mg (1 ml) IMI immediately.

If a severe reaction to the antivenom occurs and if the patient may die

(a) give adrenaline tart. 1–1000 solution 0.5 ml (1/2 ml) IV slowly over 5 minutes, i.e. 0.1 ml/minute (1/10 ml/minute) immediately.

(b) give promethazine 50 mg (2 ml) IV with another syringe immediately,

(c) give hydrocortisone 100–300 mg intravenously if it is available, and

(d) repeat the adrenaline after 5 minutes if necessary.

(e) See the instruction paper with the antivenom and a specialist reference book for further management.

8. Treat any complications in the usual way.

If paralysis occurs after you have given a repeat double dose of antivenom, or if you cannot give antivenom because of a reaction,

(a) nurse the patient on his side (head down if necessary),

(b) suck out the airway every hour (or more often if necessary – noisy breathing or snoring means a blocked airway), and

(c) give artificial ventilation if necessary.

If bleeding occurs, give fresh, whole blood; *but first give* a repeat double dose of polyvalent antivenom. Arrange urgent (emergency) transfer to hospital while you do all this.

9. Do not give morphine or pethidine (which could reduce respiration). If the patient is frightened, restless or in pain, give explanation and comfort and intranasal oxygen. If a drug is really necessary, give paraldehyde.

10. Give tetanus toxoid 0.5 ml (1/2 ml) SCI, and finish the course later if the patient is not immunised. If someone has cut the wound, and it may be infected (and the patient is not immunised), then give also tetanus immunoglobulin 250 units (1 ml) IMI.

Transfer to medical officer care

Urgently (emergency) if:
1. there is a definite bite of a known poisonous snake; *or*
2. there are symptoms or signs of envenomation (weakness or bleeding etc.);
and if also
1. there is no antivenom available; *or*
2. you cannot give antivenom because the patient is allergic to antivenom (more than just an itchy swelling of the skin which you can treat with adrenaline and promethazine); *or*
3. the patient is not cured by a repeat dose of 2 ampoules of polyvalent antivenom.

Non-urgent transfer is necessary if other complications which you cannot manage at the health centre occur.

Prevention

Teach people to be careful in areas where snakes are common. Children must not collect or play with *any* snakes. Discourage young men from climbing trees after snakes. Encourage people to wear shoes when walking at night.

Seasnake bite

The effects of a bite by a seasnake are as for landsnakes; but cell poisoning of muscle is more common. Pain and stiffness of the muscles; then severe pain if the muscles are moved; and then paralysis can occur. The urine becomes red or brown or black from myoglobin (like haemoglobin but from inside a damaged muscle)

If there are real signs of envenomation (especially if there is red or brown or black urine or paralysis), give seasnake antivenom. If there is no seasnake antivenom available, give polyvalent antivenom and other treatment, as for landsnakes, (see page 375), and transfer to a medical officer urgently.

Stonefish and other fish stings

Stonefish sting causes:
1. Severe cell poisoning in the stung limb, with very severe pain; oedema; weakness; sometimes necrosis; and later, abscesses.
2. Sometimes, paralysis of all the muscles, including those used for breathing, can occur.

Treatment includes:
1. Put the affected limb into very hot water (50°C). The heat destroys the venom. This is very effective treatment.
2. If hot water is not available apply a firm bandage and splint (see page 375) immediately.
3. Infiltrate the sting area with lignocaine 1% or 2% solution, 5–10 ml. This is also very important.
4. Put up an intravenous drip.
5. Give stonefish antivenom (with precautions as for snake antivenom – see page 376) if there is still severe pain or if general signs are present *after* the above treatment.
6. Treat any other complications in the usual way.
7. Give tetanus prophylaxis (see Chapter 25 page 364).
8. Treat any secondary bacterial infection with antibiotics.

Jellyfish sting (including Box Jellyfish or 'Sea Wasp')

Box jellyfish or sea wasp sting causes:
1. very severe pain,
2. severe skin inflammation, like third degree burns,

3. sometimes paralysis of the respiration, shock and stopping of the heart.
   Other jellyfish cause less severe conditions.

   Treatment includes:
   1. Immediately get the patient out of the water. The rescuer must take care not to be stung.
   2. If the patient's breathing is not enough, or if it stops, give artificial ventilation (see Chapter 37 page 416).
      If shock develops, treat as for shock caused by acute allergic reaction (see Chapter 27 page 308).
      If the heart stops, give external cardiac massage (see Chapter 37 page 418).
   3. Immediately 'disarm' the tentacles on the patient (i.e. stop them injecting more venom). Pour household vinegar (any brand) over the affected parts and the tentacles. Pour more on as it runs off. Leave the area covered with vinegar for a few minutes.
      Do not put spirit or alcohol (of any sort) on to the affected area (as used to be recommended). If no vinegar (i.e. 3%–10% acetic acid) is available, dry the tentacles with dirt, etc. before removing them.
      Do not put any water on to the affected area for 2 hours.
   4. Give analgesics. Try lignocaine or other local anaesthetic jelly or cream. Usually repeated small doses of IV pethidine or morphine are also necessary, because of the severe pain. A general anaesthetic with ketamine may be better for the pain than large doses of morphine (which may stop breathing).
   5. Treat the skin as for burns.

Octopus stings

Stings can cause complete paralysis and stop breathing, but usually they cause no pain. Treat with artificial ventilation (see Chapter 37 page 416) until the patient starts to breathe again.

Coneshell stings

Coneshell stings can cause:
1. pain,
2. strange sensations in the body, and
3. paralysis which can stop breathing.

Treatment:
1. Wash the wound and put on a firm bandage and splint (see page 375).
2. Infiltrate the sting area with 1%–2% lignocaine to relieve the pain.
3. Give artificial ventilation (see Chapter 37 page 416), if the patient stops breathing, until he starts to breathe again.

Scorpion stings

The effects of scorpion stings can be different from place to place. The effects are usually much more severe in children than in adults.
1. Most stings cause severe pain, often with swelling, and sometimes bleeding, at the place of the sting.
2. Some stings cause many types of severe general symptoms and signs.
3. Some stings cause paralysis and death by stopping breathing.
4. Some stings cause shock.

Treatment will depend on what type of scorpion is present in your area. Sometimes the toxin is destroyed by heat. Sometimes local anaesthetic injections are very helpful. Sometimes an antivenom is available. Treat as for Stonefish stings (page 377) (using, of course, scorpion not stonefish antivenom, if necessary).

Spider bites

Only a few spiders cause severe or fatal bites. Effects may include:
1. There may be severe pain at the place of the bite with swelling and redness developing quickly. Later on an ulcer may form.
2. The pain may soon spread all over the body and cause muscle spasm (muscles contract and are then tight all the time) and pain. Shaking and fits can occur.
3. Many different types of general symptoms and signs can occur.
4. Shock may occur.

Treatment includes:
1. Wash or clean the bite.
2. Give analgesics as necessary for the pain (see

Chapter 7 page 28).

3. Give diazepam for severe muscles pain and spasm or for fitting (see Chapter 25 page 267).
4. Give atropine 0.6 mg (1 ml) if the pulse is very slow.
5. Treat shock if it occurs (see Chapter 27 page 305).

Centipede and insect bites

These stings can cause:
1. severe pain at the bite area,
2. general symptoms and signs of cell poisoning, and
3. allergic reaction.

Treatment includes:
1. Give analgesics.
2. Comfort the patient.

3. Remove sting with the point of a needle, if it is from a bee.
4. Wash the affected area.
5. If there is an allergic reaction, give antihistamine orally or IM or IV if necessary, and adrenaline SC or IM if necessary (see Chapter 27 page 308).

Tick paralysis

The bites of some ticks can cause paralysis, if the tick stays in the body for a few days.

Remove the tick. Give artificial ventilation (see Chapter 37 page 416) if necessary. Transfer the patient urgently to a hospital if artificial ventilation is necessary.

The patient will get better if you give artificial ventilation until the paralysis goes.

34

Poisoning

Acute poisoning is almost always caused by a poison which a person swallows and absorbs through the gastro-intestinal tract. Sometimes acute poisoning is caused by a poison which a person breathes in and absorbs through the lungs; or caused by a poison which a person gets on the skin and absorbs through the skin; or caused by a poison which a person has injected.

The commonest chemicals which cause poisoning are drugs, petroleum products such as kerosene, and weed killers or insecticides.

The poisoned person often takes the poison accidentally e.g. children find and eat coloured tablets or a person drinks kerosene or weedkiller from a bottle which normally has a drink in it.

The poisoned person sometimes takes the poison to commit suicide (kill himself). People often take poisons not to really commit suicide, but to influence another person (to make him feel sorry or guilty, or to make him behave in a different way). This is called 'self-poisoning,' (and *not* 'attempted suicide') and is a form of acting out (see Chapter 35 page 390).

When a person says they have been poisoned you *must always* admit and treat the patient, even if you do not know it is true; or even if you think it is not true.

The treatment of poisoning is an emergency. *Treat the patient immediately*. If he has to wait for treatment to start, the patient is more likely to die.

You cannot treat acute poisoning by giving an antidote, because there are no antidotes for most poisons. (An antidote is a chemical which will work against a poison and stop the effects of the poison.)

But you can treat most patients who have been poisoned. You must always do two things when a patient is poisoned. If you do these two things quickly, most poisoned patients get better.

1. Stop the patient absorbing any more poison into his body.

   If the patient swallowed the poison, empty the patient's gastro-intestinal tract by making him vomit and giving him diarrhoea (see exceptions later).

   If the patient absorbed the poison through his skin, remove all his clothes and wash him all over with soap and water.

   If the patient breathed in the poison, immediately take the patient into fresh air; and give artificial ventilation and oxygen if necessary.

   If the poison was injected, put a firm bandage and a splint on the limb which was injected. The patient must not move the injected limb or walk around. (see Chapter 33 page 375).

2. Keep the patient alive by treating any symptoms and signs that develop, until his body removes the poison already absorbed.

   If the patient stops breathing, give artificial ventilation.

   If the patient develops shock, treat shock, etc. *See page 307* for more details.

   You may need to transfer the patient to medical officer care for the treatment of some symptoms and signs.

> If you do these two things:
> 1. stop the patient obsorbing any more poison, and
> 2. keep the patient alive, by treating any symptoms and signs which develop.
> then you can cure most poisoned patients.

There are two other things which you must do:
1. Give antidotes if there are any.
   The only antidote you probably have in a health centre is naloxone or nalorphine, which you give for an overdose of morphine, pethidine or codeine. The medical officer has only 2 or 3 other antidotes.
2. Stop the poisoning occuring again.

If the patient poisoned himself then you most give social or psychiatric help.

If the patient was poisoned accidentally, then you must give health education about the storage of drugs and poisons. The most common kind of poisoning is a patient who has swallowed a poison.

Poisons (and drug overdoses) swallowed

Admit for inpatient treatment all cases of suspected poisoning. Find out:

1. what the patient has swallowed, (tell a relative to bring a sample and the original container);
2. how much he swallowed; and
3. when he swallowed it.

Treatment of swallowed poisons

For *petroleum products* (e.g. kerosene) see page 382.

For *strong acids or alkalis see page 383.*

If the patient is unconscious see page 383.

For other cases treat as follows:

1. Immediately make the patient vomit (to remove the poison from the stomach), *but not if he is unconscious or has swallowed a petroleum product (e.g. kerosene) or a strong acid.* (Rub the back of the tongue and pharynx with several wooden tongue depressors held together.)
2. Make the patient drink 200 ml (1–2 cups) of milk or water, *but not if unconscious.*
   Then make the patient vomit again. *But not if the patient has swallowed a petroleum product (e.g. kerosene) or a strong acid.*
   Do this many times until he vomits only water or milk and no food or poison. (The milk or water also dilutes the poison and slows its absorption.)

> For chloroquine or quinine poisoning, the most important part of the treatment is to make the patient vomit *immediately* and then again many times (or wash the stomach out (see 3 below).

3. Wash out the stomach if patient will not vomit. Lay the patient on his side with his head lower than the rest of his body. Put a large diameter (1.5 cm or 3/4 inch) tube into the stomach. Then aspirate the stomach contents. Then wash out the stomach, by putting 200 ml (1 cup) of milk or water down the tube and then aspirating it again. Do this at least 20 times, until the aspirated fluid is clear and contains no food or drugs. (It may need over 100 times.)
4. Give a laxative e.g. magnesium sulphate (Epsom salts) 30 g (30 ml of crystals in a measuring glass or 1 tablespoonful) in two cups of water. Make the patient drink this when the vomiting is finished, or put it down the tube after the stomach is washed out. (This causes diarrhoea and removes the poison from the intestines.) Repeat the dose in 1/2 hour if there is no diarrhoea.
5. Give an antidote, if there is one (usually there is not).
6. Observe the patient every hour for level of consciousness, RR and depth of respiration, PR, BP, and any other complications which the poison may cause. Note any complications which are developing before they become severe (especially loss of consciousness, not breathing properly and shock).
7. Treat any complication in the usual way, e.g.
   • fitting – anticonvulsants (see Chapter 25 page 267)
   • unconsciousness – routine care of unconscious patient (see Chapter 25 page 264)
   • cyanosis – intranasal oxygen 2–4 litres/minute.
   • not breathing – artificial ventilation after clearing the airway (see Chapter 37 page 416)
   • shock – elevate the legs and give IV plasma volume expander (see Chapter 27 page 305)
   • pain – use *small* doses of pethidine or morphine if there is a risk of depression of respiration (usually only give for swallowed acid).
8. Transfer the patient to Medical Officer care if complications which you cannot treat at the health centre may occur (see page 382).
9. Use any case of poisoning to give health education on the proper storage and use of drugs and poisons (see page 382).
10. Check the patient's mental state. Treat any psychiatric condition. Help to solve any problem (see Chapter 35 page 391).

Transfer

Transfer a patient who has swallowed poison or drug overdose if:

1. You think dose of the poison he has swallowed is more than:
   - aspirin – 300 mg/kg,
   - chloroquine, amodiaquine ('Camoquin') and quinine – twice the normal treatment dose (*but* contact medical officer first) (see below).
   - corrosive acid (e.g. battery acid) – anything more than a little,
   - ferrous sulphate (iron) – 100 tablets (but small doses, e.g. 10 tablets are very poisonous to children),
   - methanol (methyl alcohol) – 10 ml, or methylated spirits – 200 ml,
   - paracetamol – 5 mg/kg, or
   - phenobarbitone – 20 mg/kg.
2. The patient has a dangerous level of consciousness, or respiration, or pulse or BP.
3. The patient's level of conciousness, respiration *or* BP gets worse every hour for 4 hours. Transfer the patient then before the levels of conciousness, respiration and BP etc. become dangerous.
4. Complications occur which you cannot treat properly in the health centre (especially unconsciousness which continues for more than 24 hours).
5. If you think the patient may try to commit suicide again and that you cannot stop him in the health centre.

> Aways check the patient's mental state if he tried to commit suicide

Treat with chlorpromazine and transfer the patient if he has severe psychotic depression, or you have another good reason to think that he may try to commit suicide again.

If not, try to solve the patient's problems and treat in the usual way. Do *not* supply phenobarbitone which the patient may take as another overdose.

Prevention of poisoning

Use any case of poisoning to teach people:

1. Always store all poisons and drugs away from children.
2. Never put poisons, especially kerosene, in drink bottles (soft drink or beer or wine bottles, etc.).
3 . Always put a label on all bottles which contain drugs and poisons.
4. Always throw away (into the toilet) any old medicines, tablets or the contents of any bottle which has no label.

Chloroquine, amodiaquine ('Camoquin') and quinine overdose

More than the proper treatment dose is dangerous. More than twice the proper treatment dose will probably cause death.

These drugs are absorbed very quickly and cause death usually within 1–6 hours.

The most important part of the treatment is to empty the stomach and intestines *as quickly as possible. Immediately* make the patient vomit many times or wash out the stomach. For other treatment see page 381.

If the dangerous dose of these drugs has already been absorbed, there is not much the medical officer can do, unless he has special equipment and drugs. Urgently contact the Medical Officer and ask if you should transfer the pateint urgently (emergency).

Treatment if the patient has swallowed a petroleum product (e.g. kerosene)

1. Do *not* make the patient vomit.
2. Give 1–2 cups of milk or water to drink.
3. Do *not* wash out the stomach.
4. Give 30–60 g (30–60 ml) magnesium sulphate crystals (Epsom salts) in water or milk.
5. There is no antidote.
6. Make routine observations (see page 381).
7. Treat pneumonia when it occurs. Give oxygen if it is severe.
8. Transfer if severe pneumonia develops, especially if you do not have oxygen.
9. Use the case to give health education that kerosene should never be stored in drink bottles and should always be stored away from children.
10. Treat any mental disturbance in the usual way.

Treatment if the patient has swallowed strong acids or strong alkalis

1. Do *not* make the patient vomit.
2. Give 1–2 cups of milk or water to drink.
3. Do *not* wash the stomach out.
4. Do *not* give a laxative.
5. Do *not* try to give an antidote (e.g. alkali if acid swallowed).
6. Make routine observations (see page 381),
7. Treat any complication in the usual way.
8. Transfer all patients who have swallowed any strong acid or alkali to medical officer care (urgent). Meanwhile, the patient must not eat at all or drink large volumes of fluid.
9. Use the case to give health education that no poison should be stored in a drink bottle, and that all poisons should be stored away from children.
10. Treat any mental distrubance in the usual way.

Treatment if the patient is unconscious

1. Do *not* make the patient vomit.
2. Do *not* give fluids to drink
3. Do *not* wash out the stomach.
4. Do *not* give laxatives.
5. Give naloxone 0.5–1 mg or nalorphine 5–10 mg for pethidine, morphine or codeine overdose. Do not give other antidotes or stimulants.
6. Make routine observations (level of consciousness, size of pupils, RR and depth of respiration, PR, BP).
7. Treat complications in the usual way.
   (a) Give special nursing care an unconscious patient (see Chapter 25 page 264).
   (b) Check that there is a good urine output (125 ml/hour). Give IV fluids if necessary.
   (c) Treat shock if it occurs (raise legs, give plasma volume expanders and see Shock, Chapter 27 page 305.
   (d) Give artificial ventilation and arrange urgent (emergency) transfer if the patient is not breathing enough, or stops breathing (see Chapter 37 page 416).
8. Transfer any patient whose level of consciousness or whose respiration or BP becomes dangerous. Also transfer any patient who is getting continually worse, before the levels become dangerous.
9. Use the case to give health education that no drugs and poisons should be stored in drink bottles and that all drugs and poisons should be stored away children.
10. Treat any mental disturbance in the usual way.

Poisoning from seafoods

Fish or shellfish can cause poisoning, even though the food looks good and tastes normal. Symptoms and signs include:
1. gastro-enteritis,
2. strange sensations in the body,
3. weakness which can develop into complete paralysis and death from paralysis of breathing, and
4. other symptoms and signs

Treatment is as in the 10 principles for other types of poisoning above.

If weakness of the respiratory muscles develops, treat with artificial ventilation and transfer urgently to medical officer care.

35

Psychiatric Conditions

Mental disorders and mental diseases

A person in good mental health can think, feel and act in a way his own community expects and understands. He accepts himself, is comfortable with other people and is satisfied carrying out the normal duties of life.

> A mental disorder or disease is present when a person cannot think, feel and act in the way his own society expects or understands.

Remember that:
1. What may be abnormal in one society may be normal in another sociey.
2. A criminal can behave in an a way society expects; but he chooses not to.

There are two groups of psychiatric conditions:
1. conditions with an organic cause, i.e. an alteration in the structure or function of part of the body which causes the psychiatric condition (see this page); and
2. conditons which do not have organic cause, i.e. there is no alteration in the structure or function of any part of the body which causes the psychiatric condition (see page 385).

There is also an important difference between:
1. psychotic conditions or diseases (psychoses) (see page 386); and
2. non-psychotic conditions or disorders (see page 386).

Causes of psychiatric conditions

Organic causes of psychotic diseases[1]

1.   Any disease of the brain especially
   • head injury
   • meningitis (all types)
   • cerebral malaria
   • encephalitis
   • African trypanosomiasis
   • syphilis
   • malnutrition with beri beri
   • damage to the brain at birth (mental subnormality)
   • wearing out of the brain in old age (senile dementia)
   • and others (see a specialist reference book)
2. Abnormalities in the blood going to the brain
   • alcohol, drugs, poisons
   • low oxygen from any cause, e.g. shock, anaemia, etc.
   • toxins from severe infections in the body, especially septicaemia, pneumonia and typhoid
   • toxins from the body – liver failure
   • and others (see a specialist reference book)

Organic psychoses caused by a disease of the brain or an abnormality of the blood going to the brain can be of two types:
1. an acute organic psychosis, or
2. a chronic organic psychosis.

An acute organic psychosis started recently, and the patient is confused or delirious (see later, page 388). Treatment is possible and you must give it

---

1 Note that these two lists of causes of organic psychoses are the same as the two lists of causes of unconsciousness or of convulsions etc. (see Chapter 25 page 264). An organic psychosis is only another way the brain does not work properly when there is a disease of the brain or abnormality of the blood going to the brain.

quickly, to stop brain damage which cannot be cured occurring.

A chronic organic psychosis has been present for a long time, and the patient is demented (see later, page 388). Treatment is often not possible and so urgent treatment of the organic condition is not necessary.

> Always think of an organic causes first in every patient with **any** mental disturbance.
> Always
> 1. Take a full history from the patient and his family or friends.
> 2. Do a full physical examination
> 3. Test the urine
> 4. Send blood of VDRL
> Always think of an acute organic cause first in any patient with an **acute** mental disturbance who was not mentally abnormal before.
> Always
> 1. Do a lumbar puncture
> 2. Take a malaria smear and given antimalarial drugs
> 3. Look carefully for head injury
> 4. Smell the breath
> 5. Look for malnutrition (beri beri)
>   *after* doing the above history, examination and tests 1–4.

Non-organic causes of psychiatric conditions

Non-organic causes include the experiences the patient has had. Most important are the relationships he has had with his family (especially as a child), friends, girl-friends, wife, etc. Also important are events at home, school, work, etc.

These *relationships and events can cause stress*. Two things especially cause stress. (1) Separation from people important to him. (2) A decision which the person cannot or does not make.

Stress causes anxiety. In anxiety, the brain stimulates certain nerves and the adrenalin producing gland. This causes dry mouth; sinking feeling in the abdomen; nausea and diarrhoea; palpitations; sighing or deep breathing; urinary frequency; sweating, cold hands and feet; a feeling of weakness; tightening of muscle groups (tension which can cause headache or backache if it remains for some time), etc. Anxiety is unpleasant but normal. The best way to remove the anxiety is to solve the problem causing the stress; or if this is not possible, to cope with it in a healthy mature way. If anxiety continues for a long time or if the anxiety is very great, then the stress and anxiety can cause mental disorders and diseases.

Stress and anxiety can cause non-organic non-psychotic conditions. These include:
1. *'Pathological anxiety'* or *'Anxiety state'*. This is a continuing anxiety state which can have all, (but usually has only one) of the above symptoms or signs of anxiety. Especially common is headache from muscle tension.
2. *'Psychomatic disease'*. Parts of the body may be damaged by continuing nervous or other stimulation, e.g. peptic ulcer.
3. *'Reactive depression'*. Exhaustion of the body and mind.
4. *'Acting out'*. Without knowing what he is doing, the patient 'puts on' an 'act' (play act) subconsciously hoping that people will realise he has a problem, and help him solve it.

Stress and anxiety can also start some other, very serious psychotic diseases.
1. An *acute psychotic reaction* occurs when a person's anxiety and fearful thoughts completely take over his normal thoughts.
2. *Schizophrenia and Manic Depressive Psychoses* may occur in people who have an inherited vulnerability to them. But they may not have developed the disorder if there had been no stress, e.g. schizophrenia starting at a time of great stress – young person going to school or getting married etc.

Experiences help to form a person's personality. The personality is the characteristic or normal way in which a person thinks, feels, acts. Personality depends on what the person has inherited from his parents; anything that has happened to his brain; and the experience which he has had, especially as a child. Some people have *abnormal personalities,* such as anti-social personalities, sexual deviations; and alcoholism or drug abuse. The experiences a person has are a non-organic cause of the psychiatric conditon of abnormal personality.

Psychotic or non-psychotic disorder?

Psychotic diseases (or Psychoses)

Psychoses have some important typical features. In a psychosis there is a *severe disturbance of the patient's personality*.

The patient's personality is the way he thinks, feels and acts. (His acts include his appearance, his behaviour and his speech or talk.) In normal persons, the person thinks, feels and acts in a way which other people expect him to and understand. In a normal person, thinking, feeling and acting are all co-ordinated.

In a psychosis, there is a change in the way the patient thinks, feels and acts. The person is now different. He does not think and feel and act as normal. Thinking, feeling and acting may not be co-ordinated.

1. Most commonly there is a *disorder of thought*. The patient *cannot organise his thoughts* or get them 'straight'. His thoughts may suddenly stop or jump from one thing to another. He may have *hallucinations* (see, hear, feel, smell and tasts things which are not there). He may have *delusions* (false beliefs cannot be corrected by logical argument). These delusions are aften that a person or something is trying to hurt or kill him. This delusion of persecution is called a 'paranoid delusion'.

   In organic psychoses (when the patient may not be fully conscious and cannot completely understand or remember what is happening) he may have *illusions* (wrongly understand and interpret real events and physical sensations) and may become *confused* and *delirious*.
2. There may be a *disorder of mood* (the usual 'feelings' of the person).

   He may be *manic* (too happy) or *depressed* (too sad) or seem to have *no feelings*, or the *mood may not be the usual one for the circumstances* (e.g. happy when very bad things are happening).
3. Because of the disturbance of thought and mood the *actions* (appearance, behaviour and speech) may be very *abnormal*.
4. Because of one or more of these things, the patient *loses contact with reality* (does not live in the real world; but lives in his own private world of unreal and strange thoughts and feelings).
5. The patient *loss insight* (to a small or large degree), i.e. he does not know what is happening. The patient does not know he is sick. You cannot convince him that he is sick. The patient may think he is normal and everyone else is abnormal.

Non-psychotic disorders

Non-psychotic disorders are different from psychoses. There is *no change in the patient's personality* (or the way he thinks, feels and acts). The person's anxiety makes feelings which are stronger or continue longer than in a mentally healthy person. This results in an exaggeration or lengthening of thoughts and actions. This can also occur in mentally healthy people but they can control it.

1. The patient does not have a thought disorder. He does not have hallucinations or delusions. He is not confused. His thoughts are often not normal; but you can understand them and they 'make sense' if you know about the stresses and anxiety.
2. The patient's mood is appropriate to his thoughts and circumstances. The mood is often not normal; but you can understnd it, and it 'makes sense' if you know about the stresses and anxiety and thoughts.
3. The patients actions may not be normal and they may be very disturbed; but you can understand them and they 'make sense' if you know about his stresses and anxiety and his mood and thoughts.
4. The patient does not lose contact with the real world.
5. The patient does not lose insight and he knows that he is sick. However, he may deny this; but you can convince him by logical explanation.

When you see a patient with a psychiatric disorder, you must find out
1. Is there an organic cause or not? page 384.
2. Is there a cause for stress and anxiety? page 385.
3. Is this a psychosis or not? this page.

You must do a routine history and examination of *both* physical *and* mental states to do this.

Psychiatric history and examination

Psychiatric history

When you take a normal history, also take this special psychiatric history *from the patient and other witnesses*.

1. *Admission note*
   (a) Reason for admission. (If the police bring the patient, they must give a signed statement saying why they brought the patient.)
   (b) Names and addresses of those who referred the patient.
   (c) Names and addresses of patient's relatives *and* the people who were with the patient when the illness started.
2. *Complaints and duration*
3. *History of present illness*
   (a) What does the patient say has happened? What does the patient say is the cause?
   (b) What do other people say has happened? What do other people say is the cause?
   (c) What do *you* think really happened? What do *you* think the cause really is?
4. *Specific interrogation*
   Usual questions (see Chapter 6.)
5. *Past history*
   Any previous psychiatric disorder?
   • When did it occur?
   • How long did it continue?
   • What form did it take?
   • Did the patient get completely better?
   • Has the patient been taking any treatment?
   Note espcially head injury, drugs, alcohol and the usual questions (see Chapter 6).
6. *Family and contact history*
   Any mental illness and the usual questions (see Chapter 6).

Psychiatric examination

When you do a normal examination of the patient, make these 8 observations instead of just the level of consciousness.
1. Check it the patient can communicate physically (find out if he can hear, see, talk, move, etc.).
2. Check the level of consciousness:
3. Memory
   (a) recent events – e.g. What did you eat today?
   (b) long past events – e.g. Ask a fact of local importance
4. Orientation
   (a) person – e.g. Who are you? What are you?
   (b) time – e.g. Is it morning or afternoon? What day is it?
   (c) place – e.g. What is this building? Where is the toilet?
5. Intelligence – Ask a problem suitable to the patient's education.
6. Thoughts by
   (a) speech
   (b) appearance and
   (c) behaviour
   Especially
   (a) clear logical thinking or muddled up thinking?
   (b) delusions, e.g. Do people treat you normally or in some special way?
   (c) hallucinations, e.g.
   • Are any strange things happening?
   • Do you hear voices when you can see no one there?
   • Do you see people when no one else can?
   (d) any special thing the patient thinks about all the time.
7. Mood by
   (a) speech
   (b) appearance
   (c) behaviour
   Especially
   (a) manic (too happy) ⎰ e.g. How do you
   (b) depressed (too sad) ⎱ feel in yourself?
   (c) co-ordinated with the patient's thoughts and actions or not?
8. Insight
   (a) does he think he is sick?
   (b) does he know the *real* cause of the illness?

In examination of the appearance, behaviour and speech note the points listed below.
Appearance
   • facial expression – happy, sad, or worried
   • posture
   • clothing

- hygiene
- anything odd or unusual

Behaviour
- overactivity
- underactivity
- aggression
- odd or unusual
- sensible under the circumstances
- care of bodily needs – does he eat and drink? does he rest and sleep?

Speech
- fast
- slow
- none

(shows what thoughts are and what stream of thoughts is like)

Important psychiatric conditions

Acute organic psychoses

In an acute organic psychosis the brain does not work properly as there is an *acute* (i.e. started recently) *underlying disease of the brain or abnormality of the blood coming to the brain* (see page 384).

This also causes a disturbance in level of consciousness.

These two things cause the typical features of acute organic psychosis.

1. disturbance of level of consciousness, which causes
2. poor memory (especially for recent events), and
3. loss of orientation, and

These are called 'Confusion'.

4. loss of normal level of intelligence, also
5. the patient cannot understand things that are happening and has illusions and hallucinations.

This may cause 'Delirium'.

> A patient who has recently become confused or who is delirious has an acute organic psychosis.

You can treat most causes of acute organic psychosis, and often you can cure them. But, if you do not give proper treatment quickly, then these conditions either cause death or permanent damage to the brain. A good example is acute bacterial meningitis causing acute organic psychosis. See page 384, for the list of the common causes of acute organic psychoses, and of the diagnostic procedures you must do on all patients with acute organic psychosis.

> If a patient has an acute organic psychosis you must quickly find the cause and give effective treatment.

Chronic organic psychoses

In chronic organic psychosis there is a *chronic* (i.e. did not start recently) underlying *disease of the brain*. So the brain does not work properly.

This causes the typical features of chronic organic psychosis:
1. poor memory, especially for recent events;
2. some loss of orientation;
3. loss of intelligence and can not easily learn new things;
4. changes in the mood – often irritable, and sudden changes from one mood to another.

The patient has 'dementia'. There is a long past history of the condition. Most of the causes can not be treated or cured. See page 384 for a list of the causes of chronic (and acute) organic psychoses and the diagnosic procedures you must do.

> In every case of a mental disorder always first look for an organic cause (disease in brain or abnormality in blood going to the brain). This is especially important if
> 1. The level of consciousness is not normal
> 2. Orientation is not normal
> 3. Memory for recent event is not normal
> 4. Intelligence is not normal
> 5. There are sudden changes in mood
>
> i.e. delirium or confusion or dementia
>
> These things do not occur in non-organic mental disease.

388

If these things occur the patient has an organic psychosis.

You must find and treat the cause of the organic psychosis if possible. If the condition started recently urgent diagnosis and treatment are essential.

Schizophrenia

Schizophrenia is a non-organic psychosis. You will not find an underlying disease of the brain or abnormality of the blood going to the brain.

There are *abnormal thoughts often with delusions and hallucinations* even though *the patient is fully conscious and orientated*. Mood is also often disturbed and feelings may not be co-ordinated with thoughts and actions, or the patient may appear to have no feelings. So appearance, behaviour and speech etc. may be very abnormal. The patient has little or no insight and often says he is not sick at all.

In the acute stage the thought disorders may be very severe with strange hallucinations and delusions. Especially important are paranoid delusions (thoughts that someone is trying to hurt the patient when this is not true).

The patient may even attack the person he thinks may hurt him.

In the acute stage, the patient is fully conscious, fully orientated, but has abnormal thoughts (especially delusions and hallucinations) and possibly abnormal feelings.

In the chronic stage (after many years) the patient may appear to have few thoughts, very little feeling about anything, and may behave like a child.

If a patient
1. is fully conscious and orientated with a good memory and reasonable intelligence, but
2. has abnormal thoughts especially hallucinations or delusions, and
3 . possibly has inappropriate or no feelings
then the patient probably has schizophrenia.
Check that the patient does not have an acute organic psychosis.

Manic depressive psychosis

Manic depressive psychosis is a non-organic psychosis. You will not find an underlying disease of the brain or abnormality of the blood going to the brain.

There is a *disturbance of the mood*. The patient has a definite feeling which he thinks will not stop. It may be of great happiness (mania). It may be of great unhappiness (depression). There is no real cause for this feeling in what is happening to the patient. The patient appears fully conscious and orientated with a normal memory, but he thinks and acts in co-ordination with the feelings he has; so there may be some delusions usually of being a very important person or God, in mania, or of being a very bad person or of having a terrible disease, in depression. Sometimes there are vague hallucinations. So appearance, behaviour and speech may be very abnormal. The patient has little insight and often says he is not mentally abnormal.

The abnormal mood of the patient often goes after some weeks. Sometimes the patient can change from one mood to the other, i.e. from being too happy for no reason to being too sad for no reason. (This change does not happen quickly.)

Sometimes patients who feel very depressed try to commit suicide (and sometimes also try to kill their families). People who are manic often make quick and bad decisions as they feel and think everything will be all right. They may lose their money or their lives because of these decisions.

If a patient
1. is fully conscious and orientated with a good memory and reasonable intelligence
2. has abnormal feelings (he is too happy or too sad) for which there is no real cause
3. possibly has abnormal thoughts co-ordinated with the abnormal feelings
then the patient probably has manic depressive psychosis.
Check that the patient does not have acute organic psychosis.

In the non-organic psychoses there is a disturbance in thoughts or mood. The patient **does not have**

1. disturbance in level of consciousness,
2. disturbance of recent memory,   i.e. delerium
3. disturbance of orientation,   or confusion
4. disturbance of intelligence, or   or dementia
5. sudden swings in mood.   or dementia

It the patient has any of these things, look for a disease of the brain or an abnormality of the blood going to the brain.

Acting out

'Acting out' is a name for a large group of non-organic non-psychotic mental disorders.

The patient acts out the feelings which he cannot talk about. The patient may act fits, unconsciousness, paralysis, drunkenness, physical sickness, suicide, helplessness, dangerous behaviour, etc. He pretends that this is his real problem; but the patient really has a different problem which he is hiding. The acting attracts attention which he (without realising it) hopes will then lead someone to find the real problem, and solve it.

The patient has no loss of consciousness, memory or orientation. There are no signs of physical disease on examination and tests (unless the patient is acting a physical sign).

This group of conditions includes things like 'phobias', 'obsessions', 'hysteria', etc. Chronic forms of acting out are often called 'neuroses' or 'psychoneuroses'. Underlying all these conditions is stress and anxiety, and the acting out is only a way of trying to cope with this anxiety.

Acute psychotic reation (with no organic cause)

This is any type of severe mental disturbance when these things occur:
1. The patient (who is usually young) has a problem which he cannot solve and which causes great anxiety.
2. Fear replaces clear thinking and controls the thoughts, feelings and actions of the patient. Any type of psychotic (or non-psychotic)

behaviour may result. The patient may appear to have schizophrenia or mania (i.e. a non-organic psychosis). Singing, shouting and other disturbing behaviour are common. Irritable answers to all questions are common. But hallucinations and delusions are not common.
3. Once the problem is found and solved the patient becomes normal again within days or weeks.
4. There may be repeated attacks with repeated problems; but after each attack the patient gets completely better. But the patient may not ever cope well with problems.

An acute psychotic reaction is different to a non-organic psychosis (schizophrenia or manic depressive psychoses). In non-organic psychosis:
1. the patient does not become completely normal even when his problems are found and solved, and/or
2. if the patient had a previous attack he was not completely normal before this attack.

In every patient who has very disturbed behaviour, you must try to find out if the patient has a big problem. If he does, you should try to solve it. Until you do this, you cannot know if the patient's mental disorder is caused by an acute reaction to anxiety or caused by a non-organic psychosis.

You cannot make a diagnosis of acute reaction when you first see the patient. You can only make it when the patient gets better. If the patient does not get completely better, he must have schizophrenia or another condition.

Management of patients with psychiatric conditions

Principles of management of patients with psychiatric conditons

1. Treat symptoms and signs (i.e. give symptomatic treatment).
   Control the patient, if necessary (see page 391).
   Look after the patient's bodily needs.

2. Change the patient himself by
    (a) treatment of any organic cause,
    (b) 'counselling' (talking to the patient),
    • first try to find out any cause of stress and anxiety,
    • then try to solve this cause of stress and anxiety,
    • teach the patient to talk to others about his needs and worries,
    (c) drugs, especially chlorpromazine, and
    (d) electro-convulsive therapy.
3. Change the patient's environment by:
    (a) 'counselling' (talking to the patient's family, friends and the people he lives and works with),
    • first try to find out any cause of stress and anxiety,
    • then try to solve this cause of stress and anxiety,
    • show the people how they can help the patient,
    (b) sometimes change the patient's school, work, etc., and
    (c) sometimes send the patient back to his home area, if he is away from it.
4. Follow up the patient to see if he needs further treatment or help.

Management of a psychotic patient

(Schizophrenia, Mania, Acute reaction, Organic psychosis).

Management includes 4 things
1. TREAT THE CAUSE
    (a) Treat any organic cause in the usual way.
    (b) Try to solve any cause of stress and anxiety.
    (c) Give chlorpromazine for non-organic psychosis.
2. TREAT THE PSYCHOTIC BEHAVIOUR
    (a) Admit with a helpful friend or relative. Educate the friend (see below).
    (b) Check that the patient cannot hurt himself or others (see below).
    (c) Give chlorpromazine (see below). Reduce the dose of chlorpromazine when

---

the patient improves. But, if it is a non-organic psychosis continue a maintenance dose (see below).
    (d) Give promethazine if side effects of chlorpromazine develop (see below).
3. TRANSFER SOME PATIENTS
    Most patients are best treated in the health centre.
    A few patients need transfer (see below). Before transfer, make special arrangements (see below), and give special treatment (see below).
4. CHANGE THE PATIENT'S ENVIRONMENT IF NECESSARY
    See above.
    Follow-up the patient regularly to check that he takes any chlorpromazine necessary, and to find out if he needs more treatment before the condition becomes severe again.

---

1. Treat the cause
(a) *If organic psychosis* – treat the underlying disease affecting the brain, or the condition affecting the blood going to the brain.
(b) *If acute reaction* (to stress and anxiety) – try to solve the problem causing stress and anxiety.
(c) *If non-organic psychosis* – treat with chlorpromazine (see below).

2. Treat the psychotic behaviour (the main treatment of non-organic psychoses too)
(a) *Always admit the patient with a responsible friend or relative.*
Tell the friend how to care for and comfort the patient. Check that the staff and other patients do not tease the patient.
(b) *Check that the patient cannot hurt himself or anyone else*
Nurse the patient on the floor if he is throwing himself around.
    Do not leave articles which the patient could use as a weapon, (e.g. knife, piece of wood, etc.).
    If necessary, get 4 strong men to put the patient into a chair. Two strong men can then hold him until the drugs make the patient quiet or he goes to sleep.

(c) *Give chlorpromazine* (25 mg *or* 100 mg tablets) and solution for injection 25 mg/ml (50 mg in 2 ml amps) *to produce the neuroleptisation syndrome.*

Choose a suitable oral dose (see below)
- Give this dose (1) regularly 6–hourly and
(2) hourly if necessary
- Give twice this dose (1) immediately and
(2) last dose at night

Choose a suitable IM dose if the patient refuses to take any of these oral doses. (Give the oral dose too when the IM dose settles the patient, see below.)

Increase the dose if necessary (see below).

Give chlorpromazine tablets regularly every 6 hours.

Choose the dose that will probably be necessary (from 50 mg to 200 mg).

Try 50 mg for a small, old or sick patient, and for a patient who is quiet and is not very disturbed by hallucinations or delusions.

Try 200 mg for a large or young patient, and for a patient who is violent or very active, and for a patient who is very disturbed by frightening hallucinations or delusions.

Most patients need between 50–200 mg.

Give an extra dose of chlorpromazine tablets (use the same dose as above)
- when you first see the patient,
- with the last regular dose at night,
- every hour *if necessary* for violent behaviour or very disturbed speech and thoughts that are not controlled by the regular doses.

Give chlorpromazine by injection every time the patient refuses to swallow ANY ONE of the regular 6-hourly or the 'if necessary' doses

Choose the dose that will probably be effective (50–100 mg (2 ml – 4 ml)).

Give the oral dose that was refused *also*, when the patient starts to settle after the IM dose.

Every day, note the total amount of oral and IM chlorpromazine given the day before, and divide this by 4 to give the new 6-hourly regular dose (which is also the 'as necessary' and night dose).

If the patient has schizophrenia or manic depressive psychosis

Leave him on the dose which settled him for 1 week (after he has settled well).

Then slowly reduce the dose by 100–200 mg every week to 100–200 mg every night.

Discharge the patient on 100–200 mg each night.

It may be possible to stop the chlorpromazine after 3 months.

Follow the patient up every month.

If the disease comes back soon or often after the treatment stops, then continue the treatment all the time.

Follow the patient up and give him a supply of chlorpromazine every month, (or at the least each 3 months).

You can stop chlorpromazine quickly if
- the psychosis is a reaction to a problem which is solved, or
- the psychosis is caused by an organic disease which is cured.

(d) *Give promethazine if side effects from chlorpromazine develop*

If there is shaking, muscle spasms, tongue or face spasms, eyes turned up, head bent back, limbs held in unusual positions, etc.

then give promethazine 50 mg (2 ml) IMI or IVI then promethazine 25 mg (1 tab) twice daily

and continue the chlorpromazine.

3. *Transfer*

Transfer only these patients to Medical Officer care:

(a) an organic psychosis; but you cannot find or treat the cause (urgent);

(b) a patient who is not better after 200 mg chlorpromazine every day for 3 weeks (non-urgent);

(c) a patient who is very depressed and wants to kill himself and does not quickly improve (urgent);

(d) side effects of chlorpromazine are not controlled by promethazine (urgent); or

(e) a patient who has committed a serious crime. The police are responsible for transfer.

Make the following special arrangements when transferring a psychiatric patient

1. Always send a letter to the Medical Officer

with details about the patient and the reasons for his transfer.

2. Always send a reliable friend or relative who can speak the patient's language and whom the patient trusts.

3. For medico-legal reasons, send a letter from the patient's nearest relative requesting the patient's transfer, admission and treatment.

4. Control the patient's behaviour with drugs before transfer (see page 391 and 392).

5. Send a health worker, who can physically manage and treat the patient.

Before transferring a psychiatric patient by air

1. Make sure the patient's behaviour has been controlled by chlorpromazine.

   Give another *extra* dose of chlorpromazine 150 mg orally 1½ hours before departure.

   Fifteen minutes before departure, check the patient again.

   If the patient is not *very* quiet, give chlorpromazine 50 mg (2 ml) IMI.

2. If you are worried the patient may still not be controlled, also give paraldehyde 0.2 ml/kg (usually 10 ml) IMI.

3. *Never* transfer the patient alone. There must be a health worker (and, if necessary, another person) with the patient, who can physically control the patient, if he behaves abnormally, and who has chlorpromazine and paraldehyde injections and can give them.

4. Always explain all the details to the pilot.

Management of a non-organic non-psychotic disturbance

(Anxiety state, Acting Out, Reactive Depression, etc.)

1. Do a full history and examination (See Chapter 6) and any tests necessary. Check that you look for all the causes of the patient's symptoms. If you find no cause for the patient's symptoms, think of a mental disorder and do these things;

2. Find out if the patient has a cause for stress and anxiety. See the patient often to find out. Also see relations, friends, etc. You can only diagnose mental disorder as the cause of the patient's symptoms, if you find a cause for stress and anxiety (as well as no organic cause).

3. Try to *solve the cause of the stress and anxiety*. This is the most important part of the treatment.

   You may need the help of a social worker, police, pastor, employer, teacher, family, etc. to do this.

4. Then explain to the patient how the stress and anxiety can cause the symptoms he has. (e.g. If a headache, explain how the tightening of the forehead and neck muscles for a long time causes pain in the head, just as exercising the arm or leg muscles for a long time causes pain in them.)

5. If necessary, give drugs to help reduce the anxiety.

   Use diazepam 5 mg (1 tab), or if not available phenobaritone 30–60 mg (1–2 30 mg tabs) three times a day for 1–2 weeks. If diazepam is not successful, try chlorpromazine 25–50 mg (1–2 × 25 mg tabs) three times a day for 1–2 weeks.

   Do not keep the patient on drugs. Only give the drugs for a few weeks and then stop. The patient must solve his problem to stop the anxiety. The patient must not depend on drugs (or alcohol) to control the symptoms of his anxiety.

6. Show the patient how to relax and encourage him to do this.

   Tell the patient how exercises and sports will help and encourage him to do these.

7. If the problems cannot be solved, the patient may improve just by talking to you about how he is.

8. Refer or non-urgently transfer a patient to a Medical Officer when all this doses not help the patient, and you cannot be certain that there is no organic cause for the symptoms.

Prevention of psychiatric conditions

1. You can:
   • help to improve family life in the community;
   • Help to educate parents and community leaders in good ways of bringing up children;
   • help to improve the environment in which the families live; and
   • help to meet the other real needs of families.

   These things will help children to grow up with normal ways of thinking, feeling and acting and to reduce the possibility of developing psychiatric conditions.

You can co-operate with others in doing things to improve family life.

2. Give help to people at times of stress and anxiety.

Important times of stress and anxiety include;

- leaving home – going to school,
- getting a job,
- tertiary education,
- getting married,
- having children, and
- sickness or death in the family.

If a person's problems can be solved or helped at such times, then the mental disease which may be caused by these will not develop.

You can co-operate with others in giving this help.

3. Early diagnosis and early effective treatment of psychiatric conditions will stop mild cases from becoming severe cases.

4. Effective rehabilitation of patients into the family and the community after treatment will reduce the effect of the condition on the patients, the families and the whole community.

36

Some Common Symptoms and Signs

Pyrexia of unknown origin (PUO)

(fever of unknown cause)

There are many causes of a fever. But there are usually other symptoms or signs, or positive results of tests, in the patient with the fever. These other things usually show you the diagnosis for the patient. You (and the patient) then accept the fever as part of the disease and do not worry about the fever. You treat the cause of the disease and the fever goes away with the rest of the illness.

Sometimes when you first see a patient with a fever you can find no other symptoms and signs or abnormal tests to show you the diagnosis. If you ask the patient every day about his symptoms, and if you carefully examine the patient every day, you can usually find the cause of the fever and make a diagnosis.

Sometimes you can only find the cause of a fever after all these things:
history repeated many times
examination repeated many times
blood tests at a hospital
urine tests at a hospital
biopsies at a hospital
laparotomy at a hospital
therapeutic trials of drugs, etc. at a hospital
but this is *very* unusual.

Causes of fever include:
1. infections of all types in all organs – this is the most common and important causes of a fever;
2. non-infective inflammatory diseases including:
   • rheumatoid disease and other similar diseases,
   • trauma, and
   • allergic reactions of certain types;
3. neoplasm;
4. drugs and chemicals;
5. inherited diseases; and
6. many other causes.

Infections which cause fever

There are 3 groups of infections which cause fever:
1. Infection of *a particular part of the body which is caused by one of many different organisms*. The disease is often named after the part of the body infected (e.g. pneumonia when the lung is infected; pyomyositis when the muscle is infected: enteritis when the intestine is infected). There is no one specific organism which infects these places. The organisms may be viruses or bacteria or worms etc. *These types of infections occur in all parts of the world*. See Chapters 19–32, and septicaemia in Chapter 12.
2. *A specific organism which causes a specific disease which often affects more than one part of the body*. The disease is often named after the specific organism (e.g. measles, chickenpox). No other organism causes the same disease as this specific organism does. *These types of disease occur all over the world*. See specific viral diseases in Chapter 16, malaria in Chapter 13, tuberculosis in Chapter 14, leprosy in Chapter 15 and some of the diseases in Chapter 19.
3. Another group of diseases is similar to group 2. *One particular organism causes disease*, which may affect *more than one part of the body*. But *these diseases occur only in certain parts of the world*. Diseases in this group which cause a short fever (a fever present for a week or less, although it may return) are in Chapter 17. Diseases in this group which cause longer fevers are in Chapter 18. If some of the diseases in Chapter 17 and Chapter 18 do not occur in your country, do not think of them. Think only of the diseases which the patient can possibly have.

Always include these infections in the differential diagnosis of a patient with a fever

1. A non-specific infection of a part of the body which can occur anywhere in the world
   - meningitis
   - septicaemia
   - upper respiratory tract infection, especially otitis media
   - influenza
   - pneumonia (especially in an upper lobe, where it is more difficult to find on examination)
   - gastro-enteritis
   - intra-abdominal abscess, especially pelvic inflammatory diseases, appendix absecess, and liver abscess
   - urinary tract infection
   - osteomyelitis
   - acute bacterial ('septic') arthritis
   - abscess in another place, especially pyomyositis and injection abscess

2. A specific infection which can occur anywhere in the world
   - malaria
   - tuberculosis
   - leprosy with reaction
   - measles
   - mumps
   - chickenpox

3. A specific infection which occurs in your area. If any of these occur in your area, they are likely to be the cause of your patient's fever
   - relapsing fever
   - typhus fever
   - plague
   - bartonellosis
   - dengue and related fevers
   - yellow fever, and related insect borne virus infections which cause haemorrhagic fevers
   - haemorrhagic fevers caused by other virus infections which are spread man-to-man or rat-to-man
   - typhoid fever
   - brucellosis
   - leishmaniasis
   - trypanosomiasis
   - allergic reactions to schistosomes and other worms or parasites in the body

The management of a patient with a fever of unknown cause

1. Do a full medical history.
2. Do a full clinical examination.
3. Do routine tests
   (a) Haemoglobin estimation
   (b) Urine test in *all* cases for protein, pus and bile
   (c) Others as indicated
   (d) Take tests to send to the laboratory, depending on which diseases occur in your area:
   - blood slide, for malaria and relapsing fever in all cases;
   - blood or lymph gland or other aspirate for leishmania, and trypanosomes if these occur in your area;
   - others as indicated
4. Write down a differential diagnosis of all possible causes. See list on this page for common infectious diseases.
5. Look for symptoms and signs to check for these diseases in 4.
6. Do tests to check for these diseases in 4
   (a) tuberculin test,
   (b) lumbar puncture.
   Take tests to send to the laboratory to check for these diseases in 4
   (a) sputum for AFB,
   (b) others as indicated.
7. Treat any cause you find *and/or*
   Give *all* patients antimalarial drugs as indicated (see Chapter 13.) if the patient is in or from an area where malaria occurs.
8. See the patient daily.
   Ask for new symptoms daily until the patient is cured. Examine for new signs daily until he is cured. Remember to examine the ears and do a pelvic examination at least once more. Test the urine again. If not cured in 2 days, treat as in 9 or 10.
9. *If you find no other abnormalities and the patient looks 'sick' and does not improve after 2 days (antimalarials for 2 days)*
   - Transfer to Medical Officer care.
   If transfer is not possible, and the patient gets worse
   Give IV (slow drip) or IMI quinine then 'Fansidar' if the patient is from or in an area where malaria occurs (see Chapter 13.)

Give IVI fluids

Give IVI antibiotics as for septicaemia (see Chapter 12)

• If patient is not greatly improved in 2 days, transfer.

If transfer is still not possible, and patient may die before transfer is possible, start anti-tuberculosis treatment (see Chapter 14.). (Transfer is essential later, even if the patient improves, unless positive sputum proves the diagnosis of tuberculosis.)

10. *If you find no other abnormalities, and the patient does not look 'sick' but does not improve after 3 days (antimalarials for 3 days).*

Repeat the course of antimalarials. Observe carefully to check that the drug is swallowed and absorbed (no vomiting or diarrhoea).

If the patient still has fever at the end of 1 week, take another malaria smear and send it to the laboratory to find out if the patient has drug resistant malaria.

Then treat the patient for chloroquine resistant malaria, and observe the result.

If the patient still has fever after a treatment course for chloroquine resistant malaria, transfer is essential.

11. If the fever goes after a 3 day course of chloroquine, but returns within the next 2 weeks:

Take a blood smear and send it to the laboratory to find out if the patient has chloroquine resistant malaria or relapsing fever.

Treat for chloroquine resistant malaria and observe while waiting for the result.

Malaise (Patient feels unwell)

1. Do a full medical history.
2. Do a full clinical examination.
3. Do routine tests: (a) Hb if pale, (b) urine test in *all* cases.

   Take tests to send to the laboratory for the common infectious diseases in your area (see page 396).
4. Write down a differential diagnosis of all the possible causes.
5. Look for symptoms and signs to check for these diseases in 4.

6. Do or send tests to check for these diseases in 4. Especially remember

   (a) tuberculin test,

   (b) sputum for AFB,

   (c) lumbar puncture,

   (d) blood slide for malaria and relapsing fever,

   (e) blood or lymph gland or other aspirated material for examination for leishmaniasis or trypansomiasis.
7. Treat any cause you find *and/or*

   Give *all* patients antimalarial drugs as indicated, if the patient is in or from an area where malaria occurs.
8. See the patient daily.

   Ask about new symptoms daily until he is cured.

   Examine for new signs daily until he is cured.

   Remember to examine the ears and do a pelvic examination at least once.

   Test the urine again.

   Manage as in 9, 10 or 11.
9. *If it is an acute illness and you find no abnormalities and the patient looks 'sick'*

   If it is an acute illness and does not improve after 2 days (and antimalarials for 2 days), transfer the patient.

   If transfer is not possible and the patient gets worse, treat as for pyrexia of unknown cause, 9. See page 395.
10. *If it is a chronic illness and you find no abnormalities and the patient does not improve after 2 weeks.*

    Transfer the patient.

    If transfer is not possible, send blood for Hb, white cell count (total and differential), liver function tests, urea and VDRL. Send sputum for AFB. Send urine for full examination. Do a tuberculin test. Send the appropriate tests for any other diseases common in your area. Ask for a Medical Officer to send you a *report on what the tests mean*.
11. *If you find no abnormalities and the patient does not look 'sick'.*

    Think of a mental disturbance.

    Find out if the patient has a problem or a cause for stress and anxiety.

    But diagnose a psychiatric cause only if

    (a) you find *no* organic cause and the patient does not look 'sick' *and*

    (b) a *real* cause for stress and anxiety *is*

present, or

(c) positive signs of a non-organic psychosis (see Chapter 35 page 385) are present.

Generalised oedema (Swelling of the whole body)

Do a full history and examination (see Chapter 6). Test the urine for protein, sugar, blood and pus.

1. Check that the *whole* body (legs *and* back and sometimes face) has oedema.
   Lymphoedema or elephantiasis usually affect only the limbs (usually legs) and the lymph glands are usually enlarged.
   If localised oedema, see page 399.
2. If the urine contains protein, look for:
   (a) nephrotic syndrome (*much protein (>1/8 or +) and much oedema*)
   (b) pre-eclamptic toxaemia (*female, pregnant, BP higher than 120/80, protein in urine*)
   (c) chronic kidney failure (*nausea, wasted, anaemic, BP high*)
   (d) acute glomerulonephritis (*blood in the urine, BP high, fever*)
   (e) heart failure (*see below*)
3. Look for heart failure
   (a) The signs of heart failure are:
   • *raised jugular venous pressure* ⎫ almost
   • *enlarged liver* ⎬ always
   • *oedema* ⎭
   • *fast pulse* – usually
   • *cyanosis* – often
   • *crepitations* – sometimes
   (b) You can usually find the cause of the heart failure e.g.
   • *chronic obstructive lung disease*
   • *pneumonia*
   • *severe anaemia*
   • *IV fluids given too quickly*
   • *other* see Chapter 27 page 303
4. Look for severe anaemia.
5. Look for malnutrition (unusual in an adult) or chronic disease of the gastro-intestinal tract (especially chronic vomiting or chronic diarrhoea or dysentery).
6. Look for cirrhosis (chronic liver disease)
   (a) *you can find no other cause and*
   (b) *ascites that is worse than the oedema*

(c) *very thin arms and* ⎫ the typical
shoulders ⎪ appearance of
very swollen ⎬ cirrhosis see
abdomen ⎪ Figure 24.5
moderately swollen ⎪
legs ⎭

Management

Give diuretics
Do not give diuretics if it is toxaemia of pregnancy or malnutrition.

Give hydrochlorothiazide 50 mg (1 tab) daily. Increase the dose to 100 mg (2 tabs) daily if necessary.

Also give frusemide 40 mg (1 tab) daily if necessary. Increase the dose slowly to 160 mg (4 tabs) daily if necessary.

Give potassium if necessary
1. If the patient is not eating a tuber diet (i.e. sweet potatoes, etc.), or
2. he is taking digoxn and diuretics, or
3. he is taking frusemide and hydrochlorothiazide,

then give potassium chloride slow release tablets 1200 mg (2 tabs) three times a day.

Treat the cause if possible and transfer to medical officer care if necessary
Nephrotic syndrome
Give prophylactic antimalarials (see Chapter 26 page 288.)

Give pyrantel 625 mg (5 tabs) once.

Refer to Medical Officer if the patient is not cured in 6 weeks (as some cases can be cured by other drugs).

Pre-eclamptic toxaemia
The patient must rest in bed.

If the patient not cured in 2 days or if she gets worse at any time or if she has fitting, treat (see an obstetrics book) and transfer urgently.

If she is cured, keep her in the health centre on observation or tell her to return every week for examination, until delivery.

Chronic kidney failure
The patient must drink 3 litres of fluid daily.

Give chlorpromazine 25 mg every 6 hours if

necessary IMI (1 ml)) if there is vomiting or orally (1 tab) if there is nausea.

The patient must take as much salt as possible without causing oedema or heart failure – if these develop, reduce salt until these go.

No high protein foods.

Other kidney conditions
See a medical reference book.

Heart failure
Diuretics are the most important treatment in most cases (see Chapter 27 page 304). If there is acute, severe heart failure give frusemide 40 mg (4 ml) IV.

Give oxygen if there is acute shortness of breath or cyanosis.

If there is chronic obstructive lung disease, see Chapter 20 page 171.

If there is pneumonia, see Chapter 20 page 164 and give digoxin (see Chapter 27 page 304)

If there is anaemia, see Chapter 21 page 182 and transfer for blood transfusion.

If IV fluids were given too quickly, stop or slow the drip.

If there is no cause obvious, give aneurine 50 mg (1 tab) daily for 2 weeks.

If other treatment is necessary (e.g. aminophylline, digoxin) see a specialist reference book.

Transfer to Medical Officer care *if*
1. you have not diagnosed a cause which cannot be treated, especially if the pulse is irregular, *or*
2. you have diagnosed a cause that you can treat but proper treatment does not cure it.

Severe anaemia
See Chapter 21 page 182 and transfer for blood transfusion.

Malnutrition or chronic gastro-intestinal disease
Check that the patient has a good mixed diet of enough food, at least three times a days.

Pyrantel 625 mg (5 tabs) once.

Treat any cause of vomiting or diarrhoea (see Chapter 23 page 234 and page 236).

Diuretics are not necessary.

Transfer if the patient does not improve.

Cirrhosis
Check the patient has a good mixed diet with high protein (see Chapter 24 page 245) but no salt (tinned meat and fish have too much salt).

Give pyrantel 625 mg (5 tabs) once only.

Diuretics are often necessary for the rest of the patient's life (usually a smaller dose after the ascites goes).

Transfer if the diagnosis is not certain, especially if there are masses or tenderness in abdomen.

Localised oedema (Swelling of one part of the body)

1. *Check for swelling of the rest of the body.* If generalised oedema, see page 398.
2. *Check that the swelling is oedema* and not a lump from another cause.
   Types of lumps include
   (a) Congenital (the patient was born with it)
   (b) Traumatic (caused by injury)
   (c) Inflammatory
   * infection
   * trauma
   * allergy
   * bites, stings, toxins
   (d) Neoplastic (cancer)
   (e) Degenerative. Remember especially:
   * hernia
   * prolapse
   * thrombosis (clotting) in a blood vessel
   * calcification
   * swelling caused by a blocked duct
3. *Look for causes of localised oedema*, especially:
   (a) Injury. *History. Type of lesion. Haematoma often present (bruise).*
   (b) Infection. *If acute* – red or shiny; swollen; tender; hot; the part cannot work properly.
   (c) Lymph vessel and lymph gland disease (see Chapter 22 page 196) especially:
   * acute bacterial infection
   * acute filarial inflammation
   * chronic bacterial infection
   * chronic filarial inflammation
   * tuberculosis
   * cancer.
   (d) Snakebite. *History.*
   (e) Allergic reaction. *Swelling and often redness and itch but little tenderness. Asthma and shock, sometimes.*

(f) Clots in main deep veins. *History of little recent leg movement (e.g. operation, illness, long trip) or of injury to limb or of IV injection or of infection; you can find no other cause.*

4. *Treat any cause you find.*

(a) Injury. See a surgery book.

(b) Infection. See Chapter 11 page 38

(c) Lymphatic disease. See Chapter 22 page 199

(d) Snakebite. See Chapter 33 page 374

(e) Allergic reaction. Give promethazine 25 mg (1 tab) 1–3 times daily and, if necessary, adrenaline tart. 1–1000 ½ ml each 6 hours.

(f) Clots in the main deep veins. If it is in the leg, transfer urgently to Medical Officer care. In other cases treat with sling, aspirin, heat and antibiotics.

5. *Treat the affected part.*

(a) Keep it higher than the rest of the body if possible, e.g. blocks under the foot of bed; arm in sling.

(b) protect from further injury, especially if chronic. e.g. wear shoes if the leg or the foot is affected.

Generalised wasting

Do a full history and examination (see Chapter 6).
    Test the urine for protein and sugar.
    Send sputum for AFB if there is a cough.
    Look for signs of these conditions

1. Malnutrition (history of eating – what? and how often?).

2. Chronic disease of the gastro-intestinal tract, especially if there is chronic vomiting (usually transfer) or chronic diarrhoea (treat with pyrantel (Chapter 23 page 218) and metronidazole (Chapter 23 page 225) and transfer if this does not cure it).

3. Chronic infections, especially

(a) tuberculosis (*chronic cough or enlarged lymph glands*),

(b) malaria (*attacks of fever, anaemia, large spleen*),

(c) tropical splenomegaly syndrome (*anaemia, very large spleen*),

(d) visceral leishmaniasis (*fever, very enlarged spleen, enlarged lymph nodes, anaemia, diarrhoea, skin infiltrations sometimes*),

(e) trypanosomiasis (*history of skin lesions at first, fever, enlarged lymph glands, enlarged spleen, enlarged liver, anaemia, fast pulse, nervous system disease*).

4. Repeated attacks of ordinary infections.

5. Chronic, non-infectious diseases, especially:

(a) chronic obstructive lung disease (*chronic cough, sputum AFB negative*),

(b) chronic kidney failure (*protein in urine, anaemia, nausea, BP high*),

(c) cirrhosis (*thin shoulders, some swelling of legs and back, severe swelling of abdomen, no protein in urine*),

(d) thyrotoxicosis (*eating much, staring eyes, shaking hands, fast pulse*).,

(e) diabetes (*eating and drinking much, passing much urine, sugar in urine*).

6. Cancer of any organ (*often lumps or bleeding*).

7. Others (see a specialist medical reference book).

Dehydration

Dehydration is present when there is not enough salt and/or water in the body.

The body normally contains 60% water.

If 0–5% of the body weight is lost (3 kg in 60 kg person, i.e. 3 litres) there is mild dehydration.

If 5–10% of the body weight is lost (6 kg in 60 kg person, i.e. 6 litres) there is moderate dehydration.

If 10–15% of the body weight is lost (9 kg in 60 kg person, i.e. 9 litres) there is severe dehydration which will probably soon cause shock and death.

Causes include:

1. Too much fluid lost from
   • intestines (vomiting, diarrhoea),
   • skin (sweating),
   • urine (diabetes, chronic kidney diseases)
   • lungs (fast breathing in high fever)

2. Not enough fluid taken in –
   • too sick to drink
   • unconsciousness
   • woman in labour
   • no water to drink

The most important *signs* in adults are:
• fast pulse,
• low BP,

- inelastic skin,
- little urine passed and urine dark colour,
- sunken eyes, and
- dry mouth.

Do not mistake inelastic skin from weight loss (wasting) or old age, for the inelastic skin of dehydration.

For *management* of patient with dehydration, see Chapter 23 page 223.

Loss of weight

Find out *how long* the condition has taken to develop.
1. In a few hours
   - loss of fluid (dehdration), from any cause (see page 400).
2. In a few days
   - loss of fluid (dehydration), from any cause (see page 400).
   - not taking in fluid (dehydration), from any cause (see page 400).
   - not eating
3. In a few weeks or months
   - wasting condition, from any cause (see page 400).
   - malnutrition

Note only loss of fluid can cause rapid (in a few hours) loss of weight.

Lumps (Masses)

Examination of lump

Note especially
Site
- in what tissue or organ?
- where in that tissue or organ?
Size
Shape
Surface
Consistency
Fluctuancy
Tenderness and other signs of inflammation
Fixed to surrounding tissue or not
Function of the affected tissue or organ
Regional (or nearby) lymph nodes

Types of lumps

1. Congenital
2. Traumatic
3. Inflammatory
   - infection
   - trauma
   - allergy
   - bites, stings, toxins
4. Neoplastic
5. Degenerative – remember
- Hernia
- Prolapse
- Thrombosis (clotting) in a blood vessel
- Calcification
- Swelling caused by a blocked duct

If a lump is neoplastic, these signs will usually help you to find out what type of neoplasm it is.

If it is a simple or benign lump it –	if it is a malignant lump, it –
has clear regular edges	has irregular edges
is not hard	is hard
can be moved	is fixed to other tissues
grows slowly (years)	grows fast (weeks or months)
does not grow into surrounding tissues	grows into surrounding tissues
does not spread to lymph nodes	spreads to lymph nodes
does not spread to other organs	spreads to other organs
does not form ulcers	often forms ulcers

Abscess

An abscess is a collection of pus in one part of the body.

Diagnosis of an abscess

1. There are general symptoms and signs of infection.
2. There are local symptoms and signs of inflammation.
3. There are signs of fluctuation in *two directions* at right angles; but only if the abscess is near the surface of the body. Place the index and

middle fingers of one hand on the swelling. Then press down quickly between the two fingers with a finger of the other hand. If fluctuation is present, you will feel the 2 fingers being lifted. Then put the 2 fingers at right angles (or 90°) to the first position and do the test again. If fluctuation is *again* present, then there is fluid (e.g. pus) under the 2 fingers. Note that fluctuation in one direction only does *not* mean there is fluid under the fingers (normal muscle 'fluctuates' in one direction).

Treatment of an abcess

1. Give *antibiotics* only if:
   (a) There are severe general symptoms and signs of infection (fever, fast pulse, etc.),
   (b) The infection is spreading into the surrounding tissue (cellulitis) or lymph vessels or lymph glands.
   (c) The bone may be infected (osteomyelitis) (continue for at least 4–weeks).
   (d) It is a breast abscess.
   (e) It is a hand or finger abscess.
   (f) It is a pyomyositis.
   See Chapter 11 page 40 for choice of antibiotic.
2. *Incise and drain* the abscess if:
   (a) Pus is definitely present (i.e. if fluctuant in 2 directions at right angles; or soft).
   (b) A breast abscess has not improved after 2 days of antibiotics or has already been present for 4 days when you first see it.
   (c) It is a hand abscess and patient cannot sleep for 1 night after you start antibiotics (transfer to Medical Officer is usually necessary).
   (d) It is pyomyositis or osteomyelitis. Incise immediately if it is very swollen; or after 2 days if it is not almost cured by antibiotics.

   Use anaesthetic topical spray if it is a small superficial abscess (except hand).

   Use general anaesthetic (ketamine) or lytic cocktail or regional block if it is a large or deep abscess or in the hand.

   Use these anaesthetics only if you have had special training and have all the necessary resuscitation equipment available.

Do not cut or damage other structures.

Cut the skin and subcutaneous tissues with a scalpel.

Push a closed pair of artery forceps into the abscess, and then open the forceps.

Make a hole big enough to insert your finger (except hand abscess).

Destroy all walls inside the abscess with you finger (inside a sterile glove). Feel if the bone is affected.

Leave a rubber drain in the abscess, that comes out through the skin.

Pack the wound with gauze soaked in Eusol or strong 3% saline if it bleeds much.

Apply a Eusol dressing.

3. Give *drugs for pain* if necessary See Chapter 7 page 28
4. *Dress after incision*
   Dress when necessary (at least daily, but more often if necessary).

   Use either a little acriflavine emulsion smeared on an absorbant pad soaked in strong (3%) saline or an absorbant pad soaked in Eusol.

   Remove any pack in 1 day.

   Remove the drain when there is only a little discharge (2–3 days).

   When the sore is clean and there is no more pus and slough, dress with a weak (1%) saline dressing or a vaseline gauze dressing.

   Transfer to Medical Officer any case where the abscess is deep, or near important structures in the neck, chest, abdomen, or in the hand (usually).

Abdominal pain

1. *Take a full history* (see Chapter 6).
   Ask about the pain, especially
   (a) is it a colic? (if colic, see below.)
   or
   is it a constant pain? (if constant pain, see below)
   (b) where exactly is the pain?
   Remember to ask about
   (a) recent trauma to abdomen,
   (b) the date of last normal period.
2. *Do a full examination*. (see Chapter 6).
   Remember to check carefully for:
   (a)T° (? infection)

(b) PR: BP; skin elasticity; hands and feet warm or cold; (?dehydration, ?shock)

(c) Colour (? anaemia, ? bleeding)

(d) Abdominal
- distension
- movement on respiration
- hernia and scars
- tenderness – guarding – rigidity
- masses
- enlargement of organs
- intestinal bowel sounds
- pelvic examination 'PR' or 'PV' for tenderness, masses or enlarged organs

(e) Chest disease (pain referred to abdomen)

(f) Spine disease (pain referred to abdomen)

3. *Test urine for protein, pus, bile, sugar*

Look at any vomit or abnormal stools or vaginal discharge to see what it contains.

The pain is a colic (If pain is constant, see below)

Colic is caused by obstruction or inflammation of:

(a) the GI tract (stomach or small intestine or large intestine), *or*

(b) the female reproductive tract (tubes or uterus), *or*

(c) urinary tract (ureters) (often more a constant pain with times when it is worse), *or*

(d) biliary tract (bile ducts) (unusual).

See Figure 36.1.

Causes of colic in these organs include

1. GI tract

(a) Gastroenteritis (*diarrhoea, central abdominal colic, sometimes vomiting; no definite abdominal tenderness; often dehydration and fever*).

(b) Intestinal obstruction (*constipation; central abdominal colic; vomiting; no abdominal tenderness; no fever*).

(c) Enteritis necroticans ('Pigbel') (*signs of obstruction (see above) and peritonitis* (see Chapter 23 page 213).

(d) Others

2. Genital

(a) Labour (*large, non-tender uterus; no fever or shock*).

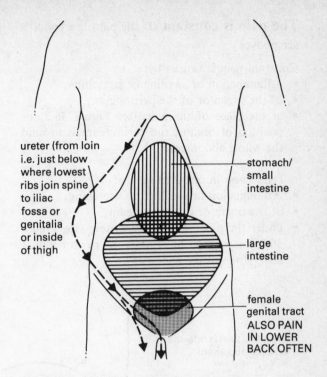

ureter (from loin i.e. just below where lowest ribs join spine to iliac fossa or genitalia or inside of thigh

stomach/small intestine

large intestine

female genital tract ALSO PAIN IN LOWER BACK OFTEN

Figure 36.1 Diagram to show the place in the abdomen where the patient feels colic from the various organs which can cause colic.

(b) Antepartum 'accidental' haemorrhage (*large, tender uterus; often anaemia and shock*).

(c) Miscarriage (*PV bleeding; uterus enlarged; no abdominal or pelvic masses or tenderness*).

(d) Ectopic pregnancy (*1–2 periods late or missed; some dark red PV bleeding; usually also constant lower abdominal or general abdominal pain and tenderness; often fainting; (see an obstetrics book)*).

(e) period pains (dysmenorrhoea) (*past history of similar pain with periods; on examination NAD*).

3. Ureters

Stones (*pain in typical place* (see Figure 36.1); *kidney sometimes tender; often bood in the urine*).

If the pain is a colic

1. Where is the pain? What organ is probably causing it? (See Figure 36.1)

2. What condition is probably affecting this organ? (see Figure 36.3)

The pain is constant (If the pain is a colic, see above)

Constant pain is caused by:
- inflammation or swelling or stretching,
- of the organ or of the peritoneum,
- at the place of the pain (see Figure 36.2 for position of organs; the peritoneum is around the whole abdomen).

Tenderness in one area means:
- inflammation or swelling or stretching,
- of the organ or the peritoneum,
- under the place of the tenderness (see Figure 36.2 for position of organs; the peritoneum is around the whole abdomen).

Tenderness all over the abdomen (generalised), often with guarding and rigidity means:
- inflammation or irritation of the whole peritoneum by,
- pus (peritonitis) (see page 406), or
- blood from trauma (see page 406), or ectopic pregnancy.

Note. Tenderness over an area is more accurate than pain over that area for diagnosing inflammation or swelling or stretching of the organ or peritoneum under that area.

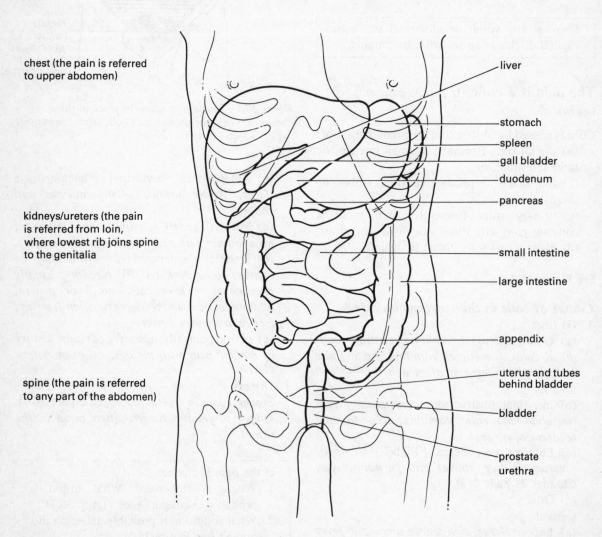

chest (the pain is referred to upper abdomen)

kidneys/ureters (the pain is referred from loin, where lowest rib joins spine to the genitalia

spine (the pain is referred to any part of the abdomen)

liver
stomach
spleen
gall bladder
duodenum
pancreas
small intestine
large intestine
appendix
uterus and tubes behind bladder
bladder
prostate
urethra

Figure 36.2 The position of organs which can cause abdominal pain.

abscess or hepatoma or hepatitis in liver; or heart failure

urinary tract infection or stone in kidney

trauma or malarial inflammation of spleen

epigastric hernia

peptic ulcer in stomach or duodenum

pigbel in small bowel

appendicitis

antepartum 'accidental' haemorrhage

pelvic inflammatory disease or ectopic pregnancy

urinary tract infection or stone or acute retention of urine in bladder

urethritis (e.g. gonorrhoea); prostatis

Figure 36.3 Common conditions of organs which cause constant abdominal pain.

Note *also* these 4 causes of constant abdominal pain.
1. All over
   – pus in peritoneum (peritonitis)
   – blood in peritoneum (trauma or ectopic pregnancy
2. Any part – spinal disease (fracture or tuberculous) with referred pain.
3. Upper abdomen – chest disease (pneumonia or pleurisy) with referred pain.
4. From where lower rib joins spine to genitalia or upper, inner thigh – ureteric colic (stones).

If the pain is constant
1. Where is the pain?
   What is the organ that is probably causing it? (See Figure 36.2.) (If the pain is all over, the peritoneum is affected)
2. What condition is probably affecting this organ? (See Figure 36.3.)

Transfer urgently to medical officer if

(but, first start treatment, see this page)
1. There is generalised peritonitis or blood in the peritoneal cavity. In both
   - *constant generalised pain*
   - *often vomitig and constipation*
   - *the abdomen is distended and does not move well on respiration*
   - *the abdomen is tender all over, often with guarding and rigidity*
   - *intestinal sounds are not present.*

   If peritonitis
   - *pulse fast, temperature raised, BP normal (later BP low and shock)*

   If bleeding
   - *pale, pulse fast, BP low (sometimes shock), usually afebrile.*
2. Localised peritonitis (e.g. appendicitis)
   - *constant pain one part of the abdomen*
   - *abdomen does not move well over affected area and is tender over affected area, often with rebound tenderness and guarding.*
   - *pulse fast*
   - *temperature raised*

   But you can treat liver abscess and hepatitis, or pelvic inflammatory disease, or splenic inflammation (not trauma), at the health centre.
3. Obstruction of intestine
   - *colicky abdominal pain*
   - *vomiting*
   - *constipation*
   - *abdomen*
     - *distended*
     - *no tenderness unless strangulation when tender over one area or over a hernia*
     - *intestinal (bowel) sounds increase when the pain comes.*
4. Ectopic pregnancy or severe 'Pelvic Inflammatory Disease'

   (a) *missed or late or irregular or heavy periods*, and

   (b) *lower abdominal pain*, and

   (c) *vaginal bleeding or discharge* and

   (d) *uterus enlarged and also tender or*
   - *a mass or tenderness next to the uterus or*
   - *tenderness of all the abdomen often with guarding and rigidity and no intestinal sounds* and

   (e) *pulse fast, BP low, pallor, normal temperature – if there is bleeding (ectopic*

miscarriage, antepartum haemorrhage) or
   - *pulse fast and temperature raised – if there is infection (septic abortion, pelvic inflammatory disease and sometimes ectopic pregnancy).*
5. Antepartum haemorrhage.
   (See an obstetrics book.)
6. Acute retention of urine that you can not cure with catheterisation of bladder and treatment of urinary infection.
7. Ureteric colic (non-urgent).

Acute 'surgical' abdomen

(Peritonitis, Bleeding into peritoneum.

Obstruction of the intestine)

1. The patient must not eat or drink.
2. Start an IV drip.

   Give IV fluids as necessary.

   If there is shock – see Chapter 27 page 305.

   If bleeding into the peritoneum is probable (you suspect if from the history, examination, progressive pallor, rising pulse, etc. in absence of evidence of severe infection) – see Chapter 27 page 305 and arrange emergency transfer for urgent blood transfusion.

   If there is dehydration – see Chapter 23 page 223.

   If only maintenance fluids are necessary – see Chapter 23 page 228.

   If you do not know if the patient is taking enough fluid and patient cannot pass urine, insert an indwelling urethral catheter and measure the urine passed every hour (it should be > 30 ml/hour). Increase the IV fluids until the urine passed is > 30 ml/hour.
3. Give chloramphenicol, unless infection is not probable.

   Give chloranphicol 2 g immediately and then 1 g every 6 hours.

   Give by IVI if there is shock or a drip running; and by IMI to other cases.
4. Give an antimalarial drug by injection as indicated (see Chapter 13 page 56).
5. Do intragastric suction if there is evidence of intestinal obstruction (repeated vomiting and distension and colic) or paralysis (repeated vomiting and distension).

   Put a tube through the nose into the stomach.

Aspirate (suck out) all the fluid and gas possible, immediately and every hour.

Leave the end of the tube open, and hang it over the side of the bed, lower than the patient. Fluid will drain from it.

Check the volume of all the fluid which comes out of the tube, and is vomited.

6. Treat the underlying condition.

Abdominal surgery will almost always be necessary. Transfer to a Medical Officer urgently for the necessary surgery.

In Enteritis necroticans (pigbel) and a few other conditions, the above treatment may be enough.

7. Treat any other conditions present, or any complications which develop, in the usual ways.

8. Transfer the patient urgently (emergency) to a Medical Officer at a hospital. First get the patient's written permission for any tests, treatment or surgery which may be necessary.

9. Give analgesics unless a Medical Office can see the patient almost immediately. (If so, do not give analgesics because they may make the tenderness and signs in the abdomen less.)

Give IM pethidine

– 75 mg (1½ ml) to a small adult (< 50 kg)
– 100 mg (2 ml) to a large adult (> 50 kg)

Abdominal tenderness – guarding – rigidity

You discover abdominal tenderness, guarding and rigidity during palpation of the abdomen.

Palpate the abdomen to discover 3 things.

1. Tenderness. If it is present, where is it?; and also, are rebound tenderness and guarding and rigidity present?
2. Are normal organs enlarged? – liver, spleen, uterus and bladder.
3. Are there masses or lumps in other places including hernia and lymph glands.

Do palpation only **after** inspection.

Palpate first for tenderness – guarding – rigidity like this:

1. Be gentle. If you hurt the patient with your first palpation, the patient may not relax again. The examination will then be difficult.

Figures 36.4 and 36.5 show the proper way to palpate an abdomen, with the palm of the hand held flat. Do not bend the fingers, or use the tips of the fingers.

Fingure 36.6 The wrong way to palpate an abdomen. *Use the palm of the hand.* DO NOT USE THE TIPS OF THE FINGERS LIKE THIS.

2. First move the *palm* of your hand gently over the whole abdomen. This helps the patient to relax. Also you can after find an area of tenderness by feeling the patient's abdominal wall muscles contract (and seeing his eyes or face muscles also contract) when your hand moves over the tender area.

3. Then palpate with the *palm* of your hand held flat and not the tips of the fingers). Again, look at the patient's face and feel the abdominal muscles contract to find tender parts.

   Palpate carefully all over the abdomen. Do not forget the loins (kidney areas at the back), or any other part.

   Start in a place which is probably normal. Palpate a place you suspect is abnormal last.

4. If you do not find any tenderness with 2 and 3, then palpate more deeply. Again, palpate all areas of the abdomen.

5. If it is difficult to decide exactly where the most tender place is, you can do a gentle 'one finger palpation' in the place where you found the tenderness. If you look at the patient's face, feel the abdominal muscles contract and ask

Finger 36.7 One finger palpation. Only do this when you have found a tender place with normal palpation, but you cannot decide which is the most tender place. Press the point of one finger gently onto different parts of the tender place like this, until you find the most tender area.

the patient where it hurts most, you can usually decide which is the most tender place with 'one finger palpation'. (See Figure 36.7.)

Causes of abdominal tenderness – guarding – rigidity

Inflammation of or swelling of or stretching of an organ or of peritoneum causes *tenderness* on palpation over the organ or periteoneum. If the condition is mild, tenderness may be the only sign that you find.

You can find *rebound tenderness* if you quickly remove the palpating hand (which is pressing firmly on the abdomen) from the abdomen. The release of the pressure on the contents of the abdomen causes movement and, therefore, pain over the inflamed or stretched organ or peritoneum (e.g. in appendicitis, if you suddenly lift your hand off the abdomen during palpation of the left iliac fossa, the patient will feel pain in the right iliac fossa, where the inflamed appendix is).

If the inflammation or swelling or stretching of the organ or peritoneum is more severe and acute then *involuntary guarding* may occur. When you do the palpation, the overlying muscles contract. This stops the palpation putting more pressure on the affected organ or peritoneum causing more pain. The patient cannot completely stop this muscle contraction, even if you help him to relax (e.g. by talking to him) or he tries himself. (This is different from voluntary guarding which is often caused by worry, and goes if the patient does not think about his abdomen when you palpate it.)

Rigidity occurs if the inflammation of or swelling of stretching of the organ or of the peritoneum is even more severe and acute. The muscles do not relax at any time.

Localised tenderness – guarding – rigidity occur over the affected organ or peritoneum. The exact

A. Anterior view   B. Posterior view

Finger 36.8   Diagrams to show the normal positions of important organs in the abdomen.

place of this tenderness usually shows which organ is affected, see Figure 36.8 (e.g. right iliac fossa, appendix, appendicitis; epigastrium, stomach/ duodenum, peptic ulcer).

Abdominal mass

To find out what an abdominal mass is, you must decide:
1. Where is the mass? or
   In which organ or structure is the mass?
2. What type is the mass? or
   Is this mass congenital or traumatic or inflammatory or neoplastic or degenerative, etc. (see Chapter 4 page 10)?

A full history and examination is necessary. A pelvic examination 'PR' and/or 'PV' is often also necessary.

It is also usually necessary to:
test the urine for protein, pus, blood and bile,
look at the stools,
look at any vomit, and
look at any vaginal discharge.

Where is the mass?

Think of all the structures and organs in the area which could be affected and could contain the mass.

Start at the skin on the anterior (front) of the abdominal wall, and think of all of the organs under it to the skin on the posterior (back) abdominal wall. See Figure 36.8.

Remember that if the patient contracts his anterior abdominal muscles (e.g. by lifting his head when he is lying on his back), any mass that you can still feel must be anterior to (in front of) the muscles. You cannot easily feel masses behind the hard contracted muscles.

If you think that a certain organ probably contains the mass, then look for other signs in history, examination and tests to show if the organ has abnormal function and disease, or not: e.g. if you think the mass is in the pelvic colon, then ask carefully about bowel colic, constipation or diarrhoea, blood in the stool, weight loss, etc.; examine for weight loss; do a careful rectal examination to try to feel if the mass is in the bowel wall; and carefully look at the stool for blood.

What type is the mass?

The mass may be congenital or traumatic or inflammatory or neoplastic or degenerative etc. in any of the organs in that area.

Some types of masses are more probable in some organs than in others (e.g. the spleen is probably enlarged by malarial inflammation or lymphomatous cancers or blood disease – other types of masses such as congenital or degenerative are not probable).

For inflammatory masses, see in Chapter 3 page 8. For neoplastic masses, see Chapter 3 page 9 and below.

You can find other signs of the type of mass in history, examination and tests, e.g. fever, fast pulse, etc. if it is an inflammatory mass; or weight loss, enlarged hard fixed lymph nodes etc. if it is a neoplastic mass.

Common causes of abdominal masses

You can find the causes of most masses if you answer these 2 questions:
1. Where is the mass or in which organ or structure is the mass? and
2. What type is the mass?
and then look for
1. other signs of disease in the suspected organ, and
2. other signs of the nature of the pathological process suspected.

Common causes of abdominal masses include:
1. generalised enlargement of:
   (a) liver,
   (b) spleen,
   (c) uterus,
   (d) bladder,
   (e) kidney, and
   (f) lymph glands on posterior abdominal wall;
2. inflammatory masses (e.g. abscesses) of:
   (a) any of the organs in 1 (above),
   (b) part of the gastro-intestinal tract, or
   (c) the peritoneum;
3. neoplastic masses of:
   (a) any of the organs in 1 (above),

(b) part of the gastro-intestinal tract, or
(c) the peritoneum.

Especially common causes of masses in the abdomen include:

In the right iliac fossa
- appendicitis/appendix abscess
- amoeboma of the intestine
- cancer of the intestine
- tuberculosis of the intestine

In the left iliac fossa
- amoeboma of the intestine
- schistosomiasis of the intestine
- cancer of the intestine

In the lower abdomen
- distended bladder
- pregnant uterus

- ectopic pregnancy
- pelvic abscess
- cancer of the ovary or uterus

In the left upper abdomen
- spleen (malaria, visceral leishmaniasis, schistosomiasis, lymphoma, etc.
- kidney tumour; or swelling caused by a blocked ureter

In the right upper abdomen
- liver (amoebic abscess, hepatoma)
- kidney, tumour; or swelling caused by a blocked ureter.

In the epigastrium
- cancer of the stomach
- liver (amoebic abscess, hepatoma, secondary cancer; but also sometimes a normal large left lobe of the liver)

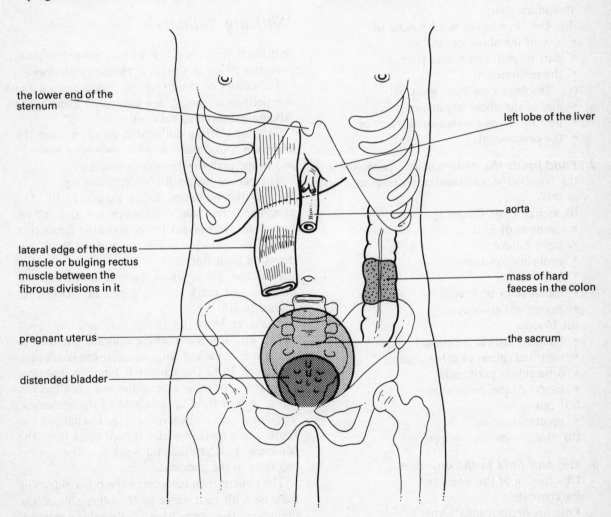

Finger 36.9 Normal structures which you may mistake for pathological masses.

411

Normal structures which you may mistake for pathological masses. (See Figure 36.9)

Generalised abdominal swelling

Causes of swelling of the whole abdomen include five groups of conditions:

1. A solid mass inside the abdomen
(a) *Generalised enlargement of any organ,* especially:
- the liver,
- the spleen,
- the uterus (or ovary or tubes),
- the bladder,
- the kidney, or
- the lymph glands on the posterior abdominal wall;

(b) *Any large inflammatory mass* of:
- any of the above organs, or
- part of gastro-intestinal tract, or
- the peritoneum;

(c) *Any large neoplastic mass* of:
- any of the above organs, or
- part of the gastro-intestinal tract, or
- the peritoneum.

2. Fluid inside the abdomen (see page 406)
(a) *Fluid in the peritoneal cavity* (ascites, blood or pus)
(i) ascites (clear fluid)
- cirrhosis of liver
- heart failure
- nephrotic syndrome
- kwashiorkor
- tuberculous peritonitis
- cancer of peritoneum
(ii) blood
- bleeding ectopic pregnancy
- ruptured spleen or other organ
- tuberculous peritonitis
- cancer of the peritoneum
(iii) pus
- peritonitis;
(b) *Fluid in an ovarian cyst.*

3. Gas and fluid in the intestines
Obstruction of the intestines
Paralytic ileus
Enteritis necroticans ('pigbel')
Peritonitis

4. Fat

5. Abdominal wall swellings
Hernia
Lipoma
Cellulitis

Inguinal swellings

Causes of inguinal swellings include:
hernia (see a surgery book),
lymph gland enlargement (see Chapter 22 page 199),
inflammation – cellulitis, abscess, etc., and traumatic swelling.

'Shifting dullness'

Shifting dullness is a sign which shows that *fluid (water or blood or pus)* is *in the peritoneal cavity.*

For *causes* of fluid (ascites, blood and pus) in the peritoneal cavity, see causes of Generalised Abdominal Swelling (above).

Test for shifting dullness in all cases when the *abdomen is distended or* when *ascites or blood or pus* in the peritoneal cavity is possible.

The patient lies on his back, facing up.
Percuss the abdomen as in Figure 36.10. The abdomen is resonant (hollow) on top and dull on both sides, as the gas in the intestine floats that part of the intestine to the top and the fluid runs down on both sides.

Find the place where resonance changes to dullness and mark it with a pen or chalk. (See Figure 36.10)

In Figure 36.11 the patient is lying on his back facing up. The place where dullness changed to resonance is marked with an unbroken chalk line. In Figure 36.12 the patient is lying on his side. Fluid from the other side of the abdomen has run down to join fluid on this side of the abdomen. The new place where dullness changed to resonance is marked with a dotted chalk line. The 'dullness' has 'shifted' (moved) up. The patient has fluid in the abdomen.

The patient then rolls on to the other side. The dullness with then move to the other side of the abdomen. The places where dullness was marked will now be resonant. The dullness will now be in

Finger 36.10 The method of percussion of the abdomen for fluid. Note that the finger on the abdomen is kept parallel to the patients bed.

Figures 36.11 and 36.12 (below) show how to find if there is fluid in the abdomen. (See text for details.)

the area posterior (behind) the line on the other side of the patient, and will also shift closer to the umbilicus.

> Note that shifting dullness only means that fluid is present in the peritoneal cavity. It does not diagnose what type of fluid is present in the peritoneal cavity. Use other symptoms and signs and tests to find out what type of fluid is causing the shifting dullness.

The main differential diagnosis is an ovarian cyst.

Bowel sounds

Intestinal or bowel sounds may be
1. normal, or
2. increased, or
3. decreased or absent.

Intestinal sounds are increased when the patient feels colic, when there is
1. obstruction of the intestine or
2. gastro-enteritis.

Intestinal sounds are decreased or absent if there is:
1. pus in the peritoneal cavity (peritonitis from any cause), or
2. blood in the peritoneal cavity (e.g. bleeding ectopic pregnancy or ruptured spleen or other organ), or
3. paralytic ileus.

Listen for at least two minutes (10 minutes if possible), before you decide that bowel sounds are reduced or absent.

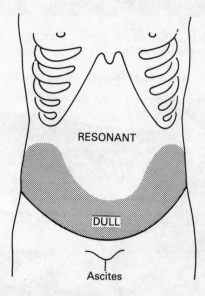

Figure 36.13 Diagrams to show one way of diagnosing an ovarian cyst or fluid in the peritoneal cavity. The patient is lying on her back facing up.

414

37

Emergency Resuscitation

the arms quickly and strongly towards the back and chest of the patient (see Fig. 37.1.). Repeat two or three times, if necessary. This is not just squeezing the patient – it is like a punch; but with the fist starting on the abdominal wall and helped by the other hand. This should force air out of the lungs through the trachea and the larynx and expel (push out) the foreign body. (See Figure 37.1.)

If the patient has fallen turn him face downwards and do the same thing.

If the patient is small, you can lift him up by the waist leaving his chest and head hanging down, and then hit him very hard on his back (between his shoulder blades) with the side of your fist. This will force some air out of the lungs and should expel foreign body.

If these methods do not work, you can sometimes get the foreign body out of the throat, if you push your fingers down deep into the back of the patient's throat and pull out what is there.

Inhaled foreign body

If the foreign body is in the larynx or trachea, it will cause obstruction of the airway which may be complete or not complete.

If the obstruction is complete the patient usually makes violent breathing movements, with indrawing of the ribs; cyanosis and death quickly occur. Sometimes complete obstruction causes only sudden unexpected unconsciousness and no breathing and then death.

If the obstruction is not complete, there is severe shortness of breath, stridor and indrawing of the ribs on breathing in.

Obstruction of the larynx or trachea may occur when the patient is eating ('food choking'). Suspect it in every case of respiratory distress or loss of consciousness which occurs during eating. It is also common if the patient had a foreign body in his mouth or if he was drunk. It is more common in patients with chronic bronchitis.

> If you suspect obstruction, act immediately.

If the patient is standing or sitting, stand behind the patient and put your arms round his upper abdomen. Make a fist of one of you hands and hold this fist with the other hand. Put the fist on the patient's anterior abdominal wall between the umbilicus and the ribs. Then pull up and in with

Figure 37.1 The method of forcing a foreign body out of the trachea or larynx.

415

Artificial ventilation (artificial 'respiration') heart stimulation and external cardiac (heart) massage

Artificial ventilation is necessary if the patient cannot breathe enough.

This occurs only when the patient is:
1. unconsciousness, *and*
2. not breathing or breathing with only a few breaths (even if deep).

Causes include:
- near drowning,
- paralysis from snake bite,
- an unconscious patient whose airway becomes blocked,
- very deep unconsciousness (especially after a drug overdose),
- sometimes after anaesthetics or operations,
- cardiac arrest (stopping of heart), and
- others.

Heart stimulation and possible external massage is necessary if the heart has stopped.

This only occurs when the patient is unconsciousness *and* the pulse is absent.

Causes include:
- electrocution,
- reaction to drugs
- shock which is not treated,
- breathing stops and no one gives artificial ventilation, and
- others.

Do artificial ventilation and heart stimulation or external cardiac massage only if the patient may recover and return to normal life. The underlying condition must be treatable. The patient must have collapsed suddenly or unexpectedly collapsed. Do not do these things if the patient is slowly getting worse, even with all possible treatment.

If the patient is unconscious and you cannot feel a pulse (even if there is some breathing) or
if the patient is unconscious and not breathing or is breathing with only a few breaths (even if you can feel a pulse)

---

then emergency resuscication is necessary. You must start artificial ventilation and, if necessary, heart stimulation or external cardiac massage within three minutes.
If you do not do this, the patient will die or have severe brain damage from which he cannot recover.

Artificial ventilation of the lungs

Clear the airway
Extend the head (or move the head back on the top of the neck). Hold the back of the neck with one hand and push the top of the head back with the other hand. This will bend the head back on the top of the neck as far as possible.

Push the angle of the jaw forward from behind *or* pull the jaw forward from under the front of the jaw.

Extract (get out) anything from the mouth or throat which could block the airway. Use your fingers (and, if necessary, a cloth).

Suck out the airway if you have a sucker (but do not leave the patient to find one).

Mouth to mouth ventilation
(a) Separate the patient's lips.
(b) Hold the patient's nostrils together,
(c) Take a deep breath.
(d) Open you mouth widely.
(e) Seal your lips around the patient's mouth.
(f) Blow your breath into the patient's lungs.
(g) Look to see if the patient's chest rises as you blow air into the patient's lungs.
(h) Then remove your mouth from the patient's mouth.
(i) Look to see if the patient's chest falls when you stop blowing air into the patient's chest.

If the chest does not rise and fall check that
- the head is extended,
- the jaw is well forward, and
- the airway is not blocked by foreign bodies,
and try the mouth to mouth ventilation again.

If the chest still does not rise and fall, turn the patient onto his side and hit the patient *hard* on the back between the shoulder blades with the side of your fist. This will force air in the lungs through the airway and expel (push out) any foreign bodies in the lower airway, which are

(a) The tongue is blocking the troat of an unconscious patient. Compare with (b). tongue

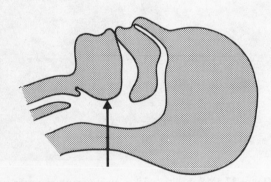

(b) Normal airway in a conscious patient

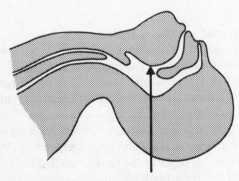

(c) The head extended and the jaw forward. In this position the tongue does not block the throat; the air passages are not obstructed, even in an unconscious patient

Figure 37.2 (a), (b) and (c). Diagrams to show how to stop the tongue blocking the airway of an unconscious person.

Figure 37.3 Patient ready for artifical ventilation. Note (1) airway cleared, (2) head extended, (3) jaw held forward, (4) nostrils held, (5) mouth open.

Figure 37.4 Health worker looking to see if the chest falls after he stopped blowing his breath into the patient.

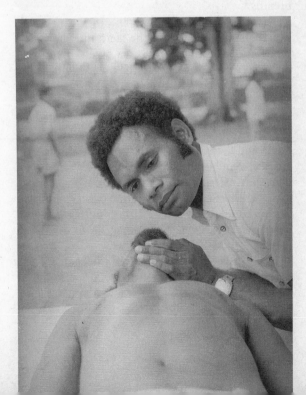

blocking the air going into the lungs. (See Figure 37.1 page 415 for another method.)

Then repeat the mouth to mouth ventilation again.

Continue artificial ventilation
Repeat the artificial ventilation 15–20 times every minute i.e. about 3–4 seconds for each breath (in and out).

Check for cardiac arrest
After 4 breaths stop and check if the patient has a cardiac arrest or not.

Stimulation of the heart and external cardiac massage

> Feel for the radial pulse. If the patient is unconscious *and* has no pulse, the heart has stopped.

Stimulate the heart
Give a single hard quick blow with the side of the fist to the middle of the patient's sternum over the heart. This may start the heart.

Continue artificial ventilation for another 4 breaths.

Then check the pulse again. If the patient's heart is still stopped, hit the sternum again, 3–4 times in 3–4 seconds; and then give 4 breaths of artificial ventilation. Check the pulse again. If the patient's heart is still stopped, repeat all this 3–4 times.

If you can transfer the patient to a Medical Officer or a hospital *within minutes* (or less than 1 hour) and there is staff at the hospital who can do artifical ventilation and external cardiac massage, then start external cardiac massage, if you cannot start the heart as above. External cardiac massage is rarely successful in a health centre because you need special drugs and equipment to treat the patient.

Even if you do not do the external cardiac massage, continue the artificial ventilation because you may not have felt a weak pulse which was there.

Figure 37.5 A health worker giving external cardiac massage. Note that the elbows are straight and that he uses the weight of his body to push down the sternum as he moves backwards and forwards (He is not pushing the sternum down by bending and straightening his elbows.)

External cardiac massage
Put the patient on a hard surface, flat on his back.

Kneel beside the patient.

Put the heel of one hand on the lower part of the sternum, and put the heel of the other hand on top of the first hand.

Hold your arms straight and move backwards and forwards, using the body weight to push the sternum in, towards the backbone. (Do not lift the hand off the sternum.)

Push the sternum down 3–5 cm (1–2 inches). You need about 20–30 kg of pressure in an adult. Do this about 70 times a minute.

If someone else is giving artificial ventilation. Give 5 cycles of external cardiac massage and stop for one cycle of mouth to mouth respiration. Then repeat.

418

If no one else is available, give 15 cycles of external cardiac massage, then 2 quick deep breaths of artificial ventilation. Repeat until someone comes to help.

Continue artificial ventilation until the patient
1. can breathe properly for himself, *or*
2. has been transfered to a Medical Officer, *or*
3. for more than 30 minutes the patient
   - has not tried to take a breath himself, and
   - has had no pulse without ECM, and
   - has widely dilated pupils, and
   - is obviously dead.

Continue external cardiac massage until the patient
1. has good pulse and BP himself *or*
2. has been transfered to a Medical Officer *or*
3. for more than 30 minutes
   - has had no pulse without ECM, and
   - has widely dilated pupils, and
   - is obviously dead.

Near drowning

Start resuscitation immediately you see the patient, even before he is brought out of the water.

Resuscitation includes:
1. Clear the airway (see page 416).
2. Give mouth to mouth ventilation, if the patient is not breathing properly (see page 416).
3. Stimulate the heart and give external cardiac massage, if the heart has stopped (see page 418).

4. Change from mouth to mouth ventilation to ventilation with a self-inflatable bag (e.g. an 'Air Viva' 'Ambu-Bag') and oxygen as soon as possible.
5. If all this does not cause return or normal respiration and heart beat, and if the patient is still alive, and if you can continue resuscitation while you transfer the patient to a hospital or Medical Officer's care; then continue resuscitation and arrange urgent (emergency) transfer.
6. If these things are not successful, and if the patient is not starting to recover within 1 hour, then stop the treatment.
7. If the patient's breathing and circulation do improve, then treat like this:
   (a) Give intra-nasal oxygen 2 litres/minute for some hours.
   (b) If the patient nearly drowned in salt water and becomes shocked, treat with plasma volume expander as in shock (see Chapter 27 page 305).
   (c) Check the urine output carefully. If there is no urine output or only a little red or brown urine with protein in it, start treatment for acute kindey failure (see Chapter 26 page 293) and arrange urgent (emergency) transfer to hospital.
   (d) Give antibiotics as if the patient had pneumonia (see Chapter 20 page 166).
   (e) Do not discharge the patient for at least 24 hours. Sometimes complications and death occur hours after the patient has seemed to have recovered.

Appendix A

Incubation Periods

Incubation periods can be misleading in areas where diseases are endemic. In practice in such areas it is probably sufficient to remember whether the incubation period is of long, medium or short duration.

Malaria
The incubation period in man (from the bite of an infected mosquito until the start of symptoms and signs of malaria) is usually about 2 weeks. However, it is often much longer. It cannot be shorter than 8 days.

Leprosy
The incubation period is usually 2–4 years; but it can be shorter or very much longer at times.

Measles
The incubation period is 1–2 weeks.

German measles
The incubation period is 2–3 weeks.

Chicken pox
The incubation period is 2–3 weeks.

Mumps
The incubation period is 2–3 weeks

Leptospirosis
The incubation period varies from 1–3 weeks.

Plague
The incubation period is usually less than a week.

Typhus
The incubation period is 1–2 weeks.

Yellow fever
The incubation period is 3–6 days.

Typhoid
The incubation period is from 3 to 60 days, but usually about 10 days.

Gonorrhoea
The incubation period is usually less than 1 week, but can be longer.

Syphilis
The incubation period is about 3 weeks until primary syphilis develops (it can be 10–90 days)

Chancroid
The incubation period is 2–5 days.

Cholera
The incubation period is from a few hours to 5 days.

Acute viral hepatitis
The incubation period is 2 to 6 weeks for Hepatitis A and between 6 weeks and 6 months for Hepatitis B.

Tetanus
The incubation period is usually about 2 weeks; but it can be much longer or shorter.

Index

Bronchopneumonia; *see*
Pneumonia
Brucellosis, 113–4
Bubo, 104
Bubonic plague, 104, 204
Bugs, reduvid, 121
Burkitt's lymphoma, 203–4

Calamine lotion, 98
Cancer, 9, 46, 125, 128, 136,
139–40, 199, 233
of lymph glands, 204–5
of neck, 175
of stomach, 216, 236
see also Neoplasm; Burkitt's
lymphoma
Candida infection, 128, 132
Cardiac:
arrest, 418
external massage, 416–9
Cardiovascular disease, 300
Carditis, 321
Cataract:
eye, 344–5, 365
Catheter:
intranasal, 167
urethral, 46, 286, 293
Carriers, 226, 227
chronic, 38
convalescent, 38
Cellular immunity, 35, 76, 77
Cellulitis, 361
Centipede bites, 379
Cerebellum, 253
Cerebral:
cortex, 253
haemorrhage, 278
tumour, 234, 278
Cerebro-vascular disease (stroke),
262–3, 268
Cervical:
glands, 66
smear, 284
Cervix, 136
venereal warts on, 138
CH, contact history, 17–18
Chagas' disease; *see*
Trypanosomiasis: American
Chancroid, 128, 133, 137–8, 295,
421
Chemicals:
and disease, 11
and inflammation, 9, 10
Chemoprophylaxis, 40
Chemotherapeutic drugs, 34, 35,
41–5

see also Chloramphenicol;
Penicillin; Streptomycin;
Sulphonamides; Tetracycline
Chemotherapy, 40–5
Chest:
auscultation of, 153–4
examination 18, 19, 179
infection, 71, 164, 165, 173,
177, 305
injury, 176
pain in, 66, 71, 152–65, 179,
300, 309
palpation of, 152
percussion, 153
X-ray, 71
Chicken pox (varicella), 98–9,
421
Childbirth, 128
Chloramphenicol, 34, 41–4, 46–7,
102, 104, 106, 113, 136, 163,
166, 167, 168, 172, 214, 224,
229, 231, 233, 246, 257, 308,
339, 406
dose, 43
ointment, 99
Chloroquine, 41, 54–5, 92, 158,
160, 164, 184, 246, 288, 382
dosage, 55–6
resistant malaria, 56, 58, 62–3
Chlorpromazine, 28, 57, 58, 220,
264, 391–3
Cholecystitis:
acute, 247
Cholera, 31, 226–30, 421
vaccine, 230
and Hartmann's solution, 224
Chorea, 321
Chronic condition:
definition of, 5
Cirrhosis:
of liver, 207, 208, 236, 243–5,
288, 398, 399
Clinical:
definitions, 2–7
sub –, 38
Clofazimine, 90–1, 95
Clostridia, 221
Clubbing:
of fingers, 174
of nails, 156
of toes, 174
Codeine:
compound tablets, 28, 29, 160,
167, 190, 320
phosphate, 28
COLD, Chronic Obstructive Lung

Disease; *see* Bronchitis: chronic
Colic, 403
biliary, 247
ureteric, 290, 328
Coma, 104, 120, 125, 264–6, 333
Common cold, 158, 175
Community:
health education, 3
Condylomata accuminata, 128,
133, 134, 138
Coneshell stings, 378
Confusion, 388
Congenital disease, 10
Conjunctivitis, 97, 108, 338,
340–1, 346
allergic, 162
conjunctivae, 336
red, 106
Consciousness:
level of, 265
loss of, 53, 56, 120, 206, 264–6,
307, 383, 416
care of, 258, 265–6
Constipation, 212, 213, 235, 237
severe, 122, 214
Contacts, disease:
sexual, 129, 135, 140–1
tracing, 74, 95
Control, of disease:
definition of, 5
Convulsions, 52, 57, 266–7
Cornea, 336
foreign body in, 338, 342,
ulcer, 338, 339, 342–3
Coronary heart disease, 309–10
Cortisone, 51, 70, 333
Cough, 71, 74, 149, 150, 159,
175–7
chronic, 66, 69, 71, 168, 172,
173, 325
treatment, 158, 175–6
see also Tuberculosis;
Whooping cough
Crepitations (crackles), 155, 165,
166, 172, 300, 308
Cretinism:
endemic, 331–2
Croup, 155
CSF, cerebro-spinal fluid, 254
blood in, 255
examination of, 277–8
test, 255–6, 257
Cutaneous leishmaniasis, 114, 116,
361
Cyanosis, 19, 52, 156, 158, 166,
167, 170, 223, 227, 300